BIOLOGY AND DISEASES OF THE FERRET

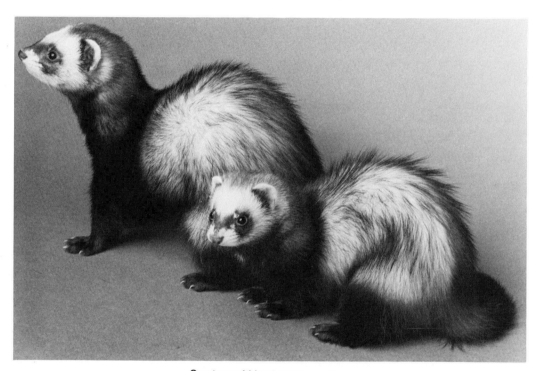

Courtesy of Marshall Farms, Inc.

BIOLOGY AND DISEASES OF THE FERRET

JAMES G. FOX, D.V.M.
Professor and Director
Division of Comparative Medicine
Massachusetts Institute of Technology
Cambridge, Massachusetts

Adjunct Professor of Comparative Medicine
Tufts University School of Veterinary Medicine
Boston and Grafton, Massachusetts

Lea & Febiger • 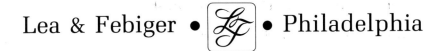 • Philadelphia

Lea & Febiger
600 Washington Square
Philadelphia, PA 19106-4198
U.S.A.
(215) 922-1330

**Cover illustration Courtesy of Ferretworld, Inc.
(Boston/Assonet, Massachusetts).**

Library of Congress Cataloging-in-Publication Data

Biology and diseases of the ferret.

    Includes bibliographies and index.
    1. Ferret as laboratory animals. 2. Ferret. 3. Ferret
—Diseases. I. Fox, James G. [DNLM: 1. Animal Diseases.
2. Carnivora. SF 997.3 B615]
SF407.F39B56 1988   636′.974447   87-26096
ISBN 0-8121-1139-7

PRINTED IN THE UNITED STATES OF AMERICA

Print No.   4 3

FOREWORD

Animals of all kinds have been drawn or painted by artists, observed in their natural habitats, domesticated, studied in laboratories, and used as beasts of burden or as food. None has been more interesting than the domestic ferret, *Mustela putorius furo.*

In this comprehensive, well-researched book, James G. Fox has assembled virtually all extant data applicable to the biology, management, and diseases of ferrets. And in so doing, a great service has been rendered to those to whom ferrets are of interest scientifically or medically.

The contents are well organized and complete, including mention even of the old sport of "ferret-legging" and the designation of the ferret as the official mascot of the Massachusetts Colonial Navy.

I recommend it to students, naturalists, veterinarians, scientists, and research libraries as the most up-to-date one-volume source of information on the domestic ferret available.

Franklin M. Loew
Dean, School of Veterinary Medicine
Tufts University

PREFACE

The European ferret, *Mustela putorius furo*, has been domesticated for over 2,000 years, although confusion exists as to its exact origin and early use as a domesticated animal. Ferrets in Europe and the British Isles were used for rabbit hunting and rodent control, and even today remain popular for hunting in some geographic locations. It wasn't until the 1900s, however, that the ferret was first formally introduced as an animal model for biomedical research, and it wasn't until the 1980s that ferrets began to appear routinely at many veterinary hospitals with anxious owners in need of veterinary care for their pets. Because the ferret was seen infrequently in the laboratory animal milieu, and even less so in the routine small animal practice, easily accessible sources of information on its biology and diseases were unavailable.

This book, therefore, is intended for veterinarians and scientists who either provide veterinary care or utilize the ferret in biomedical research. The contributing authors and I hope that the book will prove useful in introducing the ferret, and its diseases and biology, in a concise, easily assimilated format. The text is an attempt to present current information about diseases encountered in the ferret, as well as salient biologic characteristics of the animal. I realize that there are significant gaps in our knowledge regarding diseases and biology of this species, and it is hoped that this text and continued use of the ferret will help to fill existing voids in these areas.

The 19 chapters presented in this text provide information on diseases as well as history of the ferret, husbandry, nutrition, physiology, anatomy, and selected uses of this species as an animal model.

A special thanks is extended to the personnel at the Division of Comparative Medicine at MIT who, over the last decade, have shared with me the excitement and frustration of working with a species of animal whose diseases and biology are not well documented. Without their continued perseverance and dedication in documenting new diseases and instituting new husbandry, therapeutic, and surgical techniques, this text could not have been written. In addition, the financial contributions of Hoffmann-LaRouche, Inc.; Marshall Research Animals, Inc; and Pitman-Moore, Inc. are acknowledged. Dr. Chris Newcomer, Dr. Brad Brooks, Dr. Carol A. Kauffman, Dr. Alvin F. Moreland, Dr. Daphne A. Roe, and Dr. C.J. Thorns are also acknowledged for their excellent suggestions regarding the content of the text. I also want to thank Marian Walke and Lesley Zaret for their secretarial assistance. The staff of Lea & Febiger, and the foresight and fortitude of Kit Spahr, who have made the vision of this text a reality, are also greatly appreciated.

James G. Fox
Cambridge, Massachusetts

CONTRIBUTORS

N.Q. An, D.V.M., M.S.
Department of Anatomy and Radiology
College of Veterinary Medicine
University of Georgia
Athens, GA

P.L.R. Andrews, Ph.D.
Department of Physiology
St. George's Hospital Medical School
Cranmer Terrace
London SW17 ORE
United Kingdom

M.J. Baum, Ph.D.
Department of Biology
Boston University
Boston, MA

H.E. Evans, D.V.M., Ph.D.
Department of Anatomy
College of Veterinary Medicine
Cornell University
Ithaca, NY

J.G. Fox, D.V.M.
Director, Division of Comparative Medicine
Massachusetts Institute of Technology
Cambridge, MA

M.E. Pecquet Goad, D.V.M., Ph.D.
EG&G Mason Research Institute
Worcester, MA

J.R. Gorham, D.V.M., Ph.D.
Agricultural Research Service
U.S. Department of Agriculture
Department of Veterinary Microbiology and
    Pathology
College of Veterinary Medicine
Washington State University
Pullman, WA

I.N.C. Lawes, Ph.D.
Department of Anatomy and Cell Biology
University of Sheffield
Western Bank
Sheffield S10 2TN
United Kingdom

D.E. McLain, Ph.D.
Baxter Healthcare Corp.
Round Lake, IL

R.C. Pearson, M.S., D.V.M.
Department of Pathology
New York State College of Veterinary
    Medicine
Cornell University
Ithaca, NY

J.A. Thomas, Ph.D.
Academic Services
University of Texas Health Science Center
San Antonio, TX

CONTENTS

Section III. Research Applications

BIOLOGY AND HUSBANDRY

chapter 1

TAXONOMY, HISTORY, AND USE

J. G. Fox

TAXONOMY

Ferrets (*Mustela putorius furo*), like the stoat, weasel, badger, skunk, otter, and mink, are carnivores, and belong to the ancient family Mustelidae, which probably dates back to the Eocene period, some 40 million years ago (Fig. 1–1). The taxonomic groups in the family Mustelidae, as recognized by Corbet and Hill, include 67 species from North, Central, and South America, Eurasia, and Africa (Table 1-1).[1]

ORIGIN

The domestic ferret is often confused with the North American black-footed ferret, *Mustela nigripes*, so a short description of each will be provided to clarify the differences.

DOMESTIC FERRET

According to one author, ferrets (*Mustela putorius furo*) have been domesticated for over 2000 years,[2] but confusion exists

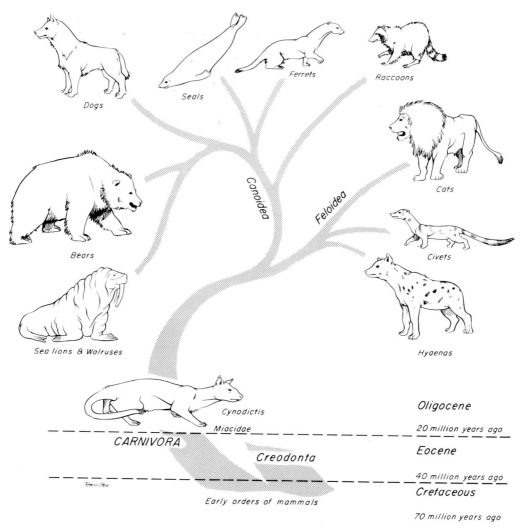

Fig. 1–1. The order Carnivora: Anatomic relatives of the ferret. (Modified from Evans, H.E., and Christensen, G.C.: Classification and natural history of the dog. *In* Miller's Anatomy of the Dog. 2nd Ed. Philadelphia, W.B. Saunders, 1979.)

because of the scarcity of written records, the use of different nomenclature in different regions, and translation difficulties from one language to another. Aristotle, in his early descriptions (c. 350 BC), stated that there existed an animal, which may have been a ferret, that could become very mild and tame.[2]

Early accounts in Greek literature from Strabo (c. 63 BC–24 AD) and Pliny (23–79 AD) noted that ferrets were used for hunting rabbits. These earlier references to ferrets are probably the basis of the belief that ferrets originated in North Africa (Fig. 1–2).[2] Evidently they were bred specifically for rabbiting (rabbit hunting), and were muzzled before being sent into rabbit burrows. This practice was later introduced into Europe, Asia, and the British Isles, where the sport is still practiced today. The first illustration of ferrets used for rabbiting occurs in a fourteenth century manuscript (Fig. 1–3).[2]

In the Linnaean classification system the ferret was named *Mustela furo*, and its identity has remained firmly estab-

TABLE 1–1. THE FAMILY MUSTELIDAE

Genus	Synonym(s)	Range	Member(s)	Number of Species
Mustela	*Grammogale, Lutreola, Putorius*		Weasel, stoat, ferret, ermine, mink, polecat	15
Vormela		Southeast Europe western China	Marbled polecat	1
Martes	*Charronia*	Eurasia, North America	Marten, fisher, sable	7
Eira	*Galera, Tayra*	Northeast Mexico to Argentina	Tayra	1
Galictis	*Grison, Grisonella*	Southern Mexico to Brazil	Grison	3
Lyncodon		Argentina, Chile	Patagonian weasel	1
Ictonyx	*Zorilla*	Senegal, Ethiopia	Striped polecat	1
Poecilictis		Sahara region	Striped weasel	1
Poecilogale		Southern Africa, Zaire, Uganda	White-naped weasel	1
Gulo		Scandinavia, Siberia, Alaska, Canada, western United States	Wolverine or glutton	1
Mellivora		Northern India, Arabia, Africa (south of the Sahara)	Ratel or honey badger	1
Meles		Europe, Japan, southern China	Eurasian badger	1
Arctonyx		Northern China, northeast India, Sumatra	Hog-badger	1
Mydaun	*Swillotaxus*	Sumatra, Java, Borneo, Phillipines	Stink-badgers	2
Tasidea		Southwest Canada to central Mexico	American badger	1
Melogale	*Helictis*	Southeast Asia	Ferret-badgers	3
Mephitis		Canada, United States, Mexico, Nicaragua	Hooded and striped skunks	2
Spilogale		North and Central America	Spotted skunks	4
Conepatus		United States to Central and South America	Hog-nosed skunks	7
Lutra	*Lontra, Lutrogale*	Eurasia; North, Central, and South America; Africa	Otters	8
Pteronura		Venezuela to Argentina	Giant otter	1
Aonyx	*Amblonyx, Paraonyx*	Africa, southeast Asia	Clawless otters	3
Enhydra		Siberia, Alaska to California	Sea otter	1

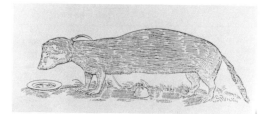

Fig. 1–2. The ferret. (From Thomson, A.P.D.: A history of the ferret. J. Hist. Med., 6:471, 1951.)

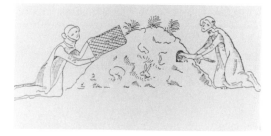

Fig. 1–3. Ferreting in the Middle Ages, about 1300 AD. (From Thomson, A.P.D.: A history of the ferret. J. Hist. Med., 6:471, 1951.)

lished since then. The word "ferret" is derived from the Latin *furonem* and the Italian *furone*, meaning thief.[2,3] The word "putorius" is derived from the Latin *putor*, a stench, which applies to the musky odor of the ferret. Today, "ferret" is also used as a verb and connotes the ferret's behavior and traits: to remove from a hiding place, to search out with keenness, or to draw out by shrewd questioning.

The ferret (*Mustela putorius furo*) has been and is now used for hunting, biomedical research, and recently in North America as a pet, and is most likely a domesticated version of the wild European ferret or polecat (*M. putorius* or *M. furo*).[2,4] Alternatively, it may be related to the steppe polecat (*M. eversmanni*), which it closely resembles in skull morphology.[5] The domesticated ferret, although introduced to North America by the early English settlers some 300 years ago, has not established feral colonies on this continent.

Behavioral differences between the domesticated ferret and the wild European polecat have been documented. The ferret is not as temperamental nor as vigorous and agile as the European polecat.[4] In addition, domesticated ferrets do not develop a fear of humans nor of unfamiliar environments, and are more tractable. The F_1 hybrids of the domesticated ferret and polecat, however, were found to develop a fear of humans when left with their mothers during a critical period between 7½ and 8½ weeks of age.[6] Imprinting may be involved in this process.

When attention response to a rustling noise was tested, the wild ferrets and the F_1 hybrids habituated more rapidly than the domesticated ferret. The F_1 hybrids' responses depended on their previous environmental history—animals raised outdoors responded differently than those raised indoors. Because the ferret's natural habitat contrasts greatly with the indoor environment, those ferrets raised indoors showed a greater response. These findings agree with Lorenz's hypothesis that the behavior of domesticated animals resembles that of juvenile individuals of their wild counterparts.[7]

The wild ferret is completely interfertile with the European polecat, thus verifying their close genetic relationship. The wild European ferret however, usually produces only one litter, while the domesticated ferret produces two or more litters yearly.[8,9] The female ferret and male stoat (*Mustela erminae*) will also produce fertile hybrids.[10] The F_1 generation of a wild polecat and domesticated ferret is also fertile. The wild polecat, or ferret native to much of the British Isles and northern Europe, is also known as the fitch, fitchew, foul marten, fitchet, or foumart.[3,4] Feral colonies of ferrets also exist in New Zealand, where they were introduced in 1882 to control wild rabbits.[4,11] They have also reportedly played a role in reducing the numbers of 20 endemic bird species, including unique flightless birds such as the kakapo and kiwi.[12] In addition, the state of Washington lists the ferret (*M. putorius*) as a feral animal on San Juan Island, where it was initially introduced together with other predators to control an excessive population of European rabbits. Because of the competition, the population of native mink (*M. vison*) on the island has been reduced in numbers.[13, 14]

NORTH AMERICAN BLACK-FOOTED FERRET

The black-footed ferret, *Mustela nigripes*, the North American representative of the Holarctic group of polecat species, was at one time prevalent on the North American plains where its main prey, the prairie dog, colonized large towns.[15] Consequently, in the first half of the twentieth century, large-scale prairie dog eradication programs resulted in placement of the black-footed ferret on the endangered species list in 1967.

In the 1960s and 1970s researchers attempted to breed the animal in captivity and to understand its biology and diseases. These attempts were basically unsuccessful, and the programs were abandoned.[16]

The species had last been sighted in South Dakota in the early 1970s, and by 1980 many believed that the black-footed ferret was extinct.[17] In 1981, however, a rancher's dog killed a weasel-like creature near Meeteese, Wyoming. Luckily, the animal was retrieved by the rancher's wife, and a local taxidermist recognized it as a black-footed ferret.[17] Biologists from the Department of Fish and Wildlife Service and from the Biota Research and Consulting Company soon converged on the area, and documented new sightings of the black-footed ferret. Because they are nocturnal and spend most of their time in underground burrows, it is difficult to track these ferrets. The 80,000-acre area of prairie dog colonies was surveyed, and it was estimated that there was a population of 60 ferrets for the summer of 1982, 88 in 1983, and 128 in 1984.[15]

Recent studies indicate that ferrets hunt over a 100-acre area, which is a large range for a small mammal. Therefore, only large prairie dog complexes (several thousand acres), made of many closely spaced prairie dog colonies, can support a successful breeding population of 100 to 200 black-footed ferrets.[18]

In the summer of 1985 the increasing black-footed population underwent a dramatic reversal. The first count, in August of 1985, estimated a dramatic decrease—only 58 ferrets. This number declined to 31 in October of the same year. Canine distemper, often reported in wild carnivores, had been introduced into the colony and, of the 12 ferrets brought into captivity, 6 died of the disease.

The past 2 years have been shadowed not only by the disastrous effects of the distemper outbreak, but also by the political maneuvering of the Wyoming Game and Fish Department. The group's director continued to block attempts to establish capture and breeding programs for the endangered black-footed ferret.[15]

A captive breeding program was finally established at Sybille, Wyoming, under the direction of Dr. Tom Thorne, a wildlife veterinarian.[19] These efforts will be closely monitored, and, it is hoped that attempts to mimic the ferrets' native habitat will produce litters of black-footed ferrets. Fortunately, the first litter was born in captivity in the summer of 1987.

USES

RODENT EXTERMINATORS

In England and the United States domestic ferrets have been used for rodent control. This practice became popular in the United States during the early part of the twentieth century, and tens of thousands of ferrets were raised and sold for this purpose. The Department of Agriculture distributed bulletins announcing the use of ferrets for rodent abatement.[20] Because rodents have an extreme fear of ferrets and will flee even their scent, only a few ferrets were needed to disperse literally hundreds of rodents from granaries, barns, and warehouses.

A ferretmeister would deploy his ferrets on an infested farm or granary, and the animal would then "ferret out" the rodents from their hiding places and nests. Men and terrier dogs, strategically located, would eradicate the rodents as they emerged from hiding. Alternatively, small farms or granaries would maintain ferrets and allow them territorial imperative for up to about 650 feet (200 m)— considered to be the ranging domain of a ferret—with an adequate food source. The introduction of commercially available rodenticides, however, has dramatically reduced the popularity of ferrets as rodent exterminators.

Historically, ferrets also have been used to control rodent populations endemic on ships. The Massachusetts Colonial Navy, the state's Revolutionary War naval militia, was organized on December 29, 1775. By an act of the Commonwealth of Massachusetts state legislature, the present unit was reactivated in 1967 to carry on the tradition of the original Revolutionary War units. At an impressive naval ceremony held at Bristol Community College on September 14, 1986, the ferret was officially proclaimed the mascot of the Colonial Navy of Massachusetts. The following is an excerpt from the ceremony (Fig. 1–4):

Today marks a milestone in the history of the Colonial Navy of Massachusetts. It gives me great pleasure to have all of you present here today, to bear witness to a unique naval ceremony, that to the very best of my knowledge, probably has not been performed since the late seventeen hundreds . . . over two hundred years ago. This was a traditional ceremony that both officers and men looked forward to with great delight. No . . . this was not a solemn change of command, nor an impressive commissioning of a new ship of the fleet . . . this joyous occasion was the "Introduction of the Ship's Mascot!"

Now in the days of the wooden men o' war there was, quite often, an uninvited population of rodents aboard ship. They were certainly a nuisance and caused many a moment of unpleasantness among the crew. Dogs were completely unsuccessful mousers and besides, their barking kept both captain and crew awake. Cats were infinitely preferred over dogs, but they were unable to chase mice into the many narrow holes and passageways aboard the ship, so more mice escaped than were caught. But . . . there was one animal the rats and mice could never escape from . . . no matter where they tried to hide . . . no matter how small a hole they ran into . . . they were doomed! This animal could find them . . . anywhere! This animal was one of man's best friends and totally fearless. They were in great demand aboard the ships of the colonial navy, and fortunate indeed were the crews that had a *ferret* for a mascot and friend.

It is with great honor . . . that today . . . the Colonial Navy of Massachusetts hereby tenders the following proclamation:

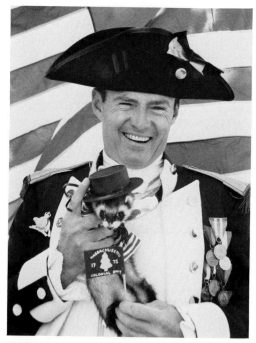

Fig. 1– 4. Frank Noble, Commodore of the Colonial Navy of Massachusetts, with Pokey the ferret, the official mascot.

Let it be known . . . that all men here and present bear witness. . . .

Whereas . . . on this day of our lord . . . the fourteenth day of September, in the year nineteen hundred and eighty-six. . . .

Whereas . . . it has been common knowledge for centuries, that you possess the unique ability to ferret out and destroy . . . all manner of mice, rats, and rodents. . . .

And whereas, by these deeds, you have infinitely improved the quality of life aboard ship. . . .

And further whereas, by your kindness, gentleness and devotion to the shipmates you so dutifully serve. . . .

It is with the utmost gratitude and pleasure . . . that the Colonial Navy of Massachusetts, does hereby and forthwith, and by the unanimous proclamation of both officers and men . . . hereby proclaim *Mustela furo*, the ferret, as its official mascot.[21]

FERRETING

Ferrets continue to be used for hunting rabbits in Britain.[22] The ferret's primary job is to chase the rabbits from their burrows into nets secured overhead. Ferrets have also been used for rabbiting in the United States but this is seldom practiced now and, in fact, is prohibited in many states. Today, in the United States and Canada, the ferret's predatory nature has been diluted by selective breeding with more docile ferrets that have been in captivity for many generations.

FERRET-LEGGING

The ferret plays an interesting and indispensable role in an English sport appropriately named ferret-legging. The contest, referred to as "put 'em down," involves a competitor who ties his trousers at the ankles, places two ferrets in them, and then secures his belt tightly. The object is to determine who can withstand the presence of the ferrets in his pants the longest. Evidently the sport has been around for centuries, but has made a remarkable comeback in the last two decades.[23] The current record, as of 1983, stands at an impressive 5 hours and 26 minutes, held by a 72-year-old Yorkshire man.

The contest requires that the ferrets have a full set of teeth. The contestant may attempt to dislodge the ferret from its biting location, but only if it is attempted from outside the trousers. According to the participants this is quite difficult, because ferrets usually maintain a strong hold for lengthy periods. Obviously, it is doubtful whether the sport will gain in popularity in other parts of the world.

PET FERRETS AND THEIR STATUS IN THE UNITED STATES

The domestic ferret is becoming increasingly popular in North America as a pet. In 1980, according to a major ferret producer, about 12,000 ferrets were sold, approximately 50% for research and the remainder for distribution as pets.[24] Small commercial breeders are now advertising locally or in ferret newsletters and, in addition, two large commercial operations produced and distributed around 30,000 ferrets for the pet industry in 1986. One estimate states that 50,000 to 75,000 ferrets are produced annually for use as pets in the United States.[13]

The pet industry is promoting ferrets in lay and trade journals, extolling the virtues of the ferret as a household pet.[25] Currently there are an estimated 400,000 ferret owners and 1,000,000 pet ferrets in the United States.[13] Also, the International Ferret Association membership now stands at 100,000, compared to 14,000 only 5 years ago.[26]

Except in two states, Alaska and West Virginia, the ferret historically has been categorized as a wild animal. Even now some states, such as New York, require a special permit to own ferrets. In California only neutered male ferrets may be owned as pets. New Hampshire, Massachusetts, Georgia, and South Carolina have banned pet ferrets. One reason cited by opponents of ferrets as pets is the lack of a Food and Drug Administration-approved rabies vaccine for ferrets, and the number of documented cases of rabies in ferrets in the United States.[24]

The United States Humane Society considers the ferret to be an exotic animal, and publicly discourages the use of ferrets as pets. This association is reportedly drafting legislation to be submitted to 46 states, proposing that pet ferrets be banned as pets.[13] There are a limited number of often cited cases in which ferrets have attacked babies or young children, inflicting serious wounds.[27,28] Although there are no data available in regard to why ferrets occasionally attack infants, case reports describe this behavior as unpredictable. Because of these attacks, one local ordinance, in Carson City, Nevada, has prohibited the sale of ferrets to house-

holds that have children under the age of 3 years. Unfortunately, no available surveys are published that compare the rate of ferret attacks with those of other pet animals.[29]

The banning of ferrets as pets is being challenged in various states by organized lobbyists, efforts that are backed primarily by ferret owners and enthusiasts. For example, in Pennsylvania, lobbying efforts at the state legislature have been successful. The state, which once required licenses from the Game Commission for ferret ownership, no longer requires such licensure, and the ferret is now categorized as a domestic animal.[25] In Alaska, which had permitted pet ferrets, the Alaska Game Commission recently issued regulations banning pet ferrets, a ruling that was subsequently challenged by a pet owner. Based on scientific information, the court ruled that the ferret was considered a domestic animal, and the ferret was removed from the jurisdiction of wildlife regulations.[25] Legislative victories for pet ownership of ferrets have also occurred in West Virginia and Maine, in which restrictions have been lifted.

The American Veterinary Medical Association Council on Public Health and Regulatory Veterinary Medicine, however, has formally discouraged the ownership of pet ferrets.[30] This announcement has created considerable controversy in the veterinary profession—in regard to whether ferrets are considered wild or exotic animals, as the Council on Public Health and Regulatory Veterinary Medicine maintains—especially in the area of rabies control. The association strongly opposes the use of wild or exotic animals as pets. Ferret breeders and owners, and some veterinarians who treat pet ferrets, argue that ferrets have been domesticated for over 2000 years and should not be considered as wild or exotic pets.[31] The controversy continues, and the Council on Veterinary Service has not issued any additional comments.

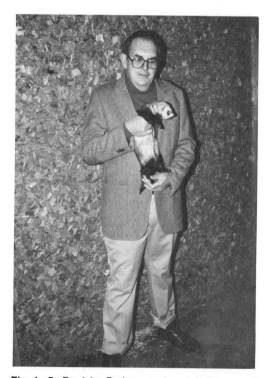

Fig. 1– 5. Dr. John Gorham, a pioneer in the use of ferrets in virology research.

FUR PRODUCTION

In North America during the early 1900s there was considerable interest in raising ferrets for their fur. European furriers were already buying and using ferret pelts. The early success of ferrets for fur production in North America was limited, partly because of the capricious behavior of fur buyers, the musky odor of the pelt, and the tendency for hair to fall from it.[20, 22] Nevertheless, commercial ferret farming for fur production has recently become more popular, and ferret farms exist in parts of the United States, Canada, certain countries in Europe, and New Zealand. Indeed, current newspaper advertisements in the United States prominently feature fitch coats for sale.

The exact genetic composition of ferrets raised for fur production varies. The F_1 generation of European polecats mated with domesticated ferrets, and the subsequent line breeding of F_1 with male European polecats, are sometimes used. In addition,

Mustela eversmanni is bred with the domestic ferret for fur production.[32]

BIOMEDICAL RESEARCH

The ferret, although domesticated for hundreds of years, was not recognized as having potential as an animal model for biomedical research until the 1900s. Early studies utilized the ferret in classic experiments with influenza virus pathogenesis.[33] Today the ferret is still the model of choice for studying the influenza virus, as well as other viral diseases (see Chap. 17, Viral Disease Models) (Fig. 1–5). Two decades later, an article detailing the use of ferrets in research cited only 26 publications.[33] Even in the 1950s and early 1960s, texts compiling data on 60 to 90 mammalian species cited the ferret infrequently. For example, in the 1956 edition of the Handbook of Biological Data, reference was made to the ferret only 11 times, and it was not cited at all

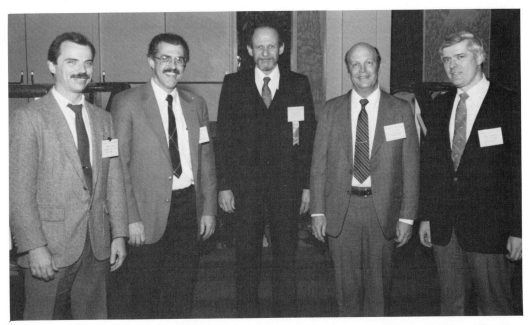

Fig. 1–6. Speakers at the 26th Annual Meeting of the Society of Toxicology. Symposium: The Use of Ferrets as an Animal Model in Preclinical Safety Studies and Biomedical Research, 1987. (*From left,* Drs. Dan McClain, James Fox, Yigal Greener, Richard Hoar, and Wayne Galbraith.)

in the Biological Handbook: Blood and Other Body Fluids, published in 1961.[7]

Literature reviews undertaken in 1967, 1969, 1973, and 1985, however, reveal an increasing appreciation for the ferret's usefulness and versatility in the study of human physiologic, anatomic, and disease mechanisms.[7,34–36] In the most recent review of research publications involving ferrets (1977–1984) using the BIOSIS data base, citations were obtained from both Biological Abstracts and Biological Abstracts/RRM.[36] In addition to 8000 journals, BIOSIS covers symposia, reviews, preliminary reports, selected institutional and government documents, and research notes. MEDLINE, from the National Library of Medicine, was also used in the literature review, and over 569 citations were identified.[36] Of the articles cited, 27% (155) involved the use of the ferret in physiology, 24% of the citations were in virology and immunology, 10.4% in pharmacology, 8.4% in toxicology, and 4% in teratology. This compendium was published as part of an entire issue of the Journal of Laboratory Animal Science devoted to the use of the ferret in biomedical research.[37] In addition, recent symposia attest to their increasing popularity for use in biomedical research (Fig. 1–6).[38,39]

The ferret's increasing popularity in research and as a pet is mainly a result of large-scale commercial production. For example, Marshall Farms, in New York, has been raising ferrets commercially for over 40 years (Fig. 1–7). Unlike scientists in Europe and the British Isles, biomedical researchers in the United States can request a specific sex, weight, and age of the animal for individual experiments. Even though the ferret is nonstandardized in regard to an exact genotype and pedigree, its routine availability in a clinically healthy state has aided immeasurably toward gaining acceptance as a research animal.

The domesticated ferret has and continues to be used extensively in studies involving virology, reproductive physiology, anatomy, and endocrinology, as well as in other areas of biomedical research. Because of the similarity of many anatomic, metabolic, and physiologic features to those of humans, use of the ferret is also being promoted as an alternative to the use of dogs and nonhuman primates in toxicology studies. A historic event regarding the use of ferrets in toxicology research was their introduction into the field of experimental teratology. This began with reports of their response to rubella virus and to chlorcyclizine, which produced cleft palates. Other substances that produce malformations in ferrets include β-aminopropionitrile, thalidomide, mustine hydrochloride, trypan blue, salicylates, and methylazoxymethanol acetate (MAM Ac). The use of MAM Ac has introduced the ferret to behavioral teratologists because it produces lissencephaly, a condition in which failure of development of cerebral gyri results in a nonconvoluted brain (of the rodent).[40] The ferret is also being used to replace the cat in neuroendocrinology and neuroanatomy experiments (see Section III: Research Applications).

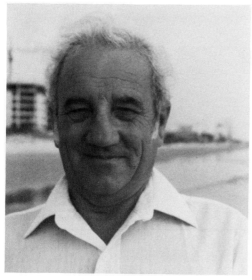

Fig. 1–7. Mr. Gilman Marshall, a pioneer in the commercial rearing of ferrets for use in biomedical research.

REFERENCES

1. Corbet, G.B., and Hill, J.E.: A World List of Mammalian Species. Ithaca, NY, Cornell University Press, 1980.
2. Thomson, A.P.D.: A history of the ferret. J. Hist. Med., 6:471, 1951.
3. Roberts, M.F.: All About Ferrets. Neptune City, NJ, T.F.H. Publications, 1977.
4. Grzimek, H.C.B., Grzimek's Animal Encyclopedia (English Ed.). Vol. 12. New York, Van Nostrand Reinhold, 1975.
5. Walton, K.C.: The ferret. *In* Handbook of British Mammals. 2nd ed. Edited by G.B. Corbet, and H.M. Southern. Oxford Blackwell Scientific Publications, 1977.
6. Poole, T.B.: Some behavioral differences between the European polecat, *Mustela putorius*, the ferret, *M. furo*, and their hybrids. J. Proc. Zool. Soc. (Lond.), *166*:25, 1972.
7. Hahn, E.W., and Wester, R.C.: The Biomedical Use of Ferrets in Research. North Rose, NY, Marshall Farms Animals, 1969.
8. Bednarz, M.: Observations on reproduction in polecat and ferret hybrids (abstr.). Anim. Breed, *30*:239, 1962.
9. Bednarz, M.: Preliminary observations on the growth and development of polecat and ferret hybrids (abstr.). Anim. Breed., *30*:239, 1962.
10. Gray, A.P.: Mammalian Hybrids. A Checklist with Bibliography. Bucks, England, Commonwealth Agricultural Bureau, 1954.
11. Andrews, P.L.R.: The ferret. *In* U.F.A.W. Handbook on the Care and Management of Laboratory Animals. 6th ed. Edited by T. Poole. Harlow, Essex, Longman Scientific & Technical, 1987.
12. King, C.: Immigrant Killers, p. 224. Oxford, England, Oxford University Press, 1985.
13. Diesch, S.L.: Pet European ferrets: A hazard to human infants. Proceedings of the 90th Annual Meeting of the U.S.H.A., Louisville, KY, 1986, pp. 364–367.
14. Stevens, W.F.: Status of Ferrets and Other Introduced Animals on San Juan Island. San Juan, San Juan Environmental Studies Report, Oct. 15, 1979.
15. May, R.M.: The cautionary tale of the black-footed ferret. Nature, *320*:13, 1986.
16. Carpenter, J.W., Davidson, J.P., Novilla, M.N., and Huang, J.C.M.: Metastatic papillary cystadenocarcinoma of the mammary gland in a black-footed ferret. J. Wildl. Dis., *16*:587, 1980.
17. Weinberg, D.: Decline and fall of the black-footed ferret. Nat. Hist., *95*:62, 1986.
18. Richardson, L.: On the trail of the last black-footed ferrets. Nat. Hist., *95*:69, 1986.
19. Pearce, M.: My friend the ferret. Wall Street Journal, p. 30. October 1, 1986.
20. Harding, A.R. Ferret Facts and Fancies. Columbus, OH, A.R. Harding, 1943.
21. Noble, Frank (Commodore, Colonial Navy of Massachusetts): Presented at Bristol Community College, Bristol, Massachusetts: September 14, 1986.
22. Wellstead, G.: Ferrets and Ferreting. Neptune City, NJ, T.F.H. Publications, 1982.
23. Katz, D.R.: Ferret legging. Outdoors, *Feb/Mar:73*, 1983.
24. Pet ferrets and rabies. C.D.C.—Veterinary Publications Health Notes, pp. 1–2. Atlanta, U.S. Department of Health and Human Services, 1980.
25. Morton, C., and Morton, F.: Ferrets, A Complete Pet Owner's Manual, p. 72. NY, Barrons, 1985.
26. Petzke, D.: The pet of the year isn't a pinup or a pup, but it is just as cute. Wall Street Journal, p. 1. April 4, 1986.
27. Diesch, S.L.: Should wild-exotic animals be banned as pets. Cal. Vet. *12*:13, 1981.
28. Diesch, S.L.: Reported human injuries or health threats attributed to wild or exotic animals kept as pets. (1971–1981). J. Am. Vet. Med. Assoc., *18*:382, 1982.
29. Pet ferret rabies. Rabies Surveillance Annual Summary, 1985, p. 9. Atlanta, Centers for Disease Control, 1986.
30. J. Am. Vet. Med. Assoc., *188*:121, 1986.
31. J. Am. Vet. Med. Assoc., *188*:1122, 1986.
32. Morton, C.: Personal communication, 1987.
33. Pyle, N.J.: Use of ferrets in laboratory work and research investigations. Am. J. Public Health, *30*:787, 1940.
34. Shump, A., et al.: A Bibliography of Mustelids. Part I: Ferrets and Polecats, p. 53. East Lansing, Michigan, Michigan Agricultural Experiment Station 6977, 1974.
35. Marshall, K.R., and Marshall, G.W.: The Biomedical Use of Ferrets in Research, Supplement I. North Rose, NY, Marshall Farms Animals, Inc., 1973.
36. Frederick, K.A., and Babish, J.G.: Compendium of recent literature on the ferret. Lab. Anim. Sci., *35*:298, 1985.
37. Ferrets in biomedical research. Lab. Anim. Sci., *35*:200, 1985.
38. Greener, Y. (Chairman): Symposium: The use of ferrets as an animal model in pre-clinical safety studies and biomedical research. Twenty-sixth Annual Meeting of the Society of Toxicology, Washington, D.C., February 23–27, 1987.
39. Fox, J.G. (Chairman): Symposium: The biology and diseases of the ferret. J. Am. Vet. Med. Assoc., *190*:1610, 1987.
40. Hoar, R.M.: Use of ferrets in toxicity testing. J. Am. Coll. Toxicol., *3*:325, 1984.

chapter 2

ANATOMY OF THE FERRET*

N. Q. An

H. E. Evans

The domestic ferret, *Mustela putorius furo*, is in the family Mustelidae of the order Carnivora. This family is thought to be the most primitive living group of terrestrial carnivores. Most family members are active carnivores, with powerful jaws and long canines. All have anal glands that are developed to some degree, giving them a musky odor. Some are arboreal, others fossorial, and a few are aquatic or marine.[1] Most are ground-dwelling, and are found in logs, crevices, and forest debris. Mustelids include diurnal and nocturnal species. The diet for most species is vertebrate prey but others will eat insects, fruit, honey, and carrion. They usually breed once a year, and several show delayed implantation. Enders has presented a classic study of reproduction in the mink.[2] General mustelid biology has been reviewed by Ewer. Kainer, Klingener, and Smith and Krasulak have described the viscera of the mink, *Mustela vison*, which are very similar to those of the ferret.[4–6]

ACKNOWLEDGMENTS

The animals used for the study presented in this chapter were provided by Marshall Farms of North Rose, NY, and included the wild type or buff-colored fitch ferret, with a black mask, and the albino or white variety.[7]

* Refer to endpaper on the front right endleaf of the book for a detailed drawing of the anatomy of the ferret.

SUPERFICIAL ANATOMY

Its body shape and short limbs enable the ferret to chase its prey through small holes or burrows large enough only for a rat. The eyes are small and the ears are short. The neck is cylindric and noticeably long, and blends gradually with the slender and elongated thorax and abdomen. The male is heavier and larger than the female, as in the mink, and there are usually more fat deposits in the inguinal region.

The body is covered by fine underfur and longer, coarser guard hairs. This combination of fine and coarse hairs provides dense insulation for the body and a very durable fur. The tail is densely furred, and aids in swimming.

SKELETON

The skeleton (Fig. 2–1) consists of axial, appendicular, and heterotopic components. Heterotopic bones are those not associated with either the axial or appendicular portions of the skeleton. Such bones may occur in the nose, heart, muscle tendons, penis, or clitoris. In the ferret the only consistently present heterotopic bones are the patella in the tendon of insertion of the quadriceps femoris, the lateral fabella in the tendon of origin of the lateral gastrocnemius, and the os penis of the male.

AXIAL SKELETON

The axial portion includes the skull and hyoid apparatus, the vertebrae, the ribs, and the sternebrae.

Skull and Hyoid Apparatus

The skull of the ferret is almost twice as long as wide and lacks sutures in the adult, making it impossible to differentiate individual bones. The facial region is short, and constitutes about a third of the length of the skull. The nasal opening is slightly constricted as compared to other mammalian skulls of similar size. The dorsal nasal concha (dorsal turbinate) is represented by a well-developed shelf on each side and the ventral nasal concha (maxilloturbinate), which occupies the maxillary sinus, has a complicated labyrinth that extends to the opening of the meatus (Fig. 2–2). The ethmoidal labyrinth attached to the cribriform plate occupies the deepest recess of the nasal cavity.

The dorsal surface of the skull is rather flat and the calvaria serves primarily for the attachment of the strong temporalis muscles, which close the lower jaw. On the median line is a sagittal crest (Fig. 2–3) that extends from the occiput to the orbits, where it flares to meet the zygomatic process of the frontal bone on each side. The brain case is disproportionately large, and caudally there is a prominent nuchal crest extending transversely from one auditory bulla to the other. The widest portion of the skull is between the zygomatic arches. Each arch is rather slender and extends from the maxilla to the temporal bone to form a large cavity on each side. This cavity is occupied rostrally by the eye and caudally by the large muscles of mastication, the masseter, temporalis, and pterygoid muscles, which attach to the ramus of the mandible. Thus, the orbit and pterygopalatine fossa are continuous. The caudal extent of the orbit is indicated by the frontal process of the zygomatic bone. There is no postorbital bar but an orbital ligament is present.

The caudoventral region of the skull is characterized by the tympanic bullae, housing the middle ear ossicles. On the lateral side of each bulla is the external acoustic meatus, where the external ear is attached. Beneath the external acoustic meatus the stylohyoid bone of the hyoid apparatus is attached along its length to the bulla (Fig. 2–4). The hyoid apparatus consists of paired stylohyoid, epihyoid,

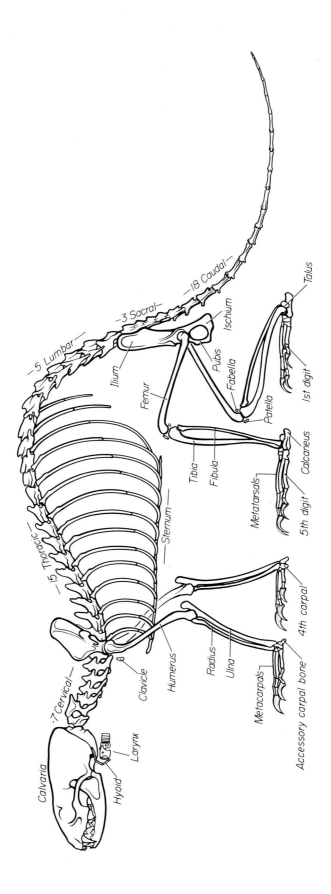

Fig. 2–1. The skeleton.

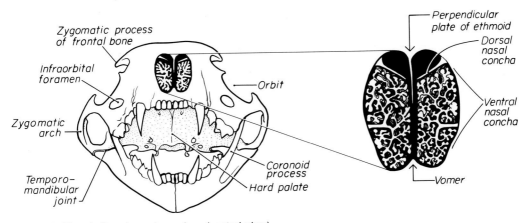

Fig. 2–2. The skull and nasal conchae (*rostral view*).

and keratohyoid bones, a median basi-hyoid, and paired thyrohyoids, which suspend the larynx.

The nasopharyngeal canal that begins at the caudal end of the hard palate is bounded by pterygoid bones caudally, which bear laterally directed hooks on the hamuli.

At the caudal end of the skull the foramen magnum is bounded by a thin shelf of the supraoccipital dorsally, with the large exoccipital condyle on each side, and the notched basioccipital ventrally.

The jaws are short and the articular condyle of the mandible fits into a transverse articular fossa that has a flange, which prevents dislocation when the jaws are opened widely, as in a killing bite. The tooth-bearing portions of the upper and lower jaws are about equal in length, but the lower arcade is narrower than the upper and thus fits within it. This provides for a shearing action when chewing. The six upper incisors are slightly longer than the six lower incisors and, when the jaws are closed, they are more prominent. There is a peculiarity in the placement of the lower incisors in that the second incisors are set back noticeably from the others, as if there were not enough room for an alveolus. The lower canines are long and pointed and close in front of the upper canines, which is characteristic for carnivores.

There are usually four premolars in the Carnivora but only three in the ferret, indicating that the first premolars of the ferret have probably been lost in development. Thus, the last upper carnassial tooth, which is the third cheek tooth, probably represents the fourth premolar, and the large lower carnassial tooth, which is a fourth cheek tooth, probably represents the first molar.

Vertebrae

The vertebral column of the ferret is quite flexible, and each vertebra is large in comparison to the size of the animal. The vertebral formula is C7, T15, L5 (6), S3, Cd18.

Cervical Region (Neck). The neck is long and the seven cervical vertebrae are more massive than the thoracics, indicating a well-developed cervical musculature to effect movement and stability of the head and neck when capturing and subduing prey. The atlas is large, with prominent wings pierced by a transverse foramen and a lateral vertebral foramen on each side. The axis has a prominent dens, a ridgelike spinous process, and large transverse processes. Cervicals 3 through 7 are similar in size, except that the transverse processes of the sixth cervical vertebra are greatly enlarged.

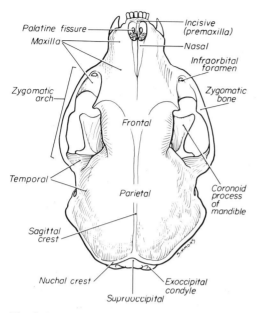

Fig. 2–3. The skull (*dorsal view*).

Thoracic Region. There are usually 15 thoracic vertebrae characterized by paired ribs. Each rib consists of a bony costal portion and a cartilaginous sternal portion that is almost as long. At the costochondral junction in the midthoracic region there is often a swelling as a result of rapid growth. These enlargements can often be palpated or seen radiographically.

Specimens have been seen with 14 ribs on both sides or 14 on one side and 15 on the other. Normally, 10 pairs of ribs attach to the sternum and the last 5 pairs join each other distally to form the costal arch. The last pair of ribs may be shorter than the others, and end unattached in the flank musculature.

The first 11 pairs of ribs articulate with the vertebral column by means of a head or capitulum, which fits into a socket between two vertebral bodies, and a tuberculum, which articulates with the transverse process of the vertebra. The remainder of the ribs each articulate on only one vertebral body.

Because the first ribs are quite short the thoracic inlet between them is restricted, barely allowing for passage of the trachea, esophagus, and great vessels. Caudally the ribs are long, and the thorax widens considerably to enclose much of the abdominal viscera.

Lumbar Region (Loin). The five or six lumbar vertebrae increase in size from the first to the last in regard to their body as well as their transverse processes. The cranial and caudal articular processes interdigitate so as to allow great dorsoventral extension and flexion, with limited lateral bending. The large transverse processes are the result of a well-developed trunk musculature.

Sacral Region (Sacrum). The three sacral vertebrae are fused as one mass, but the enlarged lateral wings of the first sacral vertebra form most of the articular face to meet the ilium. The three dorsal sacral spines are distinct, and there are two pairs of sacral foramina that open dorsally and ventrally to transmit branches of the sacral spinal nerve.

Caudal Region (Tail). The terms "coccyx" and "coccygeal vertebrae" are now restricted to the human. There are 18 caudal vertebrae in the tail, which is seven times as long as the sacrum. The first caudal vertebra is located at the level of the acetabulum, and the first three caudals form the roof of the pelvic canal. Beneath the second to fifth caudal vertebrae there are hemal arches (chevron bones) that enclose an artery and a vein. The hemal arch of the third caudal is particularly large and projects cranially, almost meeting the small arch ahead of it. The caudal vertebrae diminish in size posteriorly and become progressively more rodlike and featureless.

Sternum

The adult sternum is composed of eight bony sternebrae and a caudal cartilagi-

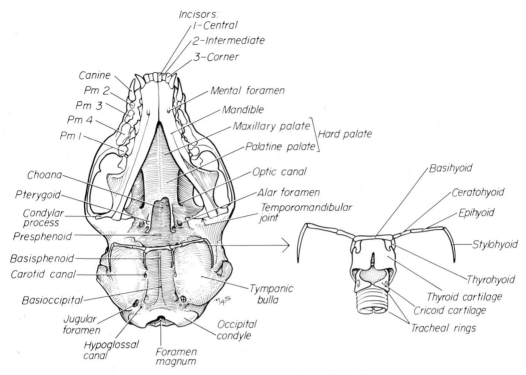

Fig. 2–4. The skull, mandible, hyoid apparatus, and larynx (*ventral view*).

nous xiphoid process. The first sternal element or manubrium is fused with the second to form a single unit longer than any of the others. The eight sternebrae are joined to each other by intersternebral cartilages. The sternal ribs attach at these joints.

APPENDICULAR SKELETON

The appendicular skeleton includes the bones of the limbs and the limb girdles. The thoracic limb or forelimb is attached to the scapula at the shoulder joint and to the skeleton only by muscles, because the clavicle is quite small in the ferret.

1. Shoulder girdle
   a. Scapula
   b. Clavicle
2. Arm or brachium
   a. Humerus
3. Forearm or antebrachium
   a. Radius
   b. Ulna

4. Forepaw or manus
   a. Carpal bones
   b. Metacarpal bones
   c. Phalanges
   d. Sesamoids of the digits

The pelvic limb or hindlimb is attached to the pelvis at the hip joint and to the skeleton via the sacroiliac joint.

1. Pelvic girdle
   a. Ilium
   b. Ischium
   c. Pubis
2. Thigh
   a. Femur
3. Leg or crus
   a. Tibia
   b. Fibula
   c. Sesamoids of the knee
4. Hindpaw or pes
   a. Tarsal bones
   b. Metatarsal bones
   c. Phalanges
   d. Sesamoids of the digits

Bones of the Thoracic Girdle and Forelimb

Scapula. The scapula or shoulder blade is roughly triangular, with a supraspinous fossa that is more than twice as wide as the infraspinous fossa. The spine of the scapula is low but expands near the neck of the scapula to form a proximally directed metacromion and a distally directed acromion process. The distal end of the scapula is enlarged and bears a glenoid fossa for the articulation of the humerus. There is a supraglenoid tubercle cranially and a coracoid process craniomedially.

Clavicle. The clavicle is a short flattened rod that lies embedded in the brachiocephalicus muscle, and is best seen from the medial side at the level of the shoulder joint. It is connected by muscle and a fascial sheet to the scapula and sternum (see Fig. 2–7). On a radiograph, it would be seen craniomedial to the shoulder joint.

Humerus. The humerus is longer than the scapula, and expanded at both ends. The head at the proximal end is large and hemispherical. A deltoid tuberosity is noticeable. The condyle at the distal end is expanded transversely, and bears a supratrochlear foramen above the enlarged medial epicondyle. The olecranon fossa is deeply excavated.

Radius. The radius is expanded and flattened distally. It is bowed slightly medially at midshaft. At the proximal end the capitular fovea lies adjacent to the medial coronoid process of the ulna, and forms a deep trochlear notch.

Ulna. The ulna is also slightly bowed and expanded at both ends. At the proximal end there is a larger olecranon and a prominent anconeal process. The anconeal process fits into the olecranon fossa of the humerus when the elbow is extended, thus stabilizing the joint. The elbow joint is deep because of the well-developed trochlear notch between the coronoid and anconeal processes.

Carpus. The carpus or wrist is formed by seven carpal bones in two rows, as in the dog. There is a large radial carpal, a smaller ulna carpal, and a palmar accessory carpal in the proximal row. In the distal row of four carpals the fourth is the largest, and probably represents a fusion of the fourth and fifth distal carpals. There is a large sesamoid bone on the distal palmar side of the radial carpal bone.

Metacarpus. There are five metacarpals, and the third and fourth are the longest. On the palmar side of each metacarpophalangeal joint there are two sesamoid bones. This is different from the dog, in which the first digit has only one sesamoid. On the palmar surface of the paw there are four metacarpal pads.

Digits. There are five clawed digits; the first is the shortest and the third and fourth are the longest. As in most mammals, the first digit has only two phalanges while the others have three. The distal phalanx at rest is normally held in overextension and there is a digital pad on its palmar surface. The base of the large claw encloses the distal phalanx completely. The ferret is plantigrade, and walks on the ventral surface of the carpus, metacarpus, and digits.

Bones of the Pelvic Girdle and Hindlimb

The pelvic girdle or pelvis consists of the two hip bones (os coxae) united with each other at the symphysis pelvis midventrally. Each hip bone is formed by the union of the ilium, ischium, and pubis. The ilium is the most cranial element and has a wing for articulation with the sacrum at the sacroiliac joint. This joint is a diarthrosis and allows for some movement. The pubis forms the cranial border of the obturator foramen, and the ischium forms the caudal border. The acetabulum for articulation of the femur is formed where the ilium, ischium, and pubis meet.

Pelvic Canal. The pelvic canal is the bony passageway between the sacrum and the pelvis. At the pelvic inlet the pubis forms the floor and walls, while the promontory on the ventral surface of the sacrum forms the roof. At the pelvic outlet the ischium forms the floor and walls while the first three caudal vertebrae serve as the roof.

Ilium. The cranial end of the narrow ilium is rounded and projects above the level of the vertebral spines. It is not possible to differentiate between a dorsal tuber sacrale and a ventral tuber coxae. This end of the ilium serves to attach the extensor muscles of the spine. The lateral surface of the ilium provides attachment for the muscles of the hip. Immediately ahead of the acetabulum there is a tuberosity for the attachment of the rectus femoris muscle, an extensor of the knee.

Ischium. The ischium forms the caudal end of the pelvis. It is expanded transversely to form a tuberosity for the origin of the thigh muscles. In the male the crus of the penis and the ischiocavernosus muscle that covers it both originate on the caudal border of the tuberosity.

The dorsal border of the ischium forms the ischiatic notch, over which the tendon of the internal obturator muscle passes. The narrowest portion of the ischium is the ramus, which meets its fellow on the midline and forms the caudal half of the symphysis pelvis.

Pubis. The pubis is very narrow and extends from the acetabulum to the symphysis. Between the pubis and the ischium is the unusually large obturator foramen. The rectus abdominis muscle, a flexor of

the spine, attaches to the cranial margin of the pubis and passes to the sternum. Overall the ferret pelvis is elongate and delicately built. It is articulated with the vertebral column only at its cranial end.

Femur. The femur or thigh bone is comparatively long and straight. It has a large head on a slightly angled neck and a large trochanter for the insertion of the hip muscles.

The distal end of the femur bears large medial and lateral condyles. Resting on the caudodorsal surface of the lateral condyle is a sesamoid bone, the lateral fabella (see Fig. 2–5), which lies in the tendon of origin of the lateral gastrocnemius muscle (see Fig. 2–10). There is no medial fabella in the medial head of the gastrocnemius (a medial fabella is always present in the dog).

Stifle or Knee Joint. This joint, between the femur and the tibia, is the most complicated joint of the limb. On the cranial surface of the knee the patella, an ovoid sesamoid bone in the tendon of insertion of the quadriceps, glides into the trochlear groove on the distal end of the femur.

Within the stifle joint, between each femoral and tibial condyle, there is a semilunar fibrocartilage or meniscus. These lateral and medial menisci are thicker at the periphery than they are within the joint, and thus act as C-shaped wedges to stabilize the joint. They are attached to the femur, tibia, and each other by ligaments (Fig. 2–5). The lateral meniscus is attached to the intercondylar fossa of the femur by a meniscofemoral ligament. Each meniscus is attached to the intercondylar area of the tibia.

The femur and tibia-fibula are held together by lateral and medial collateral ligaments on the surface of the joint capsule, and by cranial and caudal cruciate ligaments within the joint capsule. The medial collateral ligament passes from the femur to the tibia and fuses with the

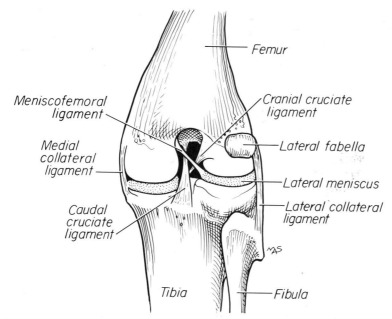

Fig. 2–5. Ligaments of the knee joint, right hindlimb (*caudal view*).

medial meniscus as well. The lateral collateral ligament attaches proximally to the femur and distally to the head of the fibula. The cranial cruciate ligament passes from the medial surface of the lateral femoral condyle and across the inter condylar fossa to the cranial intercondylar area of the tibia. It crosses the joint ahead of the caudal cruciate ligament. The caudal cruciate ligament passes from the lateral surface of the medial femoral condyle to the popliteal notch of the tibia. The cruciate ligaments are responsible for maintaining a "tight" joint.

Tibia. The tibia is the longest bone of the hindlimb. At its proximal end are the medial and lateral condyles, with an intercondylar area between. At the distal end is the tibial cochlea, which meets the trochlea of the talus. The medial part of the distal extremity of the tibia projects as the medial malleolus over the talus.

Fibula. The fibula is a slender bone that is almost as long as the tibia. Its head articu-

lates proximally with the lateral tibial condyle. Distally its lateral malleolus articulates with both the tibia and the talus.

Tarsus, Hock, or Ankle. There are seven tarsal bones, as in the dog: two large proximal bones, the talus and calcaneus; a central tarsal; and four distal tarsals.

The talus or tibial tarsal bone has a trochlea that bears the weight of the body transmitted through the tibial cochlea. The calcaneus or fibular tarsal bone is longer than the talus and has a traction process, the tuber calcanei, for the attachment of the extensor muscles of the hock.

The central tarsal is cuboidal, while the distal tarsals vary in shape. The second distal tarsal bone is the smallest and allows the second metatarsal to intercalate the distal row of metacarpal bones.

Metatarsus. There are five metatarsal bones, like the metacarpals, and the first is the shortest. Beneath each metatarsophalangeal joint there are two sesamoid bones in the tendons of insertion of the interosseous muscles. Even the first digit has two, which is unusual, because there is only one in the mink and dog. On the plantar surface there is a well-developed sesamoid bone at the base of the fifth metatarsal bone.

Digits. All the digits of the foot, or pes, bear claws that cover the terminal phalanx. The terminal phalanx at rest is in overextension. The first digit is short and has only two phalanges. All the other digits have three phalanges. The third and fourth digits are the longest.

As with the forefoot, the hindfoot is also plantigrade. It is in contact with the ground via metatarsal and digital pads from the calcaneus to the tips of the digits (see Fig. 2–1).

Heterotopic Skeleton

The male has an os penis or baculum within the elongated glans. The size and conformation of the baculum can be used for estimating age as well as for taxonomic purposes. In the adult ferret the baculum is 4.5 cm long.

MUSCLES

The muscles of the ferret are very similar to those of the mink, although differences may be seen in their delaminations and slip formation. It is not possible to say whether these differences are species-dependent, breed-specific, or merely individual variations, because muscles may vary at all levels. Williams has compared the muscles of the ranch mink, *Mustela vison*, with two genera of skunks (*Spirogale* and *Mephitis*), a marten (*Martes*), and a badger (*Taxidea*) [8] He found all of these mustelids to be quite similar, with distinctive features not present in the dog. One such feature was an angular head of the triceps brachii in addition to long, lateral, and medial heads. Another

feature was a deep rhomboideus muscle in addition to the superficial parts. He also noted that the stylohyoid muscle was absent in the mink, and it is also absent in the ferret. This muscle, which passes from the mastoid region of the skull to the basihyoid, raises the base of the tongue and thus the larynx. This muscle is also lost in some dogs, particularly in the dachshund.

The following brief muscle descriptions are based on Williams' work on the mink, modified as required for the ferret.[8]

MUSCLES OF THE JAWS

The digastricus is a fusiform muscle that functions to open the jaws. It originates on the jugular process and tympanic bulla and inserts on the ventral border of the caudal portion of the mandible. It is a combination of two muscles, and thus there are two different innervations—the rostral portion is innervated by the trigeminal nerve, and the caudal portion by the facial nerve. There is a faint tendinous inscription across the middle of the muscle as evidence of its duality.

The masseter originates on the zygomatic arch, thus forming the bulge behind the cheek. It inserts on the masseteric fossa, condyloid crest, and angular process of the mandible. It is a powerful adductor for closing the lower jaw, and some of its fibers blend with the temporalis muscle near its insertion.

The temporalis increases the size of the head, because it originates on the nuchal crest and on the frontoparietal area of the calvaria. The latter area constitutes the temporal fossa whose surface appears roughened because of the attachment of this large muscle. Insertion is on the coronoid process of the mandible. The temporalis muscle is the major adductor of the lower jaw, and is largest in the male. Both this muscle and the masseter may be delaminated into two or more muscle sheets by fascial planes.

The lateral and medial pterygoids are deep muscles that originate on the pterygoid crest and pterygopalatine fossa at the level of the choana. Insertion is on the ventral border of the mandible and on the medial aspect of the angular process. They function to assist the masseter and temporalis in closing the lower jaw for crushing and chewing.

MUSCLES OF THE TONGUE

The genioglossus is a muscle that extends the tongue and functions for lapping and cleaning. It originates on the inner surface of the mandibular symphysis, and inserts as a ventral fan into the body of the tongue.

The styloglossus originates from the stylohyoid bone and tympanic bulla, and passes to the tongue lateral to the hyoid apparatus.

The hyoglossus is the primary muscle forming the body of the tongue. It originates on the basihyoid, thyrohyoid, and epihyoid bones.

The geniohyoideus is a narrow muscle close to the midline that originates on the mandibular symphysis and inserts on the basihyoid bone. Contraction of this muscle pulls the base of the tongue forward, causing it to protrude.

The mylohyoideus passes from one mandible to the other across the midline and forms a sling that supports the tongue. It has an attachment caudally with the basihyoid bone, and tends to stabilize the base of the tongue.

MUSCLES OF THE NECK AND TRUNK

The sternomastoideus lies on the ventrolateral surface of the neck. It originates on the manubrium of the sternum and in-serts on the nuchal crest and mastoid process. The right and left muscles are fused at their origin. Contraction of only one muscle pulls the head to one side, whereas contraction of both muscles lowers the head.

The sternothyroideus is another muscle that originates on the manubrium of the sternum. It passes along the midventral surface of the neck to insert on the thyroid cartilage of the larynx.

The sternohyoideus is a third muscle from the manubrium, deeper than the others, which passes up the neck to insert on the basihyoid bone. At the manubrium, and for a short distance thereafter, the sternothyroideus and the sternohyoideus are fused with each other.

The brachiocephalicus is a compound muscle with attachments to the head, neck, and forelimb, hence its name. It is composed of three muscles that are believed to originate on the clavicle or clavicular tendon. In the ferret the clavicle is reduced to a free-floating plate within the muscle (see Figs. 2–6 and 2–7) but its position can be seen clearly from the medial side, where the clavicular tendon attaches to the medial side of the distal end of the scapula. The three components of the brachiocephalicus are as follows:

1. The cleidocervicalis (clavotrapezius, according to some authors), a broad muscle from the clavicle to the fascia, covering the neck. Its attachment extends from the level of the nuchal crest to the level of the fourth cervical vertebra.
2. The cleidomastoideus, a straplike muscle from the clavicle to the mastoid process of the skull. This muscle is hidden from view by the cleidocervicalis.
3. The cleidobrachialis (clavodeltoideus, according to some authors), which extends from the clavicle to the greater tubercle and crest of the humerus.

The action of the brachiocephalicus, with the limb fixed, is to turn the head to one side if acting unilaterally or to pull the head ventrally if acting bilaterally. When

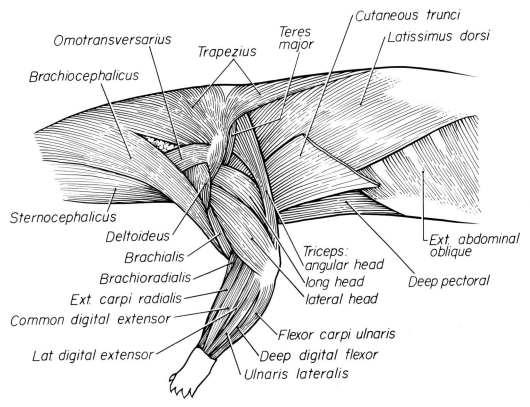

Fig. 2–6. Muscles of the trunk and thoracic limb.

the limb is not fixed on the ground the brachiocephalicus raises and advances the limb.

The neck and trunk have a series of muscles associated with the vertebral column and ribs that bend the spine. Muscles above the level of the transverse processes are extensor muscles of the spine (epaxial musculature) and those below are flexors of the spine (hypaxial musculature). If either extensors or flexors act unilaterally they will cause a bending of the spine to one side.

There are three primary groups of extensors. The most medial is the transversospinalis system, the next is the longissimus system, and the most lateral is the iliocostalis system. Each of these has muscles that span one or more vertebrae, and several of these muscles have been given specific names (e.g., splenius,

biventer, complexus, obliquus capitis, rectus capitis, and intertransversarius).

Flexors of the spine are more difficult to group because they include subvertebral muscles, scalenes, intercostal muscles, and abdominal muscles (see Fig. 2–8). An important flexor of the spine is the rectus abdominis muscle, which extends from the pelvis to the sternum. It has no attachment to the spine.

MUSCLES OF THE THORACIC LIMB

The extrinsic muscles of the limb pass from the body to the limb, whereas the intrinsic muscles are attached to parts of the limb skeleton itself (Figs. 2–6 and 2–7). In the ferret and other carnivores the thoracic limb is attached to the axial skeleton only by muscles.

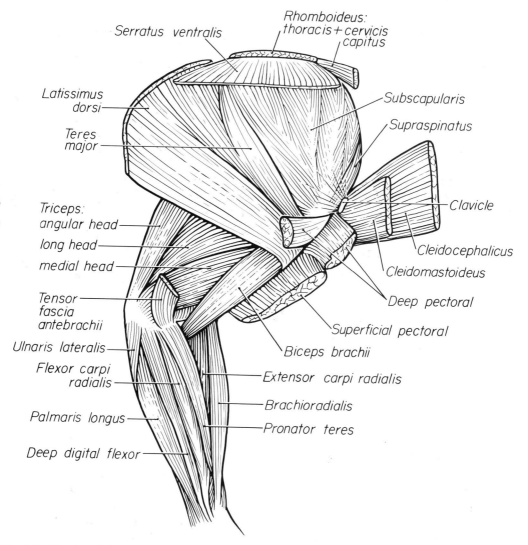

Fig. 2–7. Muscles of the thoracic limb (*medial view*).

The brachiocephalicus muscle, a three-part muscle with the vestigial clavicle, has already been discussed (see preceding discussion).

The superficial and deep pectoral muscles originate on the sternum and attach to the humerus. They serve to keep the limb under the body by adducting it. When the limb is fixed the deep pectoral muscles pull the trunk cranially. The pectoral muscles also support the weight of the body between the limbs.

The omotransversarius is the straplike muscle that passes from the wing of the atlas to the metacromion of the scapula. It can either bend the neck laterally or help advance the limb.

The trapezius is the most dorsal and superficial muscle of the shoulder. It originates on the median raphe of the neck and thorax and passes to the spine of the scapula. It functions to abduct and elevate the forelimb.

The rhomboideus is hidden from view by the trapezius. This muscle has four parts: rhomboideus capitis to the head, rhomboideus cervicis to the neck, rhomboideus profundus to the wing of the atlas, and rhomboideus thoracis to the middorsal raphe of the thorax. It elevates the forelimb and holds the scapula to the body.

The cutaneous trunci is a muscle that twitches or wrinkles the skin over the lateral body wall and flank. It is closely applied to the skin and to the latissimus muscle beneath it. Its origin is over the lumbodorsal fascia, and its final insertion is into the antebrachial fascia of the axilla.

The latissimus dorsi is a large triangular muscle behind the scapula originating on the lumbodorsal fascia and passing to the teres tuberosity of the humerus. It functions to draw the limb caudally, as in digging.

The serratus ventralis (Fig. 2–8) is a fan-shaped muscle. It extends from the serrated face on the medial side of the scapula to the transverse processes of cervical vertebrae and the ribs of the ventral thoracic wall. It acts as a sling and suspends the body between the limbs.

The intrinsic muscles of the thoracic limb that can be seen in Figures 2–6 and 2–7 are the supraspinatus, infraspinatus, subscapularis, deltoideus, teres minor, teres major, tensor fascia antebrachii, triceps brachii (long head, lateral head, medial head, and angular head), biceps brachii, brachialis, and brachioradialis.

FOREARM AND FOREPAW

The intrinsic muscles of the thoracic limb, as described and illustrated by Williams for the mink, are as follows: extensor carpi radialis, extensor digitorum communis, extensor digitorum lateralis, extensor carpi ulnaris, extensor pollicis longus et indicis proprius, abductor pollicis longus, flexor carpi ulnaris, palmaris longus, superficial digital flexor, deep digital flexor, flexor carpi radialis, pronator teres, supinator, pronator quadratus, lumbricales, abductor pollicis brevis, flexor pollicis brevis, adductor pollicis, adductor digiti secundi, abductor digiti quinti, flexor digiti quinti, adductor digiti quinti, and interossei.[8]

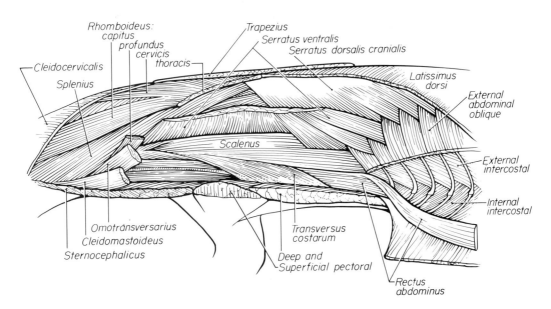

Fig. 2–8. Deep muscles of the neck and trunk.

PELVIC LIMB

All the muscles of the pelvic limb that were dissected in the ferret closely resemble those of the mink, as described by Williams and also by Smith and Krasulak.[6,8] Extrinsic muscles of the limb originate on the pelvis or vertebral column, and pass to the femur.

Muscles of the Rump

The tensor fasciae latae is a triangular muscle (Fig. 2–9) that originates on the sacrum and ilium between the sartorius and the middle gluteal. Its broad aponeurosis of insertion passes over the quadriceps and inserts on the lateral surface of the thigh. Superficially the aponeurosis blends with the fasciae latae and the superficial gluteal. Its primary function is to tense the femoral fascia and flex the hip.

The superficial gluteal is a very thin muscle originating on the sacrum and ilium and covering the middle gluteal on the rump. It blends cranially with the tensor fasciae latae and caudally with the caudofemoralis. It inserts on the trochanter tertius, thus extending the hip and abducting the limb.

The caudofemoralis is a muscle that is absent in the dog. It originates on the sacrum, passes beneath the biceps, and inserts on the caudal surface of the femur.

The middle gluteal (Fig. 2–10) is a larger and more powerful muscle that originates on the ilium beneath the superficial gluteal. It inserts on the greater trochanter and serves to extend the hip and abduct the limb.

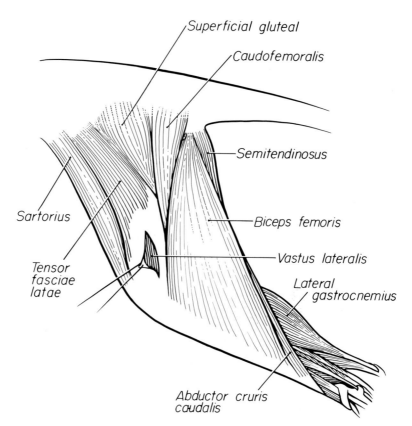

Fig. 2–9. Superficial muscles of the rump (*left lateral view*).

The deep gluteal originates on the ischiatic spine adjacent to the gemellus and inserts on the greater trochanter of the femur. A ventral gluteal muscle is peculiar to mustelids, and may be a derivative of the deep gluteal. It originates on the shaft of the ilium and inserts on the trochanter tertius.

Caudal Hip Muscles

All the caudal hip muscles function to extend the hip and rotate it outward. The internal obturator muscle originates within the pelvis and its tendon passes over the ischiatic notch, indents the gemellus muscle (Fig. 2-10), and inserts in the trochanteric fossa. It is innervated by the ischiatic nerve.

The external obturator originates on the outside of the pelvis over the obturator foramen, and also inserts in the trochanteric fossa. It is innervated by the obturator nerve.

A small quadratus femoris muscle extends from the ischium to the border of the trochanteric fossa.

Lateral Muscles of the Thigh

The quadriceps femoris lies cranial to the femur. It is composed of four heads and bellies that fuse distally as the patella tendon, which inserts on the tibial tuberosity (Fig. 2–10). The quadriceps functions as the primary extensor of the stifle. One portion, the rectus femoris, originates on the ilium and thus also flexes the hip. The other three, the vastus lateralis, vastus intermedius, and vastus medialis, originate on the proximal end of the femur. All heads are innervated by the femoral nerve.

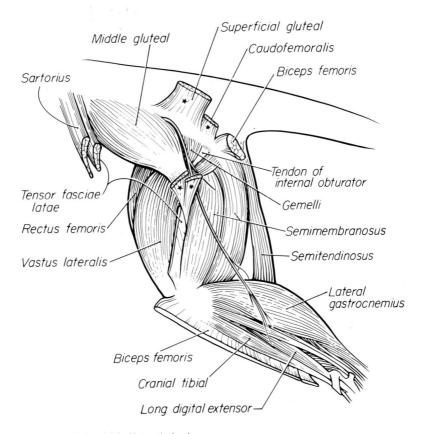

Fig. 2–10. Deep muscles of the thigh (*lateral view*).

The biceps femoris is the largest muscle of the thigh. It originates on the ischiatic tuberosity and fans out to blend with the aponeurosis of the tensor fasciae latae and the patella fascia cranially. As in the dog, there is a deep fascial slip that continues to the tuber calcis as part of the calcanean tendon. Beneath the biceps femoris is a narrow band of muscle with a similar origin that becomes superficial distally, where it inserts as part of the biceps on the distal end of the tibia. This slip of muscle is called the tenuissimus in the cat and the abductor cruris caudalis in the dog and ferret. The biceps functions as an extensor of the hip, as both an extensor and flexor of the stifle (depending on the fixation of the limb), and as an extensor of the hock.

Medial Muscles of the Thigh

The sartorius is a narrow band of muscle along the cranial border on the medial surface of the thigh (Fig. 2–11). It originates on the wing of the ilium and inserts over the medial surface of the patella onto the tibial crest. It flexes the hip and may extend the stifle. It is innervated by the femoral nerve.

The gracilis originates from the craniopubic ligament and inserts on the femur. It functions to adduct the limb and flex the stifle. Innervation is by the obturator nerve.

The pectineus is a short muscle between the adductor and the vastus medialis. It arises from the craniopubic ligament and inserts on the femur, and functions as part of the adductor.

The adductor is a compound muscle whose components, magnus et brevis and longus, are not clearly separable. The muscle originates along the length of the pelvic symphysis and inserts on the caudal surface of the femur at midshaft. It functions to adduct the limb and extend the hip. Innervation is from the obturator nerve.

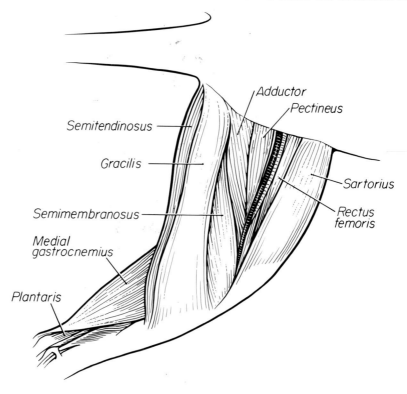

Fig. 2–11. Superficial muscles of the thigh (*medial view*).

The semimembranosus (Figs. 2–10 to 2–12) lies caudal to the adductor and beneath the gracilis. It is a large muscle that originates on the ischiatic tuberosity and inserts on the tibial crest. It functions to extend the hip.

The semitendinosus is the most caudal thigh muscle. It originates on the ischiatic tuberosity and inserts on the tibia distal to the gracilis and semimembranosus. It extends the hip and flexes the stifle.

CRUS AND FOOT

The muscles of the crus and foot (Figs. 2–9 to 2–12) include the medial and lateral gastrocnemius, popliteus, plantaris, soleus, deep digital flexor, long digital flexor, caudal tibial, peroneus longus, peroneus brevis, long digital extensor, cranial tibial, extensor hallucis longus,

extensor digitorum longus, flexor digitorum brevis, quadratus plantae, abductor metatarsi quinti, lumbricales, interossei, and digital adductors.

THE DIGESTIVE SYSTEM

MOUTH AND ASSOCIATED STRUCTURES

The mouth opening is wide, the oral cavity is extensive, and the labial commissures extend farther caudally than the carnassial teeth.

The upper lip is longer than the lower and has a distinct philtrum. There are sinus hairs or "whiskers" on the cheek, upper and lower lips, and above the eyes. The follicles of these hairs extend nearly to the mucocutaneous junction. The orbicularis oris muscle is moderately well developed. The lower lip is closely at-

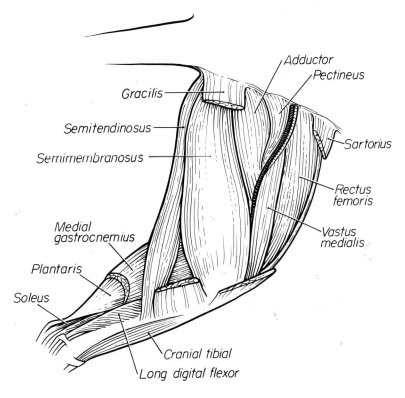

Fig. 2–12. Medial muscles of the thigh (*medial view*).

tached to the gum, and exhibits little flexibility. The upper and lower lips unite at a point opposite the third premolar teeth.

The cheeks are narrow and cannot be considered capacious. The vestibule is shallow, and the opening of the parotid duct is at the level of the third molar tooth of the upper jaw. The zygomatic salivary gland on each side opens by several ducts into the vestibule opposite the upper molar teeth. The submandibular ducts open as sublingual papillae on each side of the frenulum of the tongue.

The roof of the mouth is formed by a hard palate that is continuous caudally with the soft palate. The hard palate presents six or seven ridges, the first four of which curve across the entire width. The remaining ridges are separated by a median sulcus that becomes larger and deeper caudally. There is a distinct incisive papilla bearing two minute incisive ducts, which lead to a vomeronasal organ.

The oral mucous membrane is a delicate pink color in life, and presents a smooth surface.

Vascularization. The muscles and skin of the upper lip are supplied by a ventral branch of the infraorbital artery and by the superior labial branch of the facial artery. The muscle and skin of the lower lip are supplied by the rostral and middle mental arteries and by the inferior labial branch of the facial artery. The palate is supplied by the major palatine arteries to the hard palate and the minor palatine, as well as by ascending pharyngeal arteries to the soft palate. Blood is drained from the palate through a palatine plexus. Lymphatics pass to the retropharyngeal lymph nodes.

Innervation. The innervation of the upper and lower lips is via dorsal and ventral buccal branches of the facial nerve. The hard palate is innervated by sensory fibers in the major palatine branches of the maxillary division of the trigeminal nerve, while the soft palate is supplied by minor palatine branches of the same nerve. Branches of the glossopharyngeal and vagus also pass to the soft palate.

TONGUE

The tongue of the ferret is long and freely movable (Fig. 2–13). It is thick at the root and becomes thinner and narrower toward the round thin apex. A median

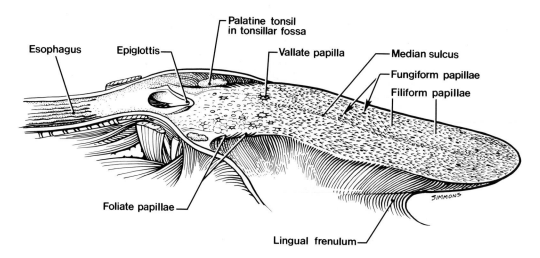

Fig. 2–13. The tongue (*dorsolateral view*).

sulcus on the dorsum is deepest over the body, and fades out at the apex.

The ventral surface is smooth and slightly convex, and flattens near the apex. The groove on the ventral surface of the body extends to the apex. The frenulum is extensive enough to permit good mobility of the tongue. There is no evidence of a lyssa.

The dorsal surface of the tongue bears numerous papillae and lingual glands. The presence of both serous and mucous salivary glands on the tongue is similar to findings in other mammals.

There are four types of papillae on the ferret's tongue. Filiform papillae are located on the dorsum of the rostral three-fourths of the tongue, and are arranged symmetrically in a row radiating outward and forward from the median sulcus. The filiform papillae are rather complex, consisting of primary, secondary, and tertiary serrations with their tips inclined caudally. Blood vessels and nerves reach the papillae through dermal pores. Only the lingual nerve, a branch of the trigeminal, innervates the filiform papillae.

Fungiform papillae are scattered, in a lesser number than the filiform papillae, over three-fourths of the dorsal surface of the tongue. They are shorter and broader than the filiform papillae. Taste buds are frequently observed on the dorsal surface of the papilla, which is covered by cornified stratified squamous epithelium. Fungiform papillae receive innervation from the chorda tympani to the taste buds and from the lingual nerve to the epithelium.

Vallate papillae are arranged in a V shape at the base of the tongue, with the base of the V directed caudally. There are from four to seven, arranged on both sides of the median sulcus. Each vallate papilla is surrounded by a moat, which in turn is surrounded by modified mucosal papillae. Taste buds are found only toward the bottom of the moat. The associated serous glands of von Ebner are also present at the base of the vallate papillae. Lymphatic aggregates are associated with the ducts of the von Ebner glands.

On the basal quarter of the ferret tongue there are many vallatelike papillae. They vary in number and are irregularly arranged, and their function is unknown.

Foliate papillae are leaflike, and are arranged in elongated groups that lie in the fold just in front of the tonsil and medial to the anterior pillars of the soft palate. Foliate papillae are covered by cornified stratified squamous epithelium, and may well contain several taste buds whose pores empty into the diverticuli.

Most of the lingual muscles do not differ appreciably from those of the dog except for the styloglossus, which is more massive in the ferret. The styloglossus originates not only from the stylohoid but also from the lateral surface of the tympanic bulla.[4]

Vascularization. The arterial supply to the tongue is mainly via the paired lingual arteries. The genioglossus and geniohyoideus muscles also receive some collateral blood supply from the sublingual artery. Blood is drained from the tongue through the lingual vein.

Innervation. The tongue is innervated by lingual (trigeminal), chorda tympani (facial), glossopharyngeal, and hypoglossal nerves. The lingual nerve is the principal sensory nerve to the rostral three-fourths of the tongue. The chorda tympani innervates the taste buds and secretory motor fibers to the lingual gland.

The glossopharyngeal nerve innervates the vallate and foliate papillae of the caudal one-fourth of the tongue. The general visceral efferent component of the glossopharyngeal nerve sends sensory and vasodilator fibers to the lingual glands located at the base of the tongue. The hypoglossal nerve is motor to the intrinsic muscles of the tongue.

TEETH

The ferret has 30 deciduous teeth and 34 permanent teeth.

Permanent Teeth

The formula for the permanent dentition of the ferret is

$$2 \left(I\, \tfrac{3}{3},\ C\, \tfrac{1}{1},\ Pm\, \tfrac{3}{3},\ M\, \tfrac{1}{2}\right) = 34$$

where I is incisor, C is canine, Pm is premolar, and M is molar.

The permanent teeth erupt between 50 and 74 days of age (Table 2–1). The upper and lower canines and lower first molar erupt first; the upper first molar erupts at 53 days; the second, third, fourth, upper premolar, and second lower premolar erupt at 60 days; the third lower premolar erupts at 67 days; and the fourth premolar and second molar of the lower jaw erupt at 74 days.

Incisors are small nipping teeth. In the upper jaw the first and second incisors are approximately the same size, while the third incisor is noticeably larger. The first lower incisor is small, while the second and third are equal in size. Lower incisors are smaller than the upper ones.

The incisors meet when the mouth is closed, and the lingual surface of the uppers overlaps the labial surface of the lowers. The crown of each upper third incisor is deflected laterally. An incisor tooth has a single root.

Canines are large and slightly curved. The length of the canine root exceeds the length of the crown, which is demarcated by a groove on the concave surface of the tooth. The upper canine is larger than the lower canine. When the mouth is closed the lower canine occupies the space between the upper canine and the corner incisor tooth. The lower canine passes rostral to the upper and lies in a groove on the lateral surface of the upper jaw. The upper canines project slightly beyond the upper dental arcade and extend superficially to the lower lip.

Premolar teeth increase in size from the first premolar to the third. The premolars have two roots except for the upper third premolar, which has three roots. The upper premolars are the sectorial or shearing teeth, with each having a large middle cone, two small anterior cones, and a posterior cone. The upper third premolar is the largest cheek tooth and has three roots. It is known as the carnassial tooth of the upper jaw.

TABLE 2–1. INTERVALS OF ENAMEL FORMATION AND TOOTH ERUPTION OF PERMANENT TEETH IN THE FERRET

Jaw	Tooth (Canine)	Enamel Formation (Days After Birth)	Eruption (Days After Birth)
Upper	C	4	50
	Premolar 2	20	60
	Premolar 3	20	60
	Premolar 4	10	60
	Molar 1	10	53
Lower	C	4	50
	Premolar 2	20	60
	Premolar 3	20	67
	Premolar 4	20	74
	Molar 1	4	50
	Molar 2	37	74

(Adapted from Berkovitz, B.K.B., and Silverstone, L.M.: The dentition of the albino ferret. Caries Res., *3*:369, 1969.)

The upper molar has an irregularly quadrilateral shape, and its long axis is transverse. There is a depression on its masticating surface that divides the crown into a larger lingual part and a smaller buccal part. It has three roots.

The three lower premolars and the first lower molar are also sectorial teeth. They resemble the first and second upper premolars, with each having a large middle cone and two anterior and posterior cones. All lower premolars have two roots. The second lower molar is a small tooth with a flattened crown and only one root.

When the mouth is closed, the first and second upper premolars occupy the spaces between three lower premolars. The third upper premolar overlaps the lower first molar. The posterior cone of the lower first molar rests on the depression on the occlusal surface of the upper molar.

Deciduous Teeth

The formula for the deciduous teeth is

$$2 \left(I \frac{4}{3}, C\frac{1}{1}, P\frac{3}{3} \right) = 30$$

The deciduous teeth erupt between 20 and 28 days, or 3 to 4 weeks of age. The canine and third and fourth deciduous molars erupt first, and the upper and lower second molars follow.

For more information about the dentition of the ferret, refer to articles by Berkovitz and colleagues.[9–12]

SALIVARY GLANDS

There are five pairs of major salivary glands in the ferret, the parotid, mandibular, sublingual, molar, and zygomatic glands (Fig. 2–14). Poddar and Jacob have determined that the parotid gland in the ferret is seromucous and the mandibular gland is predominantly mucous.[13] The sublingual gland is mucous, while the molar and zygomatic glands are predominantly mucous but contain a few serous cells in the form of demilunes.

Parotid Gland

The gland measures about 2.7 cm across the base, about 1.6 cm from base to apex, and is approximately 0.65 cm thick. It is irregularly pyramidal in shape, pale buff-colored, and lobulated. The lobules are loosely connected.

Topography. The gland lies at the junction of the head and neck between the mandibular salivary gland and the parotid lymph node. The apex of the gland is directed ventrally while the base is related closely to the basal portion of the auricular cartilage. The linguofacial and external jugular veins unite near the caudal end of the caudoventral border.

The parotid duct is about 2.8 cm long. It is formed by the union of two to three converging branches that leave the ventral part of the rostral border of the gland. The duct first crosses the superficial surface of the masseter muscle, and then goes under the facial vessels. It perforates the cheek and opens into the buccal cavity in the vestibule opposite the upper third molar tooth.

Vascularization and Innervation. The parotid artery, a branch of the external carotid, supplies the parotid gland. The venous drainage is via parotid radicles of the superficial temporal and great auricular veins. Lymph drains to the parotid and medial retropharyngeal lymph nodes. The autonomic innervation of the gland is composed of parasympathetic fibers from the auriculotemporal branch of the trigeminal nerve, while the sympathetic fibers are from the external carotid plexus.

Mandibular Gland

The mandibular gland (Fig. 2–14) of the ferret is ovoid, about 1.8 cm in diameter

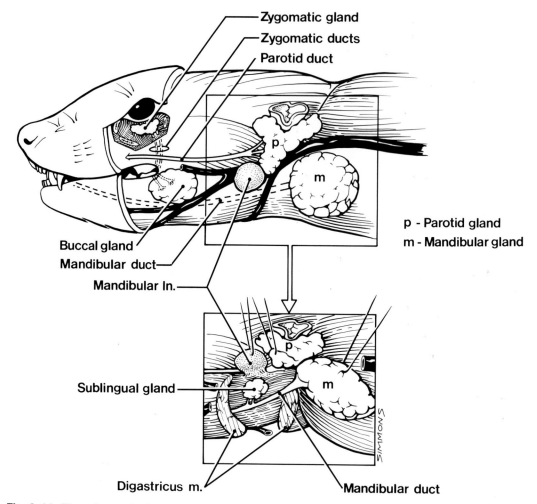

Zygomatic gland
Zygomatic ducts
Parotid duct

p - Parotid gland
m - Mandibular gland

Buccal gland
Mandibular duct
Mandibular ln.

Sublingual gland

Digastricus m.
Mandibular duct

Fig. 2–14. The salivary glands.

and 0.60 cm thick. It is gray in color. The gland lies in a depression bounded by the digastricus and sternohyoid muscles and by the tendon of insertion of the sternomastoideus dorsocaudally. Rostrodorsally it is related to the mandibular lymph node, and medially to the medial retropharyngeal lymph node and larynx.

The mandibular duct is about 3.0 cm long. It emerges from the deep surface of the gland at its rostral border. The initial portion of the duct runs rostrally between the masseter muscle medially and the digastricus muscle laterally.

On reaching the lateral part of the pharyngeal mucosa, it arches forward and runs in the intermuscular septum between the styloglossus and mylohyoideus muscles. The terminal part of the duct receives several ductules from the sublingual gland and opens on a sublingual papilla.

The mandibular gland is supplied by a branch of the facial artery, and drains to the lingual vein. Its parasympathetic fibers are from facial nerve branches. Its sympathetic fibers come from a perivascular plexus around the glandular artery. The lymphatics drain into the medial retropharyngeal lymph node.

Sublingual Gland

The sublingual gland (Fig. 2–14) is smaller than the mandibular gland. It is somewhat quadrangular and flat, measuring about 0.75 cm in length and 0.50 cm in width. It has a pinkish color, which resembles the color of muscle.

The sublingual gland lies between the caudomedial border of the masseter muscle, deep to the digastric muscle, and the dorsal border of the mylohyoid muscle.

The sublingual duct, formed by several ductules that leave the gland, subsequently joins the mandibular duct.

A branch of the facial artery and sublingual artery supply the sublingual gland. They are accompanied by satellite veins. Lymphatics drain into the medial retropharyngeal lymph node.

Molar (Buccal) Gland

The molar gland (Fig. 2–14) is irregular, pyramidal or wedge-shaped. It measures about 0.8 cm in length and 0.7 cm in width, and is pale in color.

The gland lies in a depression on the border of the masseter muscle. The lateral surface of the gland is covered by superficial fascia and by some fibers of the orbicularis oris.

The molar duct opens into the vestibule of the oral cavity just opposite the lower molar teeth.

Zygomatic Gland

The zygomatic gland (Fig. 2–14) is roughly pyramidal and similar in size to the molar gland. It is lobulated and gray in color. The gland lies deep to the masseter, caudoventral to the orbit and ventral to the zygomatic arch. It opens by several ducts into the vestibule of the oral cavity opposite the upper molar teeth.

The arterial supply to the zygomatic gland is from the first branch of the infraorbital artery as it enters the infra-

orbital canal. The venous drainage of the gland enters the deep facial vein.

PALATE

The soft palate continues caudally from the hard palate, which ends at the level of the last upper molar teeth (see Fig. 2–15). It measures 1.5 cm long, 0.7 cm wide, and 0.1 cm thick. Caudolaterally on each side a thin elliptic fold forms the wall of the tonsillar sinus. Caudally the free border of the soft palate is overlapped by the epiglottis. On each side the lateral extension of the free border forms a fold that crosses the lateral wall of the pharynx as the caudal pillars of the soft palate. These pillars meet dorsally at the entrance of the esophagus. The ventral surface of the soft palate has a sulcus.

The arterial supply of the soft palate is from the minor palatine, ascending pharyngeal, and major palatine arteries. There is an extensive palatine plexus of veins in the soft palate. The lymphatics drain to the medial retropharyngeal lymph node.

The main sensory supply to the soft palate is the minor palatine branch of the maxillary nerve. Branches from the glossopharyngeal and vagus enter the soft palate to supply its muscles.

PHARYNX

The pharynx extends from a transverse plane through the head at the level of the orbits to another plane through the axis. The conformation of the ferret pharynx is similar to that of a dolichocephalic dog. It consists of three parts, the nasal, oral, and laryngeal pharynges.

The nasopharynx is that part of the respiratory passageway above the soft palate. The choanae open into the pharynx at the intrapharyngeal opening. This opening, or pharyngeal isthmus (Fig. 2–15),

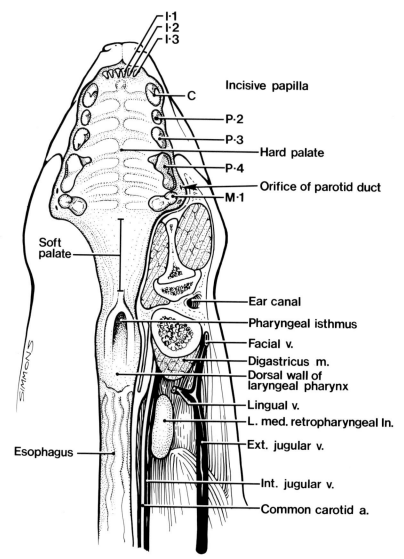

I·1
I·2
I·3
Incisive papilla
C
P·2
P·3
Hard palate
P·4
Orifice of parotid duct
M·1
Soft palate
Ear canal
Pharyngeal isthmus
Facial v.
Digastricus m.
Dorsal wall of laryngeal pharynx
Lingual v.
L. med. retropharyngeal ln.
Ext. jugular v.
Esophagus
Int. jugular v.
Common carotid a.

Fig. 2–15. The pharynx and associated structures.

opens over the soft palate into the oral and laryngeal parts of the pharynx. The pharyngeal tonsils and the openings of the auditory tubes lie on each side of the pharyngeal isthmus. The isthmus of the fauces in the ferret is well defined. It is bounded laterally by the palatoglossal arch, ventrally by the tongue, and dorsally by the soft palate.

The oropharynx, for the passage of food, is the continuation of the oral cavity into the isthmus of the fauces. It is bounded dorsally by the soft palate, ventrally by the root of the tongue, and laterally by the tonsillar fossa, which contains the palatine tonsils—these are very prominent in the ferret.

The laryngopharynx is that part of the pharynx that lies dorsal to the larynx and extends to the beginning of the esophagus. It functions in both respiration and alimentation, but its main function is in swallowing. The cricopharyngeal and thyropharyngeal muscles are the main constrictors of the laryngopharynx. Other intrinsic and extrinsic muscles of the pharynx and soft palate aid in shortening and constricting the pharynx for deglutition.

ASSOCIATED STRUCTURES OF THE PHARYNX

Structures associated with the pharynx include the palatine tonsil, thyroid, and esophagus.

Palatine Tonsil

The palatine tonsil (see Fig. 2–13) of the ferret is a flattened ovoid measuring about 6.5 cm long, 0.25 cm wide, and 0.01 cm thick. It lies in the tonsillar fossa lateral to the ventral sulcus of the soft palate.

The pharynx receives its arterial supply via pharyngeal branches of the cranial thyroid and ascending pharyngeal arteries. The palatine tonsils receive blood through tonsillar arteries that are branches of lingual arteries. The lymphatics of the palatine tonsils drain to the medial retropharyngeal lymph node.

Thyroid Gland

The thyroid gland of the ferret is bilobed, connected by an isthmus ventral to the middle portion of the trachea. In ten ferrets the average size was found to be 1.3 cm long, 0.3 wide, and 0.1 thick. It weighs about 0.6 g. It is brown in color, with the isthmus being lighter. Each lobe lies lateral to the trachea and medial to the jugular vein and carotid artery. The gland spans from the third to the eleventh tracheal rings. It lies about 0.77 cm behind the cricoid cartilage.

Vascularization. The cranial and caudal thyroid arteries provide an extensive vascular network to the gland. They are the first major branches from common carotid arteries. The blood drainage of the gland is via cranial and caudal thyroid veins, which join the internal jugular vein. Lymphatics drain to the caudal lymph node.

Innervation. The innervation of the thyroid gland is from the thyroid nerve via fibers from the cranial cervical ganglion and the cranial laryngeal nerve.

Esophagus

The esophagus extends from the pharyngoesophageal demarcation, above the cricoid cartilage, to the cardia of the stomach (Fig. 2–16). The total length is 17 to 19 cm. It passes caudally dorsal to the trachea and gradually descends to the left side. There are three parts, cervical, thoracic, and abdominal.

The cervical part is about 6.5 cm long and, at the level of C4, is enclosed in the carotid sheath. At the level of the thoracic inlet it lies lateral to the trachea.

The thoracic portion is approximately 11 cm long. It passes to the right, crossing deep to the left subclavian artery, and continues under the aortic arch. On reaching the diaphragm it passes through the esophageal hiatus, accompanied by dorsal and ventral vagus nerve trunks. The esophageal hiatus lies just under the level of T14.

The abdominal segment of the esophagus below the diaphragm is about 1.5 cm long and extends through the ligament of the left lateral lobe of the liver, and ending at the cardia of the stomach. Topographically the esophagus of the ferret resembles that of a dog.

The lumen of the esophagus shows three sites of constriction: at its origin; where it is crossed by the left bronchus; and just before passing through the diaphragm. The mucous membrane lining the esophagus, when not dilated, ap-

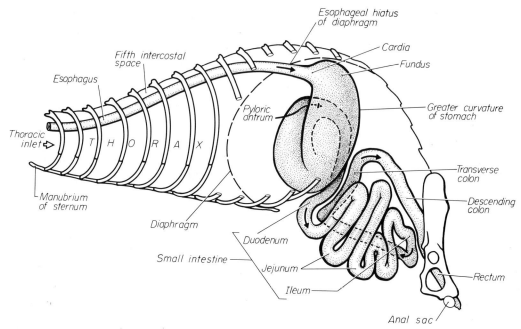

Fig. 2–16. Topography of the digestive tract (*left lateral view*).

pears as several longitudinal folds that end abruptly at the gastroesophageal junction.

Vascularization. The cervical part of the esophagus is supplied primarily by small branches from the cranial and caudal thyroid arteries. The thoracic part of the esophagus is supplied by the broncho-esophageal artery to its cranial three-fourths, and the rest is supplied by dorsal intercostal arteries. The venous drainage of the esophagus is via satellites of the arteries that supply it except for the thoracic portion, which drains into the azygos vein. The lymphatics drain into the medial retropharyngeal, deep cervical, cranial mediastinal, bronchial, portal, splenic, and gastric lymph nodes.

Innervation. The cervical part of the esophagus is innervated by motor fibers from the small pharyngoesophageal nerve and by the recurrent laryngeal nerve branches of the vagus.

ABDOMINAL VISCERA

The abdominal viscera include the stomach, small intestine (duodenum, jejunum, and ileum), pancreas, and large intestine.

Stomach

The ferret has a simple stomach similar in shape to that of the dog (Fig. 2–17). It is the largest dilatation of the alimentary canal. It is roughly J-shaped and lies in a transverse position to the left of the median plane. The stomach varies greatly in size and shape, depending on the quantity of food it contains.

Cranially the stomach contacts the liver and diaphragm. Caudally it contacts the spleen on the left and the intestine (usually descending colon) ventrally. The entrance to the stomach is the cardia, the middle portion is the body, and the exit to the duodenum is the pyloric antrum and pylorus. Externally the stomach has two

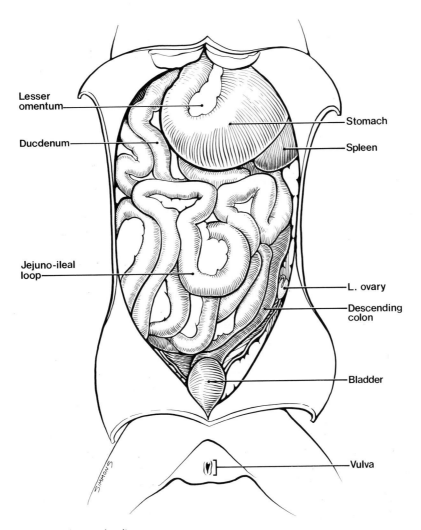

Fig. 2–17. Abdominal viscera, in situ.

surfaces and two curvatures: the greater curvature is the embryonic dorsal surface and the lesser curvature is the embryonic ventral surface.

Topography. The stomach lies in the cranial abdominal region within the thoracic cage. When the stomach is empty the cranial limit is the transverse plane, which passes through the eleventh thoracic vertebra, and the caudal limit is a plane passing through the first lumbar vertebra. The parietal surface of the stomach faces to the left, cranially as well as ventrally. The visceral surface is in direct contact with the left limb of the pancreas, which is enclosed in the visceral leaf of the omentum. The left half of the greater curvature is related to the visceral surface of the spleen. Along the greater curvature the gastrosplenic ligament joins the two organs, and contains gastrosplenic vessels and nerves. The lesser curvature faces craniodorsally and is recessed in the gastric impression of the liver. It is separated from the papillary process of the caudate lobe of the liver by the lesser omentum. The lesser omentum extends from the lesser curvature of the stomach to the portal fissure of the liver. When the stomach is filling its size, shape, and position vary. When the fundus is full it may lie caudoventrally in contact with the abdominal wall. The full stomach occupies the entire parachondriac region and pushes the intestinal mass to the right. The posterior border of the stomach may contact the left kidney at the level of a transverse plane passing through the second lumbar vertebra.

The shape and position of the stomach have been illustrated (see Figs. 2–16 and 2–17). On a left lateral radiograph the stomach inclines on a transverse plane at about 45°. On the ventrodorsal view the stomach is J-shaped and its cranial border is in contact with the transverse plane that passes through the thirteenth thoracic vertebra. The sphincter of the pylorus is moderately developed. The pyloric opening is directed craniodorsally.

Vascularization. The main arteries to the stomach are the left and right gastric arteries along the lesser curvature, and the left and right gastroepiploic arteries along the greater curvature. The veins from the stomach are satellites of the arteries to the stomach. The left gastric and left gastroepiploic veins are tributaries of the gastrosplenic vein, while the right gastric and right gastroepiploic veins are tributaries of the gastroduodenal vein.

Innervation. The stomach is supplied by parasympathetic fibers from the vagus nerve and sympathetic fibers from the sympathetic trunk via the celiacomesenteric plexus. The ventral vagal trunk, after passing through the esophageal hiatus, sends fibers to the pylorus, liver, and lesser curvature of the stomach. The dorsal vagal trunk also sends fibers to the lesser curvature and parietal surface of the stomach.[14]

Small Intestine

The small intestine (Fig. 2–16) extends from the pylorus of the stomach to the junction with the colon. It is the longest part of the digestive system, and measures from 182 to 198 cm in adult ferrets with a body length varying from 36 to 41 cm. The ratio of the length of the small intestine to the length of the body is 5:1. Poddar and Murgatroyd have cited similar intestinal measurements in the ferret.[15] The small intestine consists of the duodenum, the jejunum, and the ileum.

Duodenum. The proximal loop of the small intestine, the duodenum, is relatively short, approximately 10 cm in length. The duodenum consists of three portions. The cranial portion is about 2 cm long, and lacks a definite sigmoid loop. The cranial duodenal flexure turns abruptly to the left and then passes caudally, forming a duodenal bulb that lies opposite the thirteenth and fourteenth ribs. Ventrally the cranial portion of the duodenum is separated from the stomach by the greater omentum. Dorsally and laterally it is in contact with the liver and medially with the pancreas.

The descending portion is about 5 cm long and continues caudally to the right of the median plane. Cranially it is in contact with the body wall and the right lateral and right medial lobes of the liver. Dorsally the descending portion lies in contact with the pancreas, the caudate lobe of the liver, and the left kidney. Medially the descending portion is related to the ascending portion of the colon and separated from it by a fold of greater omentum. The descending portion has two flexures, one with the cranial portion and the other with the ascending portion, producing a C shape.

The ascending portion is about 3 cm long and runs cranially from the caudal duodenal flexure. It lies in the median plane and ends at the duodenojejunal flexure, which is located immediately cranial to the root of the mesentery and is marked by a slight constriction. The ascending portion is related dorsally to the ureter, sympathetic trunk, caudal vena cava, and aorta. Ventrally it is related to the coil of the jejunoileum on the left of the descending colon.

The mesoduodenum encloses the right limb of the pancreas, a continuation of the lesser omentum cranially. Caudally the mesoduodenum connects the descending and ascending portions to the root of the mesentery. A duodenocolic fold passes caudally from the ascending portion and continues with the mesocolon.

The major duodenal papilla, which is a common opening of the bile and pancreatic ducts, opens into the dorsal wall of the descending portion of the duodenum about 3 cm from the pylorus.[15] A minor papilla, when present, is not prominent.

Jejunum and Ileum. In the ferret the jejunum and ileum are not distinguishable externally. Poddar and Murgatroyd could find no sharp demarcation internally either.[15]

The jejunoileum (Fig. 2–18) begins at the duodenojejunal flexure and ends at the ascending colon. Its length is about 140 cm. It forms a coil of intestine that is connected to the root of mesentery by the fat-filled mesojejunoileum. The coil of the small intestine is covered by the greater omentum, and thus is separated from the abdominal wall. The coil is related dorsally with the duodenum, spleen, liver, colon, pancreas, and kidneys. Caudally the coil is related to the urogenital organs.

Vascularization. The arteries that supply the duodenum are the cranial and caudal pancreaticoduodenal arteries. The cranial pancreaticoduodenal artery is a branch of the hepatic artery from the celiac artery, whereas the caudal pancreaticoduodenal artery is a branch of the cranial mesenteric artery. The veins that drain the duodenum are satellites of the arteries. There are about 10 to 12 jejunoileal veins that drain into the cranial mesenteric vein, which drains blood into the portal vein. The lymphatics of the duodenum, jejunum, and ileum drain primarily into right and left mesenteric lymph nodes, which are prominent in the ferret.

Innervation. Nerves to the small intestine come from the vagus and sympathetic trunk by way of the celiac and cranial mesenteric plexus.

PANCREAS

The pancreas (Fig. 2–18) is V-shaped, elongated, and lobulated. It is light pink to bright red in color in fresh specimens. The gland is divided into right and left limbs (lobes) united by a body that lies close to the pylorus.

The left limb of the pancreas extends caudosinistrally dorsal to the visceral surface of the stomach and medial to the spleen. It is enclosed in the mesoduodenum. This limb is biangular in cross section. Dorsally it is related to the portal vein, left kidney, and left adrenal gland. Ventrally it is related to the transverse colon and the jejunoileum.

The right limb of the pancreas is more extensive than the left limb. It lies dorsomedial to the duodenum and follows the descending part. At the caudal duodenal flexure the right limb of the pancreas turns over itself, so that the entire right limb is located to the right of the root of the mesentery. Dorsally it is related to the caudal vena cava, right and left renal vessels, aorta, caudate lobe of the liver, right kidney, and right adrenal gland. The ventral surface of the right limb is related to the intestinal coil.

Pancreatic Ducts. The pancreatic secretion drains by many radicles into a large

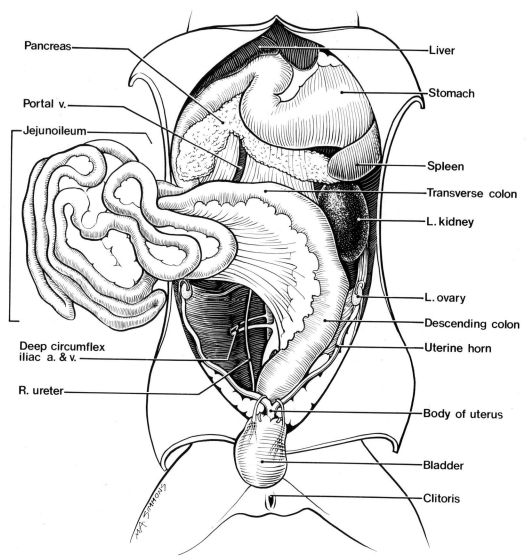

Fig. 2–18. Abdominal viscera, intestine displaced.

pancreatic duct from each limb. The ducts of the left and right limbs usually connect to form a common pancreatic duct that joins the bile duct. The opening of the duct into the lumen of the duodenum is on the major duodenal papilla, about 2.8 cm caudal to the cranial duodenal flexure. An accessory pancreatic duct and minor duodenal papilla may be present (in our study only one was seen in 40 specimens).

Vascularization. The cranial and caudal pancreaticoduodenal arteries are the main supply to the right lobe, while a pancreatic branch of the splenic artery is the primary artery that supplies blood to the left limb. Blood drains from the pancreas by satellite veins of arteries, and have the same names. Lymphatics from the pancreas drain into duodenal lymph nodes, if present, and into hepatic, splenic, and mesenteric lymph nodes.

LARGE INTESTINE, COLON, RECTUM, AND ANUS

The large intestine (Fig. 2–16) of the ferret is about 10 cm long and 0.6 cm in diameter. The length of the colon, rectum, and anus average, respectively, 7, 2, and 1 cm in length. Because a cecum is absent, the ileocolic junction is impossible to identify by gross dissection. The level of this junction can be inferred, however, by the pattern of the jejunal artery, which anastomoses with the ileocolic artery.

Anatomically, physiologically and histologically, it has been shown that there is a functional large intestine (refer to the work of Bueno and colleagues for further information).[16]

The last portion of coiled jejunoileum crosses the descending part of the duodenum ventrally and makes a flexure as it approaches the lower end of the medial surface of the spleen. Beyond this the intestine increases in diameter and passes caudally to the left flank of the abdomen. The colon begins here at the ileocolic junction, and terminates as the rectum within the pelvis. When the rectum passes through the pelvic canal it terminates as the anal canal and sphincter. The colon is suspended from the body wall by a short mesocolon.

The colon is divided into three parts— ascending, transverse, and descending. The three portions unite by two flexures, the right colic flexure and the left colic flexure. The ascending colon begins at the ileocolic junction, runs cranially, and ends at a right angle with the right colic flexure. The transverse colon runs from right to left, cranial to the cranial mesenteric artery and the root of mesentery. The descending colon is the largest segment of the colon. It is the continuation of the transverse colon at its left colic flexure and ends at the junction with the rectum at the level of the pelvic inlet.

Topography. The ascending colon lies close to the mesoduodenum and right limb of the pancreas dorsally, and the right kidney ventrally. The transverse colon is related cranioventrally with the stomach and craniodorsally with the left limb of the pancreas. Ventrally and caudally it lies in contact with the small intestinal coil. The descending colon is bound to the right of the root of the mesentery. It follows the curvature of the left abdominal wall and contacts the iliopsoas muscle dorsally. It also contacts the ventral surface of the left kidney. The uterus and the bladder lie ventral to the terminal part of the descending colon.

An external and an internal sphincter of the anus are present. The internal sphincter is the smooth muscle that is the thickening of the muscular wall of the anal canal. The external sphincter is a voluntary muscle that encloses the anal sacs, which have openings that lie on either side of the anal canal. The anal sacs or glands are ovoid in shape, about 1.2 to 1.5 cm in diameter. They secrete an oily, pungent, musky fluid. Their anatomy and surgical removal has been discussed by Creed and Kainer.[17]

The histology of the digestive system has been thoroughly studied by Poddar and Murgatroyd.[15]

Vascularization. The ascending and transverse colon are supplied by the ileocolic, right colic, and middle colic arteries, which are branches of the cranial mesenteric artery. The descending colon is supplied by the left colic artery, which is a branch of the caudal mesenteric artery. The rectum is supplied primarily by the cranial rectal artery, which is also a branch of the caudal mesenteric artery. The anus is supplied primarily by the caudal rectal artery, which is the last branch of the internal pudendal artery.

Veins draining the large intestine are satellites of the arteries and have the same names. The cranial rectal, left colic, middle colic, and right colic veins drain into the portal vein. The caudal rectal vein drains blood to the internal pudendal vein, which is a branch of the common iliac vein. The lymphatics drain to cranial and caudal mesenteric, left colic, sacral, and internal iliac lymph nodes.

Innervation. The nerve supply to the colon is via autonomic fibers from the vagus and from the cranial and caudal mesenteric plexus. Around the anal canal, the external sphincter muscle is supplied by anal branches of the pudendal nerve. The internal sphincter is smooth muscle, so it is supplied by autonomic fibers from the pelvic plexus.

HEPATIC COMPONENTS

The hepatic structures include the liver and gallbladder.

Liver

Compared to an average body weight of 800 to 1150 g the ferret has a relatively large liver (Fig. 2–19), ranging from 35 to 59 g. The ratios of liver weight to body weight are 4.3% in the ferret and 3.4% in the dog.

The liver presents two surfaces, the diaphragmatic and visceral. The diaphragmatic surface has a curved contour that follows the diaphragm and the visceral surface is irregular, made up of the impressions of the duodenum, stomach, pancreas, and right kidney. Six lobes of the liver are recognized in the ferret.

The left lateral lobe is the largest of the six lobes. Its visceral surface lies on the parietal surface of the stomach and on the part of the caudate process of the caudate lobe. Two-thirds of its diaphragmatic surface contacts the diaphragm, and is attached to it by the left triangular ligament. On the dorsal border the caudate process forms a notch for the esophagus.

The left medial lobe is smaller. It lies almost entirely to the left of the median plane. It is attached to the diaphragm by the falciform ligament, which in turn is the continuation of the thin coronary ligament around the hiatus of the caudal vena cava.

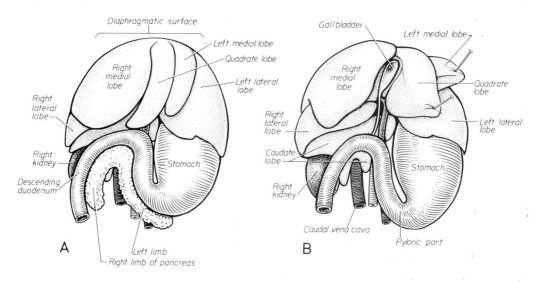

Fig. 2–19. Liver, stomach, and associated structures (*ventral view*). A, Organs in situ. B, Liver reflected and pancreas removed.

The quadrate lobe is medial to the left medial lobe. It lies almost entirely to the right of the median plane and contacts the right median lobe on the right. The left coronary ligament attaches this lobe to the diaphragm.

The right medial lobe is the second largest. Its parietal surface is related to the gallbladder, the quadrate lobe, the cystic duct, the left lateral lobe, the cranial portion of the duodenum, and the right lateral lobe. It attaches to the diaphragm by the left triangular ligament.

The right lateral lobe is smaller than the left medial lobe. It is related to the diaphragm and the right medial lobe. Its parietal surface is related to the descending portion of the duodenum, to part of the jejunoileum, and to the caudate process of the caudate lobe.

The caudate lobe is well developed and irregular in shape. Its papillary process lies along the cranial half of the lesser curvature of the stomach. This process is loosely covered by the lesser omentum, and lies entirely to the left of the median plane. The papillary process contacts the esophagus and the cardia of the stomach. With the right lateral lobe, it forms a fissure for the portal vein and bile duct. The caudate process is larger than the papillary process, and has one or two fissures subdividing it into smaller lobes.

The visceral surface of the caudate lobe has a deep cavity for the cranial portion of the right kidney and for the cranial portion of the descending duodenum. The caudate process attaches to the body wall by the continuation of the left triangular ligament, and attaches to the right kidney by a hepatorenal ligament.

The falciform ligament, a remnant of the ventral mesentery, contains the obliterated umbilical vein of the fetus. It becomes a thin fold that extends from the dorsal end of the fissure between the right and left lobes of the liver to the xiphisternal process of the sternum.

The caudal vena cava is deeply embedded in the dorsomedial portion of the caudate lobe, and continues cranially in the right lateral and left lateral lobes.

The portal fissure is located at the convergence of the right lateral and caudate lobes. The portal fissure contains the following:

1. The hepatic artery, a branch of the celiac artery
2. The portal vein, which brings blood to the liver from the stomach, intestine, pancreas, and spleen
3. The bile ducts, which come from the liver

Gallbladder

The ferret gallbladder (Fig. 2–19B) is pear-shaped. Its volume is about 0.5 to 1.00 ml, averaging 2 cm in length and 1 cm in width. The gallbladder is located in a fossa that is formed by the quadrate lobe on the left and the right medial lobe on the right. The cranial, dorsal, and lateral surfaces of the gallbladder attach to the quadrate process and the right lobe by thick connective tissue. When the gallbladder is distended it may separate the two lobes but it never extends through the liver to contact the diaphragm, as it does in the dog. Its neck is narrow and, after making a small bend, it continues as a cystic duct that is joined by three hepatic ducts (right, left, and central) to form the bile duct. The bile duct opens into the lumen of the duodenum at the major duodenal papillae, in common with the pancreatic duct. Some variations of the hepatic ducts have been described by Poddar, who also studied the histology of the liver.[18]

Vascularization. The central veins of hepatic lobules constitute the beginning of the outgoing venous system of the liver. Adjacent central veins fuse to form interlobular veins, which finally unite with each other to form the hepatic veins. The hepatic veins empty into the caudal vena cava.

The portal veins bring the functional blood to the liver from the stomach, intestines, pancreas, and spleen, while the hepatic arteries proper bring the nutritional blood.

The lymphatic vessels of the liver anastomose with those of the gallbladder and drain into hepatic and splenic lymph nodes.

Innervation. Autonomic nerves are supplied to the liver from the celiac plexus.

SPLEEN

The spleen (Fig. 2–18) of the ferret is crescent-shaped. Its length, width, and thickness are, respectively, 5.10, 1.80, and 0.80 cm. It is gray-brown in color and is firmly attached to the stomach and liver by the gastrosplenic ligament, a portion of the greater omentum.

Topography. The spleen is located in the left hypogastric region, approximately parallel to the greater curvature of the stomach. The location of the spleen is dependent on the size and position of the stomach. The visceral surface of the spleen is related to the greater curvature of the stomach, left limb of the pancreas, and colon. Its caudal border is related to the left kidney and left ovary in the female.

Vascularization. Blood vessels to the spleen are branches of the splenic artery from the celiac artery. The splenic vein drains into the gastrosplenic vein and then into the portal vein.

Innervation. The nerve supply to the spleen is from the celiac plexus, and consists chiefly of postganglionic sympathetic axons. The vagus also sends fibers to the spleen.

RESPIRATORY SYSTEM

The respiratory system is comprised of the nose and nasal passages, larynx, trachea, and the lung and related structures.

NOSE AND NASAL PORTION OF THE PHARYNX

The skin of the nose is bare and pigmented in a standard ferret. A vertical groove divides the nose into right and left portions. This groove extends downward and is continued by the philtrum of the upper lip.

The nasal cavity is the facial portion of the respiratory pathway. It extends from the nostril to the choanae, and is divided into right and left chambers by the nasal septum (see Fig. 2–2). The nasal cavity is connected to the pharynx by the nasopharyngeal opening. It is separated from the cranial cavity by the cribriform plate of the ethmoid bone.

The nasal portion of the pharynx or nasopharynx extends from the choanae to the interpharyngeal ostium. It is bounded by the hard palate ventrally, the vomer dorsally, and the palatine bones bilaterally. The hard palate is continued by the soft palate, which is mobile. On the wall of the nasopharynx there is a slitlike auditory tube opening to each side, which connects to the middle ear cavity.

LARYNX

The larynx (Fig. 2–4) serves as a passageway for air, as an aid for vocalization, and as a device to close the airway for raising intra-abdominal pressure or for preventing foreign objects from entering the trachea. Its valvular function by means of the glottis, assisted by an epiglottis, is vital for regulating the passage of ingested materials and air into their proper channels from the laryngopharynx.

Laryngeal Cartilages. The thyroid cartilage is the largest cartilage of the larynx. It forms the major portion of the laryngeal skeleton, and opens dorsally. The rostral border articulates on each side with the thyrohyoid bone, which in turn articulates with the median unpaired basihyoid.

The epiglottic cartilage is attached to the basihyoid and rostral border of the thyroid cartilage, and supports the flap-like structure known as the epiglottis. The normal position of the epiglottis allows it to rest above the soft palate so that air can enter the larynx more directly.

The cricoid cartilage is ring-shaped, with its widest portion dorsally. The paired arytenoid cartilages articulate on its rostral border.

The arytenoid cartilages are somewhat irregular in shape and articulate with the rostrodorsal border of the cricoid cartilage. These cartilages serve as attachments for the vocal folds and for muscles that can close the glottis.

The sesamoid cartilage and interarytenoid cartilage lie in interarytenoid muscles.

During normal breathing the vocal cords remain relaxed, and the opening between them appears as a slit.

Vascularization. Arteries that supply the muscles of the larynx are branches of the cranial thyroid artery, which is the first branch of the common carotid artery. Veins of the larynx are satellite veins that are tributaries of the external jugular veins.

Innervation. Nerves of the larynx are cranial and caudal laryngeal branches of the vagus. The cranial laryngeal nerve is primarily sensory. It leaves the vagus at the level of the nodose ganglion.

The caudal laryngeal nerves are the motor supply to the intrinsic muscles of the larynx except the cricothyroideus. This is the terminal segment of the recurrent laryngeal nerve.

TRACHEA

The trachea extends from the larynx to the bifurcation of the bronchi. It is made of C-shaped hyaline tracheal cartilages. Its length is about 9.0 cm long, and about 0.5 cm in diameter. There are from 60 to 70 rings. The gap between the dorsal borders of the hyaline cartilage is filled by smooth tracheal muscles.

LUNG AND ASSOCIATED STRUCTURES

The thoracic cavity is narrow cranially and continues to widen caudally, making it cone-shaped (Figs. 2–20 to 2–22). The rib cage consists of 14 ribs and 9 sternebrae. The last several ribs do not meet the sternum. The mediastinum can be divided into a cranial, middle and caudal portion.

At the level of the fifth intercostal space, the trachea bifurcates into a left and right bronchus, the bronchial tree (Fig. 2–7). Each bronchus subdivides into lobar or secondary bronchi, and these further divide into small lobules of the lung.

Lung

The ferret lung has a slightly concave base that lies adjacent to the diaphragm and an apex that lies in the thoracic inlet (Figs. 2–20, 2–21, and 2–23). The right and left apices of the lung are at the same level. In an embalmed animal the lung extends from the first and second intercostal spaces to the tenth and eleventh intercostal spaces.

The left lung is composed of cranial and caudal lobes. The cranial lobe is compressed transversely, with one-third of the distal part adjacent to the heart. Its medial border is related to the thymus, esophagus, and trachea. The cranial and caudal lobes are separated from each

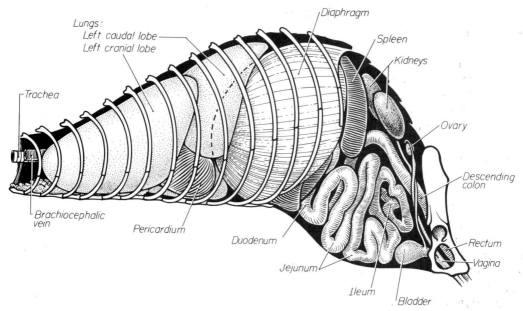

Fig. 2–20. Thoracic and abdominal viscera (*superficial left lateral view*).

other by an oblique fissure. The caudal lobe is somewhat pyramidal in shape and extends from the sixth or seventh intercostal space to the tenth or eleventh intercostal space.

The right lung is composed of cranial, middle, caudal, and accessory lobes separated by fissures. The right cranial lobe is similar to the left cranial lobe but is smaller. Its ventral border is concave and, in conjunction with the middle lobe, it forms a cardiac notch. The dorsomedian border of the right cranial lobe is related to the cranial vena cava, azygos vein, and trachea. The middle lobe lies cranial to the heart, and has a pyramidal shape. The right caudal lobe is similar to the left caudal lobe, except that it is smaller. Caudally it lies adjacent to the diaphragm and the accessory lobe of the lung. Medially it is related to the caudal vena cava. The accessory lobe is the most irregular in shape. It conforms to the dome shape of the diaphragm and curves around the caudal vena cava. It also forms a notch for this vessel and for the right phrenic nerve.

All lobes of the lung are attached to the vena cava by a strong ligament.

Pulmonary Vessels

Pulmonary arteries carry nonoxygenated blood from the right ventricle of the heart to the lung for oxygenation. Pulmonary veins return oxygenated blood from the lungs to the left atrium of the heart. The pulmonary trunk continues from the fibrous pulmonary ring, bifurcates into left and right pulmonary arteries, and ramifies in the left and right lungs (Fig. 2–24).

The right pulmonary artery is longer than the left. It runs caudolaterally, ventral to the right lobar bronchus and dorsal to the left lobar vein. The artery divides into small branches that ramify to the right cranial, middle, caudal, and accessory lobes.

The left pulmonary artery curves dorsally and gives branches to the left cranial and caudal lobes. The veins from all lobes compose most of the ventral part of the root of the lung, and are larger in size than those of the arteries.

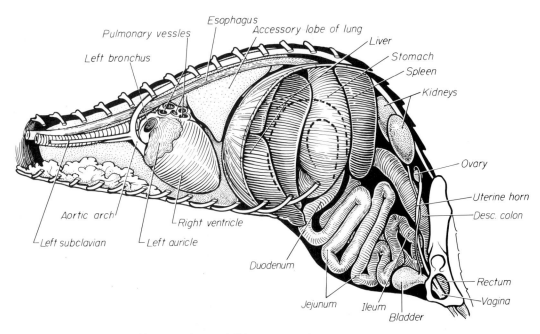

Fig. 2–21. Thoracic and abdominal viscera, left lung removed.

Pulmonary Veins. There is at least one vein for each lobe. Two veins may be present in the left and right cranial lobes.

Bronchial Arteries. The arteries that supply blood to the parenchyma of the lung arise from the first intercostal artery, which is close to its origin from the aorta. The bronchoesophageal artery also supplies branches to the esophagus, bronchi, and tracheal nodes.

HEART, MAIN VESSELS, AND ASSOCIATED STRUCTURES

Within the narrow thorax, cranial to the diaphragm and between the lungs, lie the heart, thymus gland, and great vessels covered by pericardial mediastinum.

THE HEART

The heart of the ferret (Fig. 2–25) is cone-shaped, and is obliquely placed in the thoracic cavity. The apex is directed ven-trocaudally and is connected to the sternum by a ligament that is laden with fat. It is approximately 1 cm from the diaphragm. The remaining part of the heart is largely covered by the lungs (Fig. 2–10).

Size and Weight. Truex and associates studied 12 male ferrets that had a mean body weight of 1102 g and a mean heart weight of 5.00 g (0.45% of total body weight).[19] Among 10 female ferrets studied the mean body weight was 780.8 g and the mean heart weight was 3.7 g (0.47% of total body weight). In the dog the ratio of heart to body weight is 8.10:1000 g body weight in males (0.81%) and 7.92:1000 g body weight in females (0.79%).

Topography. Covered by its pericardium, the heart extends from the sixth rib to the caudal border of the seventh or eighth rib. The longitudinal axis forms an angle of about 73° with the vertical plane. Dorsoventrally the heart axis forms an angle of about 26° with the median plane. The apex is directed to the left of the median plane. The cardiac notch is greatest on

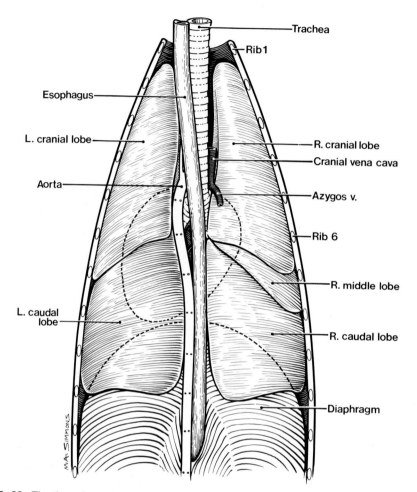

Fig. 2-22. The thoracic cavity (*dorsal view*).

the right and extends from the sixth to the tenth ribs which allows a greater exposure of the heart on the right side.

Vascularization. The coronary sinuses and their venous myocardial tributaries correspond to the pattern observed in the cat.[19] The left coronary is dominant, and the paraconal interventricular branches are easily observed when the heart is exposed. The right coronary artery may be absent.

Innervation. Andrews and co-workers have studied the vagal innervation of the ferret heart.[20] In the neck, the vagosympathetic

trunk travels in close proximity to the common carotid artery and is situated slightly dorsolateral to it. At the level of the thoracic inlet, the vagus nerve separates from the sympathetic trunk and the middle cervical ganglion. (The sympathetic trunk ascended from thoracic nerves via the cervicothoracic (stellate) ganglion and ansa subclavia. The right recurrent laryngeal nerve leaves the vagus at the level of the middle cervical ganglion. It loops around the subclavian artery, passes cranially, and ascends to the larynx in the tracheoesophageal groove.

The main vagal trunk continues caudally in the thoracic cavity. It lies close to

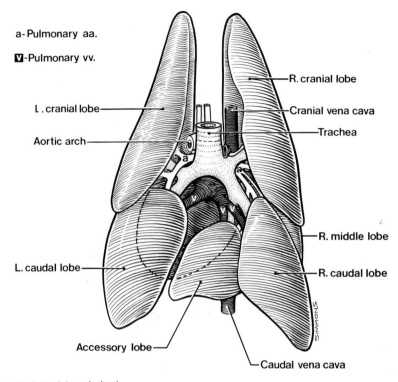

a-Pulmonary aa.

V-Pulmonary vv.

L . cranial lobe

Aortic arch

L. caudal lobe

Accessory lobe

R. cranial lobe

Cranial vena cava

Trachea

R. middle lobe

R. caudal lobe

Caudal vena cava

Fig. 2–23. Lobes of the lung (*dorsal view*).

the trachea and is slightly dorsolateral. The vagus gives a few small branches to the trachea along its course. At the level of T4 to T6 the vagus sends several branches that travel on the ventral surface of the trachea. Several of these branches may be joined by small branches that are given off by the sympathetic trunk as it leaves the vagus. The combined sympathetic-vagal branches travel on the ventral surface of the trachea until they reach the heart. They then appear to penetrate the wall of the right atrium close to the entry of the cranial vena cava. When it passes under the root of the lung, the right vagus gives rise to a branch that passes under the azygos vein to reach the wall of the right atrium.

On the left side, the left sympathetic trunk separates from the vagus in a similar pattern to that of the right. The left recurrent laryngeal nerve leaves the va-

gus at the level of T4, and travels parallel with the vagus until reaching the arch of the aorta. It passes under the arch and ascends to the larynx in the tracheo-esophageal groove. Vagal branches at about the level of T4 run as far as the aorta, at which point they are lost in a fine plexus under the arch of the aorta. The vagus also gives off two or three branches that travel to the right atrium.

DIAPHRAGM

The ferret diaphragm forms a large dome-shaped partition that separates the thoracic and abdominal cavities. It is composed of an entirely fleshy part, a central tendinous portion, and two crura.

The circumference has three parts, sternal, costal, and dorsal. The sternal portion is attached above the xiphoid cartilage

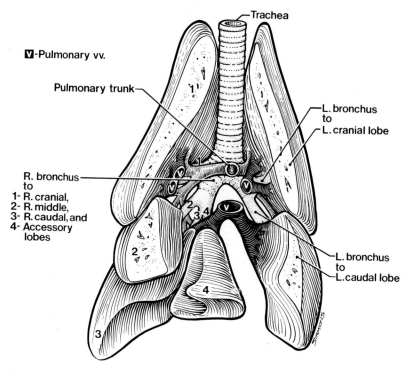

Fig. 2–24. Pulmonary vessels and bronchi (*ventral view*).

and to the cartilage of the last five ribs. The costal part is inserted as serrations to the ribs, which interdigitate with internal abdominal muscle slips. The dorsal part is attached by two tendinous crura to the dorsal wall as far as the level of the last lumbar vertebra.

The diaphragm presents three openings for the passage of the caudal vena cava, the esophagus, and the aorta. The foramen for the caudal vena cava is about 1 cm in diameter and is situated on the left of the median plane. The esophageal hiatus and the aortic hiatus are in the median plane.

Innervation. The phrenic nerve arises from the fifth, sixth, and seventh cervical nerves, and occasionally a small twig arises from the fourth. The phrenic nerve passes caudally adjacent to the external jugular vein at the level of the thoracic inlet. It lies ventral to the subclavian artery, and at this point is joined by a tiny branch from the cranial cervical ganglion. It continues caudally over the trachea on the lateral surface of the pericardium within the mediastinum to reach the diaphragm. The right phrenic nerve runs on the caudal vena cava.

THYMUS GLAND

The size of the thymus gland varies depending on the age of the animal. It lies in the cranial mediastinum of the thoracic cavity just within the thoracic inlet. Medial to the thymus are the trachea, esophagus, and vessels.

MAIN VESSELS OF THE HEART

The main vessels include veins and arteries cranial and caudal to the heart.

Arteries Cranial to the Heart

1. The aortic arch gives rise to two major branches, the brachiocephalic and the left subclavian arteries (Figs. 2–25 and 2–26).
2. Coronary arteries emerge from the base of the aortic arch and are distributed to the wall of the heart. The left coronary is dominant, and the paraconal interventricular branch is easily observed when the thoracic cavity is opened. The right coronary artery may be absent.[19]
3. The brachiocephalic artery is about 1.5 to 2.0 mm in diameter and ascends for 25 to 30 mm ventral to the trachea. At the level of the third rib it supplies a twig to the thymus. At the level of the thoracic inlet it divides into

the right and left common carotid arteries and a right subclavian artery. A small branch, the caudal thyroid artery, arises from the brachiocephalic artery at this level.
4. The left subclavian artery has a diameter of 0.50 to 0.75 mm, and runs lateral to the trachea to the level of the first rib. It gives rise to five branches—the vertebral, costocervical, superficial cervical, axillary, and internal thoracic arteries. The right subclavian artery divides into five branches, like those of the left side.
5. The common carotid artery, before branching into internal and external carotid arteries just posterior to the larynx, gives rise to the cranial thyroid branch, which supplies the thyroid.

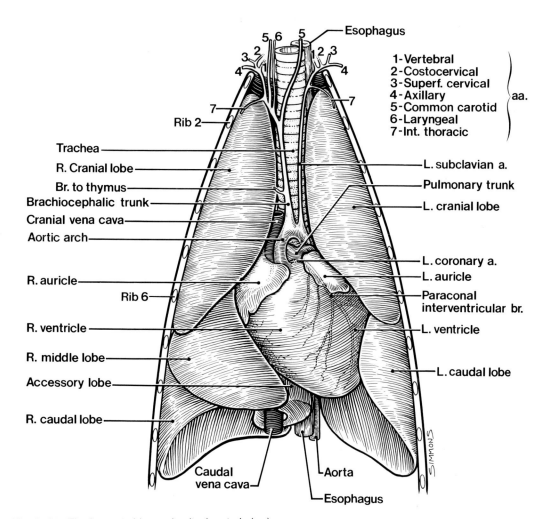

Fig. 2–25. The heart and lungs, in situ (*ventral view*).

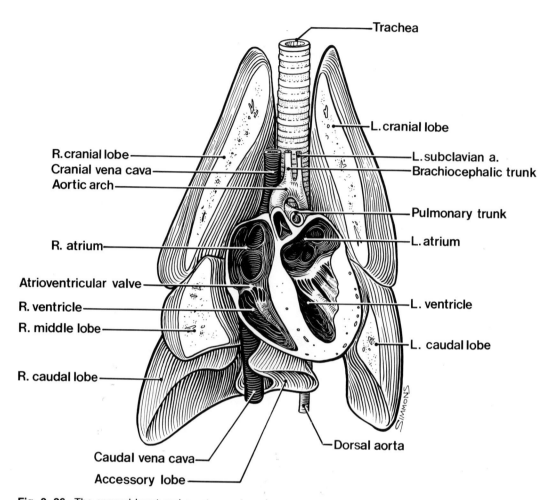

Fig. 2–26. The opened heart and great vessels.

6. The thoracic aorta is a continuation of the aortic arch in the thoracic region.
7. The intercostal arteries are branches of the thoracic aorta to the intercostal muscles.
8. The costocervical trunk is the main blood supply to the muscles at the base of the neck, cranial thorax, trachea, larynx, esophagus, thyroid gland and the cranial vena cava.
9. The internal thoracic artery branches from the subclavian artery at the same level as the costocervical trunk and passes to the inner thoracic wall adjacent to the sternum.
10. The superficial cervical artery is a large vessel that branches from the subclavian artery near the first rib, and serves neck and shoulder muscles, lymph nodes, salivary glands, skin, and skin muscles.
11. The vertebral artery passes dorsally to the transverse foramen of the sixth cervical vertebra and cranially through the transverse foramina of the cervical vertebrae. The two vertebral arteries join to form the basilar artery, which passes through the foramen magnum and contributes to the circulation of the brain.
12. The axillary artery supplies muscles of the thoracic limb.

Veins Cranial to the Heart

1. The cranial vena cava has a diameter of 3 to 3.5 mm and enters the right atrium.
2. The subclavian vein joins the internal and external jugular veins to form the cranial vena cava (refer to the article by Florczyk and Schurig[21] for more information about jugular catheterization).

3. The azygos vein, on the left of the aorta, drains the intercostal veins into the right atrium by arching around the root of the right lung and entering the cranial vena cava.

Arteries Caudal to the Heart

1. The abdominal aorta is a continuation of the thoracic aorta after passing through the aortic hiatus of the diaphragm.
2. The phrenicoabdominal vein is a small branch to the diaphragm and body wall muscles.
3. The celiac artery, the first large unpaired branch of the abdominal aorta, branches into the hepatic, left gastric, and splenic arteries.
4. The hepatic artery gives rise to the gastroduodenal and hepatic branches.
5. The left gastric artery, from the celiac artery, supplies the lesser curvature of the stomach, while the splenic artery supplies the spleen.
6. The gastroduodenal artery gives rise to the right gastroepiploic artery on the greater curvature, the cranial pancreaticoduodenal artery, and the right gastric artery to the lesser curvature of the stomach.
7. The cranial pancreaticoduodenal artery runs caudally along the duodenum and supplies the pancreas and duodenum.
8. The right gastric artery passes to the lesser curvature of the stomach and anastomoses with the left gastric artery.
9. The right gastroepiploic artery runs to the greater curvature of the stomach and anastomoses with the left gastroepiploic artery from the splenic artery.
10. The cranial mesenteric artery, the second unpaired branch of the abdominal aorta, branches into the ileocolic, caudal pancreaticoduodenal, and jejunoileal arteries. It supplies the small intestine and anastomoses with the cranial pancreaticoduodenal artery and the colic arteries.
11. The renal arteries supply the kidneys.
12. The testicular arteries in the male, or the ovarian arteries in the female, arise immediately caudal to the renal arteries.
13. The deep circumflex iliac artery supplies the flank.
14. The lumbar arteries branching from the aorta supply the epaxial muscles and body wall caudal to the thorax.
15. The caudal mesenteric artery is an unpaired vessel to the colon and rectum.
16. The external iliac artery to the hindlimb gives rise to the pudendo-epigastric and deep circumflex iliac arteries before leaving the abdominal cavity.
17. The internal iliac artery courses to the scrotum, prostate gland, and penis in the male, to the uterus and vagina of the female, and to the perineal area and rectum of both sexes.
18. The femoral artery, a continuation of the external iliac artery, supplies the hindlimb.
19. The median caudal artery is the termination of the aorta in the tail.

Veins Caudal to the Heart

1. The caudal vena cava returns blood from the caudal two-thirds of the body.
2. The phrenicoabdominal veins drain blood from the diaphragm and adjacent muscles to the caudal vena cava.
3. The portal veins drain blood from the gut to the liver.
4. The pancreaticoduodenal vein drains blood from the pancreas and duodenum to the portal vein.
5. The gastroepiploic vein drains blood from the greater curvature of the stomach to the portal vein.
6. The gastrosplenic vein drains blood from the lesser curvature of the stomach and spleen to the portal vein.
7. The caudal mesenteric vein drains blood from the large intestine to the portal vein.
8. The renal veins drain blood from the kidneys. The renal veins and all the following (9–12) empty into the caudal vena cava before reaching the heart.
9. The suprarenal branch drains from the adrenal gland to the renal branches.
10. Ovarian veins in the female drain blood from the ovary to the caudal vena cava. In the male, the testicular veins drain blood from the testicles to the caudal vena cava.
11. The common iliac veins are formed by the union of the femoral and hypogastric veins. The latter drain blood from the pelvic viscera.
12. The femoral vein, from the hindlimb, passes through the vascular lacuna and empties into the common iliac vein.

UROGENITAL APPARATUS

The urogenital structures include the kidneys, ureters, and urinary bladder, and the female and male reproductive organs.

KIDNEYS

The kidney of the ferret is bean-shaped and weighs about 4.5 g in the male and 3.7 g in the female. The ratio of kidney weight to body weight is 0.27–0.38%. The kidney in a ferret averages 2.40 to 3.0 cm in length, 1.20 to 1.35 cm in width, and 1.10 to 1.35 cm in thickness.

Topography. Both kidneys are retroperitoneal in the sublumbar region, lying on either side of the vertebral column, aorta, and caudal vena cava (Fig. 2–27). Their dorsal surfaces are in contact with sublumbar muscles while their ventral surfaces are covered by peritoneum. They

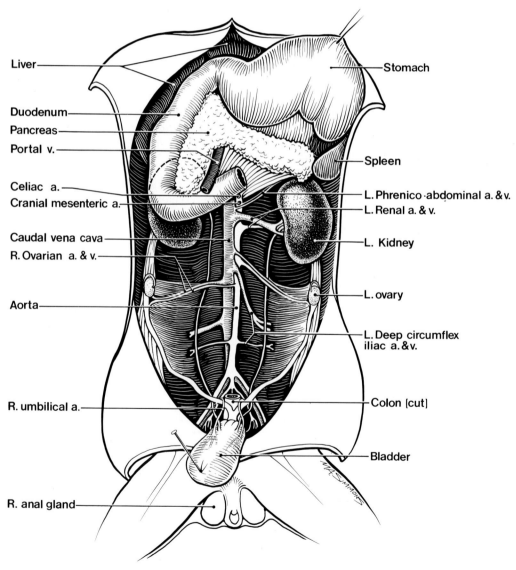

Fig. 2–27. Abdominal cavity, intestine removed.

are invested with a fibrous capsule, and the right kidney is firmly attached to the body wall and the liver.

The craniolateral surface of the left kidney is related to the dorsal end of the medial surface of the spleen, the greater curvature of the stomach, and the greater omentum. Dorsally it is related to sublumbar muscles. Caudally it contacts the descending colon and mesovarium of the female, while in the male the renal peritoneum is reflected on the dorsal body wall as parietal peritoneum. Cranially it is related to the pancreas and left adrenal gland (see Holmes's work for a more detailed discussion of the adrenal gland).[22] Medially it is related to the descending colon, mesocolon, and ascending duodenum. The cranial extremity of the left kidney lies about 0.20 cm caudal to the first lumbar vertebra.

The cranial extremity of the right kidney is embedded in the fossa of the caudate lobe of the liver. This pole is at the level of T14, and the right adrenal gland is related to this pole. Medially it is related to the caudal vena cava. Ventrally it contacts the right limb of the pancreas and ascending colon. The renal sinus of the kidney contains a renal pelvis, fat, renal vessels, ureter, and nerves.

Vascularization. The kidney is a highly vascular organ. Blood enters from the aorta through the renal artery. Blood leaves the kidney via the renal vein to enter the caudal vena cava. Capsular and parenchymal lymphatics are connected to interlobular plexuses, which pass into a lymphatic trunk that leaves the kidney at the hilus, as in the dog.

Innervation. Renal nerves are composed of myelinated and unmyelinated fibers from the sympathetic and parasympathetic systems. They form a dense plexus around the renal blood vessels. They also innervate the renal tubule and the musculature of the renal pelvis.

URETERS

These tubes carry urine from the kidney to the urinary bladder. The ureter begins at the renal pelvis and runs caudoventrally along the ventral surface of the psoas muscle. It passes dorsal to the ureter-ovarian artery in the female or to the internal spermatic artery in the male. At the caudal portion, before passing through the pelvic inlet, it runs dorsal to the external and internal arteries. It enters between the two layers of peritoneum that make up the lateral ligament of the bladder before reaching the dorsolateral surface of the bladder just caudal to the neck of this organ. The ureter enters the bladder and opens within the bladder as a slitlike orifice.

The ureter is supplied by a branch of the renal artery and by a twig of the prostatic artery in the male or by the vaginal artery in the female. The veins that drain the ureter are satellites of the arteries.

The ureters are innervated by autonomic nerves from the celiac and pelvic plexuses.

URINARY BLADDER

The urinary bladder (Fig. 2–28; also see Fig. 2–30) of the ferret varies in shape and size, and its cranial position depends on the quantity of urine it contains. The bladder stores the urine, which is brought by the ureters, and the contents are disposed of through the urethra. An empty bladder in the ferret measures about 1 cm in diameter and 2 cm in length.

Topography. Ventrally the bladder is related directly to the abdominal wall just cranial to the pelvic inlet. It is separated from the latter by two layers of peritoneum. Dorsally it is related to the jejunoileal coil, the descending colon, the uterine horn in the female, and the deferent ducts in the male.

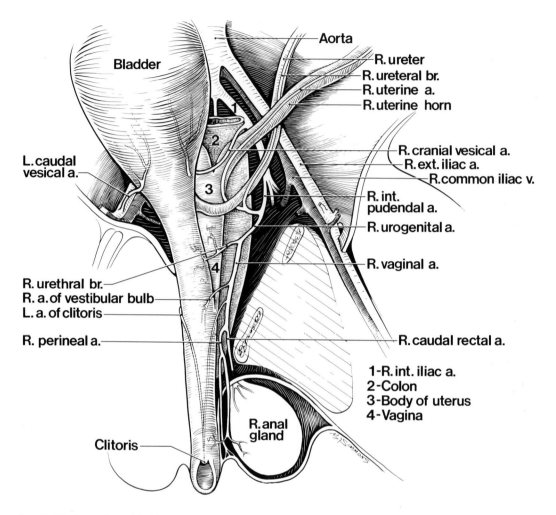

Fig. 2–28. The urinary bladder and associated structures.

The urinary bladder is fixed to the abdominal wall by three ligaments, the right and left lateral ligaments and the middle ligament of the bladder.

Vascularization. A branch of the umbilical artery, called the cranial vesical artery (Fig. 2–30), supplies blood to the organ. This branch anastomoses with the caudal vesical artery, which comes from the urogenital artery.

Blood drains from the bladder by the internal pudendal vein to the common iliac vein. The lymphatics of the bladder drain to the hypogastric and lumbar lymph nodes.

Innervation. The bladder is innervated by parasympathetics of the sacral segment of the spinal cord, and by sympathetics from the hypogastric plexus. The latter is distributed to the bladder wall.

FEMALE GENITALIA SYSTEM

Ovaries

The ovaries of the ferret are paired ovoid organs located caudal to the kidneys (Fig. 2–27). In a 600- to 800-g ferret, the ovary averages 0.45 cm in length, 0.55 cm in width, 0.21 cm in thickness, and 94 to 183 mg in weight. Chang has studied egg transfer in relation to the age of the corpora lutea in the ferret.[23]

Topography. In a sexually mature ferret (average, 600 to 800 g), the left ovary is located about 4.30 to 4.50 cm caudal to the middle of the fourteenth rib and about 0.85 cm caudal to the left kidney.

The left ovary, together with the uterine tube and cranial part of the uterine horn, lies between the abdominal wall and the descending colon. The right ovary is located about 4.30 to 4.50 cm caudal to the middle of the last rib and about 1.47 cm caudal to the right kidney.

Uterine Tube

The uterine tube or oviduct is located between the peritoneal layers of the mesosalpinx. In the ferret, the tube varies in length from 10 to 15 mm, and its external diameter is about 1.00 mm in the ampulla and 0.6 mm in the isthmus. The infundibulum at the ovarian extremity of the tube is funnel-shaped. The fimbria are slightly developed, and the ovarian bursa is almost closed.

Broad Ligament

The ovaries, oviducts, and uterus are attached to the dorsolateral wall of the abdominal cavity and to the lateral wall of the pelvic cavity by a fold of peritoneum called the left and right broad ligaments.

Cranially the ovary is attached by the suspensory ligament, which attaches to the body wall at the level of the distal third of the last rib. The ovary is attached to the uterine horn by the proper ligament of the ovary, which is so short that the ovary is fixed in the immediate proximity of the uterotubal junction.

The broad ligament at the level of the vagina reflects onto the rectum dorsally and to the urethra and bladder ventrally. Laterally the round ligament of the uterus extends to the body wall to pass through the inguinal canal along with the vaginal process.

Uterus

The ferret has two long tapering uterine horns, which fuse immediately in front of the cervix and form a short body (Fig. 2–29). In a mature ferret the uterine horn averages from 4.20 to 4.30 cm in length and 0.22 cm in diameter. The uterine body is 1.70 cm in length and 0.11 to 0.25 cm in diameter. The neck or cervix averages 1.70 cm long and 0.36 cm in diameter. A complete account of reproduction in the mink has been given by Enders.[2]

Vascularization. The ovaries, oviducts, and uterus are supplied with arterial blood via the ovarian and uterine arteries. The two vessels anastomose near the cranial extremity of the uterine horn. The veins are satellites to the arteries.

Both ovarian arteries arise directly from the aorta. The left ovarian artery and vein arise at the level of the third lumbar vertebra, and are embedded in the broad ligament ventral to the uterus. The right artery and vein arise at a lower level than that of the left.

The uterine artery is the main branch of the vaginal artery (Fig. 2–30) on each side. It enters the mesometrium at the level of the cervix, and runs cranially along the border of the uterine horn. Branches of the uterine artery supply both sides of the uterine horn.

The lymph from numerous lymphatic channels of the mesosalpinx and ovary drain to lumbar lymph nodes.

Innervation. The nerve supply to the ovary, uterine tube, and uterine horn is by way

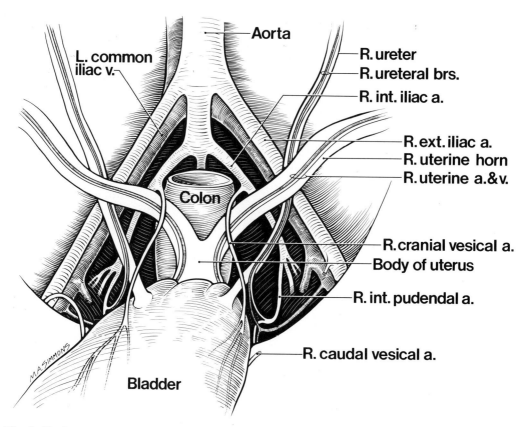

Fig. 2–29. Deep pelvic structures of the female.

of sympathetic axons from the aortic and renal plexuses.

Vagina

The vagina of the ferret is a highly dilatable canal. Cranially the blind pocket or fornix lies beneath the cervix, which is the entrance of the vagina into the body of the uterus. Caudally the vagina ends just cranial to the urethral opening. In a mature ferret the vagina is about 1.50 to 1.80 cm long and 0.36 cm in external diameter.

The cranial portion of the vagina is covered dorsally by peritoneum that reflects onto the colon and ventrally onto the bladder. The caudal half of the vagina is retroperitoneal, and is connected dorsally with the rectum and ven-

trally to the urethra by loose connective tissue.

Vulva

The vulva is the last portion of the female genital tract, also called the external genitalia. It consists of a vestibule, clitoris, and labia. The vestibule is continuous with the vagina from the external opening. The clitoris is the homologue of the male penis. It is well developed in the ferret and is located in a small pocket, the fossa clitoridis. The oval labia forms the external boundary of the vulva.

In the mature ferret the vulva is covered with hair, and averages 1.40 cm in length and 0.36 cm in diameter. The external opening is 0.65 cm in length and 0.50 cm in width.

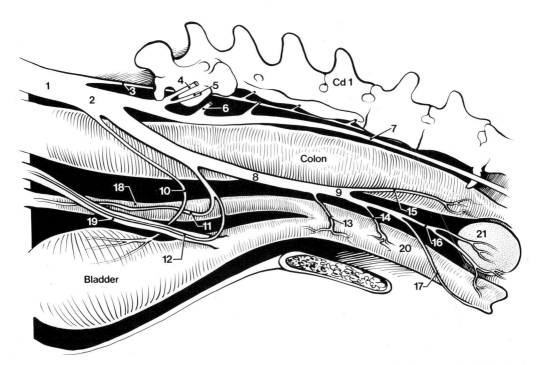

Fig. 2–30. Pelvic viscera of the female (*left lateral view*) (*1*, internal iliac artery; *2*, internal pudendal artery; *3*, medial sacral artery; *4*, iliolumbar artery; *5*, cranial gluteal artery; *6*, caudal gluteal artery; *7*, lateral caudal artery; *8*, urogenital artery; *9*, vaginal artery; *10*, cranial vesical artery; *11*, uterine artery; *12*, ureteral branch; *13*, urethral artery; *14*, artery to vestibular bulb; *15*, caudal rectal artery; *16*, perineal artery; *17*, artery of the clitoris; *18*, uterine horn; *19*, ureter; *20*, vagina; *21*, anal sac; *22*, body of the uterus).

Female Urethra

The female urethra originates from the urinary bladder at or near the cranial edge of the symphysis pelvis. It extends caudally to meet the genital tract at the vaginovestibular junction (Fig. 2–28). Its dorsal wall is in close apposition to the ventral wall of the vagina. The female urethra opens into the floor of the vagina at the urethral orifice.

Topography. The female urethra is located in the pelvic cavity. It is related to the rectum dorsally.

Vascularization. The external genitalia and urethra of the female ferret are supplied with blood by the vaginal and urethral arteries and by the artery of the clitoris. All are branches of the internal pudendal artery.

Blood from the external genitalia and urethra drain to the caudal vena cava through the internal pudendal vein. The latter unites with the caudal gluteal vein to form the common iliac vein. The two common iliac veins join to form the caudal vena cava.

Innervation. The somatic nerves, which innervate the external genitalia, arise from the pudendal and genital nerves. The autonomic innervation of the external genitalia and urethra is via the hypogastric and pelvic nerves.

MALE UROGENITAL SYSTEM

The scrotum is a pouch of skin, beneath the base of the penis, that is divided into two cavities, each of which contains a testis and an epididymis. The epididymis is composed of a mass of convoluted spermatic duct. The part that receives the efferent ductules as they leave the testis is called the head, followed by a larger mass of convoluted duct more caudally that is referred to as the body. This in turn becomes a simple duct, or tail, which passes cranially as the deferent duct (ductus deferens, or vas deferens) through the inguinal canal to join the urethra.

The testis and its vessels, nerves, and duct are wrapped by a pouch of peritoneum, called the vaginal sac, which extends through the inguinal canal prior to the descent of the testis. The testis descends through the inguinal canal to one side of this vaginal pouch, and the resulting wrappings are called tunics. Between the internal or visceral tunic and the external or parietal tunic is the remnant extension of the peritoneal cavity. The spermatic cord is composed of the deferent duct, the deferent artery and vein, and the testicular artery and vein. All are carried through the inguinal canal by the descent of the testis. In a cryptorchid (undescended testes) only the vaginal sac passes through the inguinal canal.

The deferent duct loops over the ureter to join the urethra through the prostate gland. The ureters join the neck of the bladder more cranially.

The penis is formed by two crura that originate on the tuber ischii as the corpora cavernosa. Each corpus is covered by a muscle, the ischiocavernosus, which has the same origin. The two corpora fuse with each other as they turn cranially to become the body of the penis. The cavernous sinus within each crus and corpus remains distinct, however, and is supplied with blood via the deep artery of the penis. The urethra, surrounded by a corpus spongiosum, exits the pelvic canal and passes between the crura. At this level there is an expansion of the spongiosum to form the bulb of the penis, a cavernous sinus that fills with blood via the artery of the bulb. The bulb of the penis is covered by the transverse fibers of the bulbospongiosus muscle. Both the ischiocavernosus muscle and the bulbospongiosus muscle are under hormonal control, and function in ejaculation. The corpus spongiosum around the urethra extends the entire length of the penis. At the distal end, beyond the termination of the corpus cavernosum, the corpus spongiosum expands as the glans. Within the glans there is an *os penis*, which lies dorsal to the urethra. The glans is supplied with blood by the dorsal artery of the penis. The base of the os is attached to the termination of the corpora cavernosa. The function of the os is to stiffen the penis for intromission, and possibly to dilate the cervix of the female. The primary drainage of blood from the glans is via the dorsal veins of the penis.

The prepuce is a fold of skin reflected over the penis, which is hairy on the external surface but bare within the fold. For intromission the glans is extended, and the prepuce becomes the covering skin of the corpus penis. Both the scrotum and prepuce are vascularized by the external pudendal artery and vein, and innervated by the genitofemoral nerve.

A prostate gland is present at the base of the bladder surrounding the urethra. It is not very distinct in young males. At the level of the prostate gland, the ductus deferens of each side opens into the urethra. The prostate gland is vascularized by the prostatic artery that arises from the internal pudendal artery. Blood from the gland drains into prostatic and urethral veins. Innervation of the prostate is from the hypogastric (sympathetic fibers) and pelvic nerves (parasympathetic fibers).

REFERENCES

1. Corbet, G.B., and Hill, J.E.: A World List of Mammalian Species. Ithaca, NY, Cornell University Press, 1980.
2. Enders, R.K.: Reproduction in the mink (*Mustela vison*). Proc. Am. Phil. Soc., *96*:691, 1952.
3. Ewer, R.F.: The Carnivores. Ithaca, NY, Cornell University Press, 1973.
4. Kainer, R.B.: The gross anatomy of the digestive system of the mink: I. The head gut and the fore gut. II. The mid-gut and hind gut. Am. J. Vet Res., *15*:82, 1954.
5. Klingener, D.: Laboratory Anatomy of the Mink. Dubuque, IA, Brown & Co., 1972.
6. Smith, A.A., and Krasulak, C.G.: Manual of Mink Anatomy: An Illustrated Guide to Dissection. Minneapolis, MN, Burgess Publishing, 1979.
7. Marshall, K.R., and Marshall, G.W.: The Biomedical Use of Ferrets in Research, Supplement I. North Rose, NY, Marshall Research Animals, 1973.
8. Williams, R.C.: The osteology and myology of the ranch mink (*Mustela vison*). Master's Thesis Cornell University, Ithaca, NY, 1955.
9. Berkovitz, B.K.B., and Silverstone, L.M.: The dentition of the albino ferret. Caries Res., *3*:369, 1969.
10. Berkovitz, B.K.B.: Supernumerary deciduous incisors and order of eruption of the incisors teeth in the albino ferret. J. Zool. (Lond.), *155*:445, 1968.
11. Berkovitz, B.K.B., and Thompson, P.: Observations on the etiology of supernumerary upper incisors in the albino ferret (*Mustela putorius* L.). Arch. Oral Biol., *18*:457, 1973.
12. Berkovitz, B.K.B., and Poole, D.F.G.: Attrition of teeth in ferrets. J. Zool. (Lond.), *183*:411, 1977.
13. Poddar, S., and Jacob, S.: Gross and microscopic anatomy of the major salivary glands of the ferret. Acta Anat., *98*:434, 1977.
14. Andrews, P.L.R., Grundy, D., and Lawes, I.N.C.: The role of the vagus and splanchnic nerve in the regulation of intragastric pressure in the ferret. J. Physiol. (Lond.), *307*:401, 1980.
15. Poddar, S., and Murgatroyd, L.: Morphological and histological study of the gastrointestinal tract of the ferret. Acta Anat., *96*:321, 1976.
16. Bueno, L., Fioramonti, J., and More, J.: Is there a functional large intestine in the ferret? Experientia (Basel), *37*:275, 1981.
17. Creed, J.E., and Kainer, R.A.: Surgical extirpation and related anatomy of anal sacs of the ferret. J. Am. Vet. Med. Assoc., *179*:575, 1981.
18. Poddar, S.: Gross and microscopic anatomy of the biliary tract of the ferret. Acta Anat., *97*:121, 1977.
19. Truex, R.C., Belej, R., Ginsberg, L.M., and Hartman, R.L.: 1973. Anatomy of the ferret heart: An animal model for cardiac research. Anat. Rec., *179*:411, 1973.
20. Andrews, P.L.R., Bower, A.J., and Illman, O.: Some aspects of the physiology and anatomy of the cardiovascular system of the ferret (*Mustela putorius furo* L.). Lab. Anim., *13*:215, 1979.
21. Florczyk, A.P., and Schurig, J.E.: A technique for chronic jugular catheterization in the ferret. Pharmacol. Biochem. Behav., *14*:255, 1980.
22. Holmes, R.L.: The adrenal gland of the ferret (*Mustela putorius*). J. Anat., *95*:325, 1960.
23. Chang, M.C.: Development of transferred ferret eggs in relation to the age of corpora lutea. J. Exp. Zool., *171*:459, 1969.

chapter 3

THE NEUROANATOMY OF THE FERRET BRAIN

I. N. C. Lawes

P. L. R. Andrews

The first section of this chapter is a macroscopic description of the major dissectable structures in the ferret brain, which should act as a guide for researchers whose work involves lesioning, neurophysiology, and the removal of portions of the brain for biochemical or other analysis. The second section is a brief review of some published literature on the anatomy of the ferret brain.

EXTERNAL APPEARANCE

The ferret brain is approximately 36 mm long and 24 mm wide. Viewed from above it has an almost triangular gyrencephalic forebrain, which overlaps the cerebellum (Fig. 3–1). All abbreviations are given in Table 3–1. Caudal to the cerebellum part of the medulla is visible. On the ventral surface the forebrain, midbrain, hindbrain, and lateral aspects of the cerebellar hemispheres are visible (Fig. 3–2). The terminology used in the following account generally follows that in published works on the ferret.

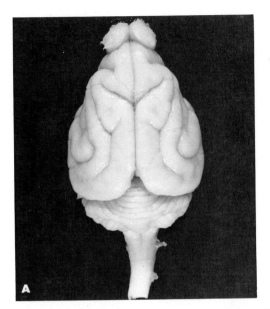 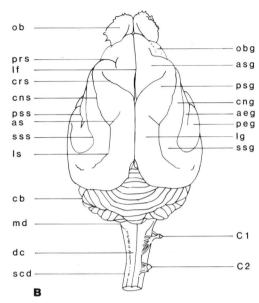

Fig. 3–1. Dorsal view of ferret brain shown in photograph (*A*, × 1.4) and line drawing (*B*). See Table 3–1 for key.

FOREBRAIN

The forebrain is composed of the telencephalon and diencephalon.

Telencephalon

The olfactory bulbs are flattened rostrocaudally, but elongated dorsoventrally (Fig. 3–3). They are widest dorsally, and immediately ventral to the widest part there is a deep groove (Figs. 3–3 and 3–4) on each side leading back to the rhinal fissure and to the lateral margins of the lateral olfactory tract. This groove corresponds to a shelf of bone in the lateral part of the cribriform plate. A large number of olfactory nerve fibers enter the dorsal as well as the rostral surfaces of the bulbs. The olfactory bulbs can be gently raised from the orbital (presylvian) gyrus to reveal a deep wedge-shaped olfactory sulcus that separates the gyrus rectus from the more laterally placed orbital gyrus (Fig. 3–3). On the ventral surface, the olfactory bulb is connected to the olfactory tubercle and to the prominent pale lateral olfactory tract (Fig. 3–2). The

medial olfactory tract has fewer fibers than the lateral, and cannot be seen from the surface.

The cerebral hemispheres are narrowest between the presylvian sulcus and the frontal pole (Fig. 3–1). Posteriorly they are widest at the posterior part of the ectosylvian gyrus. From there the edge of the hemisphere sweeps dorsally and caudally to meet the cerebellum and then continues around to the midline, where the two hemispheres meet at the longitudinal fissure.

The cruciate sulcus passes laterally and rostrally over the dorsolateral surface approximately two-fifths of the distance between the frontal pole and the caudal end of the longitudinal fissure (Figs. 3–1 and 3–4). On the medial surface, which can be seen by gently prying the longitudinal fissure open, the cruciate sulcus continues ventrally for a short distance before meeting the splenial sulcus (Fig. 3–5). The splenial sulcus runs caudally above the corpus callosum on the medial surface of the hemisphere, separating the lateral (or spleniocruciate) gyrus from the more ventral cingulate

TABLE 3–1. KEY TO ABBREVIATIONS

Abbreviation	Definition	Abbreviation	Definition
ac	anterior commissure		
aca	anterior cerebral artery	hb	habenula
acap	anterior commissure, anterior part	hc	habenular commissure
acba	anterior cerebellar artery	hcc	hippocampal commissure
acm	anterior communicating artery	hp	hypophysis
acpp	anterior commissure, posterior part	hpc	hippocampus
aeg	anterior ectosylvian gyrus	hs	hypothalamic sulcus
af	amygdaloid fissure	ht	hypoglossal trigone
aica	anterior inferior cerebellar artery	hy	hypothalamus
alc	anterior lobe of cerebellum		
alv	alveus	ic	inferior colliculus
am	amygdala	ica	internal carotid artery
anl	ansiform lobe	icp	internal capsule
ap	area postrema	inf	infundibulum
as	ansinate sulcus	ipn	interpeduncular nucleus
asa	anterior spinal artery	ipd	inferior cerebellar peduncle
asg	anterior sigmoid gyrus	ivf	interventricular foramen
ba	basilar artery	la	labyrinthine artery
bic	brachium of inferior colliculus	lc	locus ceruleus
bn	bed nuclei of stria terminalis and of anterior commissure	lf	longitudinal fissure
		lg	lateral gyrus
		lgb	lateral geniculate body
br	brachium/superior cerebellar peduncle	lgd	lateral geniculate body, pars dorsalis
		lgv	lateral geniculate body, pars ventralis
c	caudal	ln	lentiform nucleus
C1	first cervical nerve	lot	lateral olfactory tract
C2	second cervical nerve	ls	lateral sulcus
ca	cerebral aqueduct		
cb	cerebellum	mb	mamillary body
cbp	cerebellar peduncles	mca	middle cerebral artery
cc	corpus callosum	md	medulla
ccb	crus cerebri	mdb	midbrain
cd	caudate	mgb	medial geniculate body
cg	cingulate gyrus	mi	massa intermedia
cgl	cingulum	ml	molecular layer
chp	choroid plexus	mlf	medial longitudinal fasciculus
cng	coronal gyrus	mp	mamillary peduncle
cns	coronal sulcus	mpd	middle cerebellar peduncle
crs	cruciate sulcus		
cst	corticospinal tract	na	nucleus accumbens
		ndb	nucleus of diagonal band
d	dorsal	ndl	nodule
db	diagonal band		
dc	dorsal columns	oa	ophthalmic artery
dcn	dorsal column nuclei	ob	olfactory bulb
dg	dentate gyrus	obg	orbital gyrus
		obx	obex
ecp	external capsule	oc	optic chiasma
		oft	olfactory tubercle
fc	facial colliculus	og	olfactory groove
ff	forceps frontalis (minor)	ol	olive
fm	fimbria	on	optic nerve
fo	forceps occipitalis (major)	os	olfactory sulcus
fx	fornix	ot	optic tract
		ots	occipitotemporal sulcus
gl	gyrus lunaris	pca	posterior cerebral artery
gn	genu	pcm	posterior communicating artery
gr	gyrus rectus	peg	posterior ectosylvian gyrus
grl	granular layer	pf	paraflocculus

TABLE 3–1. *Continued.*

Abbreviation	Definition	Abbreviation	Definition
pfs	parafloccular sulcus	ss	splenial sulcus
pg	pineal gland	ssg	suprasylvian gyrus
pica	posterior inferior cerebral artery	sss	suprasylvian sulcus
pl	piriform lobe	st	stria terminalis
plc	posterior lobe of cerebellum	th	thalamus
pmf	primary fissure		
pml	paramedian lobe	v	ventral
pms	paramedian sulcus	va	vertebral artery
pn	pons	vm	vermis
prs	presylvian sulcus	vn	vestibular nuclei
ps	pineal stalk	vt	vagal trigone
psg	posterior sigmoid gyrus		
pss	pseudosylvian sulcus	wm	white matter
py	pyramid	III	oculomotor nerve
		IIIv	third ventricle
r	rostral	IV	trochlear nerve
rf	rhinal fissure	IVv	fourth ventricle
rss	retrosplenial sulcus	V	trigeminal nerve
		Vm	trigeminal nerve, motor root
sb	subiculum	Vs	trigeminal nerve, sensory root
sc	superior colliculus	VI	abducens nerve
scd	spinal cord	VII	facial nerve
sl	sulcus limitans	VIII	vestibulocochlear nerve
sm	stria medullaris	IX	glossopharyngeal nerve
sn	septal nuclei	X	vagus nerve
sp	splenium	XI	accessory nerve
spd	superior cerebellar peduncle	XII	hypoglossal nerve

gyrus (Fig. 3–6). It then continues onto the inferior surface, where it becomes the retrosplenial sulcus. If the cerebrum is separated from the cerebellum, the retrosplenial sulcus can be seen running rostrally toward the posterior limit of the pyriform lobe. Here it is replaced by a shallow groove that travels on the lateral boundary of the pyriform lobe, eventually joining the rhinal fissure. Lateral to the retrosplenial sulcus is a shallow groove, the occipitotemporal sulcus, which begins at the dorsocaudal limit of the ventral surface and runs rostrolaterally to end close to the retrosplenial sulcus.

The anterior sigmoid gyrus, rostral to the cruciate sulcus, meets the orbital gyrus medial to the end of the presylvian sulcus (Fig. 3–4). These two gyri produce a marked dorsal elevation between the frontal pole and the cruciate sulcus. The presylvian sulcus passes ventrally into the rhinal fissure, thus demarcating the

orbital gyrus. Caudal to it, the anterior and posterior sigmoid gyri become continuous at the lateral end of the cruciate sulcus and, together with the anterior part of the coronal gyrus, they produce an elevation on the dorsolateral surface of the hemisphere (Fig. 3–1). Apart from these two elevations, the dorsolateral surface of the hemisphere is of relatively uniform curvature.

The pseudosylvian sulcus runs dorsally and caudally from the rhinal fissure just rostral to the widest part of the brain (Fig. 3–4). Around it are the anterior and posterior ectosylvian gyri. Neither an anterior nor a posterior ectosylvian sulcus is present. Curving around the pseudosylvian sulcus is the suprasylvian sulcus, bounding the anterior and posterior ectosylvian gyri. Between the suprasylvian sulcus and the cruciate sulcus lies the coronal sulcus, which divides the coronal gyrus caudally from the posterior sigmoid gyrus rostrally.

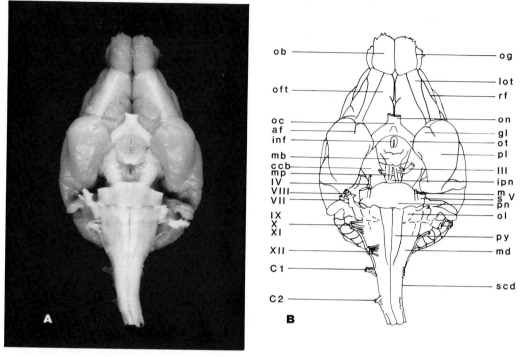

Fig. 3–2. Ventral view of brain after removal of blood vessels, shown in photograph (*A*, × 1.5) and line drawing (*B*). See Table 3–1 for key.

The lateral sulcus is a caudal continuation of the coronal sulcus, sometimes called the coronolateral sulcus.[1] Their point of union is marked by the ansate sulcus, which runs medially and rostrally and demarcates the posterior sigmoid gyrus from the lateral gyrus. The lateral gyrus lies medial to the lateral sulcus, separated by it from the more lateral suprasylvian gyrus. The lateral gyrus has also been termed the "spleniocruciate gyrus."[1] The lateral sulcus runs caudally and then curves laterally and ventrally, where it fades into the posterior sylvian sulcus. This is poorly marked on the ferret brain.

On the ventral surface, the hemispheres also appear triangular (Fig. 3–2). The lateral olfactory tract is wide rostrally but becomes rapidly narrower as it runs over the olfactory tubercle toward the pyriform lobe. Just before it terminates in the pyriform lobe, it is crossed by the middle cerebral artery (Fig. 3–7). The prominent pyriform lobe is separated from the rudimentary temporal lobe by the rhinal fissue. The cortical nucleus of the amygdala produces an elevation, the gyrus lunaris, rostromedially on the pyriform lobe. A shallow sulcus, the amygdaloid sulcus, separates the cortical nucleus of the amygdala from a more lateral and caudal elevation produced by the entorhinal cortex. The lateral part of the pyriform lobe has been designated the anterior and posterior olfactory cortex,[2] which merges indistinguishably with the angular cortex caudally. Caudal to the amygdala are the subiculum and retrosplenial area, but these are not well marked.

Diencephalon

Little of the diencephalon is visible externally (Figs. 3–2 and 3–7). The optic

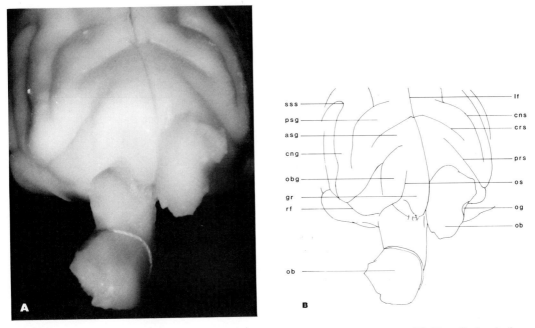

Fig. 3–3. Rostral view of forebrain, shown in photograph (*A*, × 2.8) and line drawing (*B*). The olfactory bulb on the ferret's right has been retracted to show the olfactory sulcus. See Table 3–1 for key.

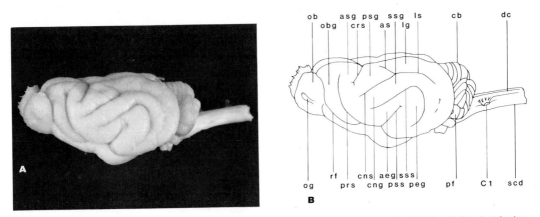

Fig. 3–4. Lateral view of ferret brain, shown in photograph (*A*, × 1.1) and line drawing (*B*). See Table 3–1 for key.

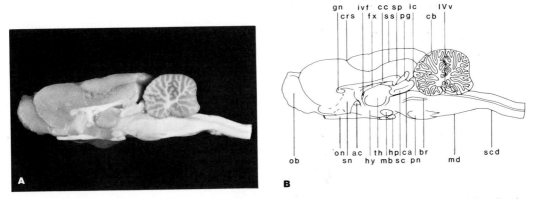

Fig. 3–5. Medial view of ferret brain after sagittal bisection, shown in photograph (*A*, × 1.2) and line drawing (*B*). See Table 3–1 for key.

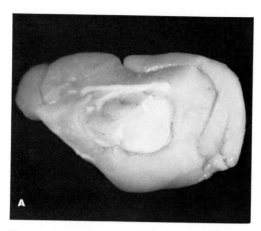
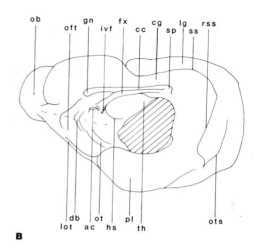

Fig. 3–6. Ventromedial view of ferret brain after sagittal bisection and coronal transection through the junction between midbrain and forebrain, shown in photograph (*A,* × 2) and line drawing (*B*). See Table 3–1 for key.

nerves converge at the optic chiasma and then diverge sharply as the optic tracts to run under the pyriform lobe, where they are concealed from view. Caudal to the chiasma is the flattened hypophysis. The caudal limit of the diencephalon is indicated by the well-marked mamillary bodies, which are visible once the hypophysis has been removed. The fornix can be seen penetrating the rostral part of the mamillary body.

The internal carotid arteries give off thick posterior communicating arteries, which turn caudally and unite with the vertebrobasilar system. The internal carotid arteries divide into the anterior and middle cerebral arteries. The middle cerebral arteries run laterally across the lateral olfactory tracts, and the anterior cerebral arteries cross the optic nerves dorsally (Fig. 3–8), turning medially to anastomose with each other as they enter the longitudinal fissure. The anastomosis is the anterior communicating artery.

MIDBRAIN

The crus cerebri (Figs. 3–2 and 3–7) consists of thick cords of descending axons running on the venral aspect of the cere-

bral peduncles from the cerebrum to the pons. The basilar artery divides into the posterior cerebral arteries between the crura. After giving off the anterior cerebellar arteries (Fig. 3–8), these anastomose with the posterior communicating arteries and then turn laterally to circumvent the midbrain on their way to the medial surface of the cerebral hemispheres.

In between the crura is the interpeduncular fossa (Fig. 3–2). The oculomotor nerve emerges from the midbrain here and runs slightly laterally before penetrating the meninges en route to the orbit. Medial to the oculomotor nerve is a ridge running caudally to a small swelling; the ridge is the mamillary peduncle and the swelling is produced by the interpeduncular nucleus. Between the mamillary peduncle and the crus cerebri the gray matter of the medial terminal nucleus of the accessory optic tract and the ventral tegmental area can be seen but are not labeled. The unlabeled posterior perforated substance, marking the entrance of blood vessels, is almost hidden by the mamillary bodies.

Dorsally, the cerebrum has to be separated from the cerebellum to reveal the tectum, consisting of the superior and inferior colliculi (Fig. 3–9). The superior

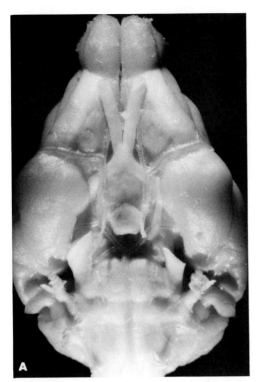
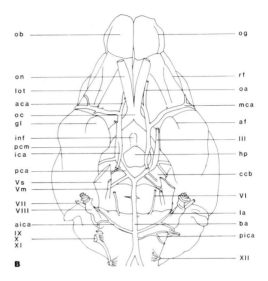

Fig. 3–7. Rostral part of ventral view of ferret brain demonstrating the vascular system and rostral cranial nerves, shown in photograph (*A*, × 2.4) and line drawing (*B*). See Table 3–1 for key.

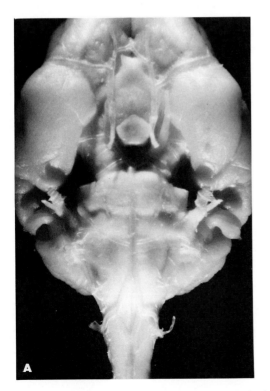
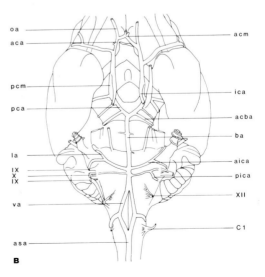

Fig. 3–8. Caudal part of ventral view of ferret brain demonstrating the vascular system and caudal cranial nerves, shown in photograph (*A*, × 2.4) and line drawing (*B*). See Table 3–1 for key.

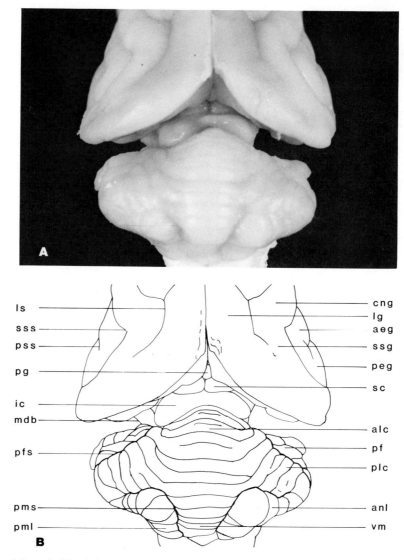

Fig. 3–9. Dorsal view of midbrain between cerebellum and cerebrum, shown in photograph (*A*, × 2.7) and line drawing (*B*). See Table 3–1 for key.

colliculus is more hemispherical, whereas the inferior colliculus is closely applied to the anterior lobe of the cerebellum and conforms to it in shape. The two inferior colliculi are joined across the midline by a well-developed ridge. If the cerebellum and inferior colliculus are separated, the delicate trochlear nerve can be seen emerging from the caudal limit of the inferior colliculus and then passing rostrally around the midbrain (Fig. 3–2).

HINDBRAIN

The hindbrain is composed of the pons and medulla.

Pons

The pons is well demarcated from the midbrain rostrally, but has a very short rostrocaudal extent (approximately 4 mm) and fades almost imperceptibly into the medulla (Figs. 3–2 and 3–7). The basilar artery runs over its ventral surface. The most noticeable feature is the very large sensory root of the trigeminal nerve, marking the point at which the pontine fibers become the middle cerebellar peduncle. Medial to the sensory root is the smaller motor root of the trigeminal nerve.

Medulla

The medulla can be distinguished from the pons by the pale corticospinal tracts descending through the pyramids on its ventral surface (Fig. 3–2). In the ferret the pyramids are elongated structures. On the lateral aspect of the medulla the facial nerve and, more dorsally, the vestibulocochlear nerve, emerge from the pontomedullary junction. The cochlear nuclei form a prominent elevation on the ventral aspect of the inferior cerebellar peduncle, which enters the cerebellum just dorsal to the vestibulocochlear nerve.

The vertebral arteries unite to form the basilar artery on the ventral surface of the medulla (Fig. 3–8), and they also give off the anterior spinal artery, which is almost as large as the basilar artery.

The olive (Fig. 3–2) is a very slight prominence situated between the cochlear nuclei and the pyramids in the most rostral part of the medulla. Near it a very fine abducens nerve may be seen and, caudally, somewhat lateral to the pyramids, several fine rootlets emerge from the medulla before collecting together to form the hypoglossal nerve (Fig. 3–8).

Caudal to the cochlear nuclei is a long shallow elevation on the dorsolateral aspect, the tuberculum cinereum, which is formed by the spinal tract of the trigeminal nerve and its nucleus. On the lateral aspect of the medulla, ventral to the tuberculum cinereum, can be found the rootlets of the glossopharyngeal, vagal, and cranial accessory nerves, with a well-developed spinal accessory nerve running rostrally from the spinal cord to join them (Fig. 3–8).

The dorsal columns are visible on the dorsal aspect of the ferret medulla, terminating in large but shallow elevations, the dorsal column nuclei (see Figs. 3–28 and 3–30). If the cerebellum is gently elevated, the U-shaped area postrema can be seen just rostral to the obex, where the caudal limit of the fourth ventricle is to be found.

CEREBELLUM

On the rostral surface of the cerebellum, the anterior lobe is demarcated from the posterior lobe by the primary fissure (Fig. 3–10). This can be recognized by its greater depth, by the secondary fissures in its walls (Fig. 3–11), and by the fact that it runs laterally and then turns rostrally, whereas adjacent fissures in the anterior lobe run laterally and those in the posterior lobe run rostrolaterally. Apart from blood vessels, only a shallow groove marks the junction of the vermis and hemispheres on the rostral surface of the cerebellum.

On the caudal surface of the cerebellum, the vermis is clearly separated from the hemisphere by a deep paramedian sulcus (Fig. 3–12). The cortex of the hemisphere curves medially from the dorsolateral aspect, forming the short limb of a symmetric inverted J on each side. More medially the cortex continues caudally, forming the long paramedian limb of the J. The direction of the folia gives the impression that the cortex is turning back on itself. The short dorsolateral limb of the J, the ansiform lobule, is continuous laterally and rostrally with the rest of the posterior lobe. The longer more medial limb of the J is the paramedian lobule. Ventrally, the posterior lobe is separated from the paraflocculus by the parafloccular sulcus, which runs perpendicular to the general direction of sulci in this vicinity (Figs. 3–12 and 3–13). Part of the paraflocculus lies in a deep fossa in the

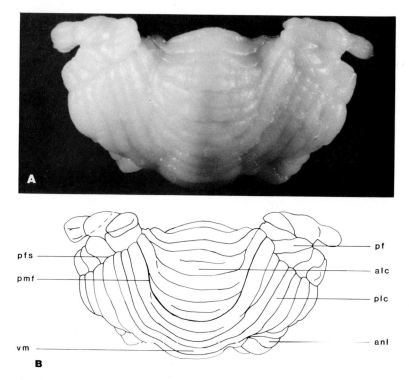

Fig. 3–10. Rostral surface of detached cerebellum, shown in photograph (*A,* × 3.4) and line drawing (*B*). See Table 3–1 for key.

petrous bone and tends to be damaged during removal of the brain unless special care is taken. The most caudal part of the vermis, overlying the obex, is the uvula. The small flocculus can be seen ventral to the paraflocculus. It is conventional to number the folia of the vermis (Fig. 3–11). The first five lobules are rostroventral to the primary fissure on the rostral surface. Lobules VI and VII lie dorsally, and the remaining three lobules continue on the caudal surface.

INTERNAL APPEARANCE

FOREBRAIN

The gray matter of the gyri can be removed using a blunt instrument to reveal the white matter below, particularly the short arcuate fibers (Fig. 3–14). The ease with which this can be done permits the separate analysis of gray and white matter, if required. The white matter forms wide troughs formerly occupied by the sulci, and narrow ridges in the place of gyri. The predominant fibers on the surface of the white matter are short arcuate fibers. These run from one ridge in the core of a gyrus, across the troughs deep to the sulci, and into the next ridge in the core of a neighboring gyrus. They lie perpendicular to the long axis of the associated sulcus.

When the short arcuate fibers are carefully removed, the next layer of white matter forms a smoother, continuous sheet of axons (Fig. 3–15). These axons run in a radial direction from most of the dorsolateral surface of the cortex to converge on the internal capsule, just dorsal to the pseudosylvian sulcus. Thus, they form a fanlike structure whose edges are the lateral, medial, and caudal limits of the cortex, and whose "handle" is the most

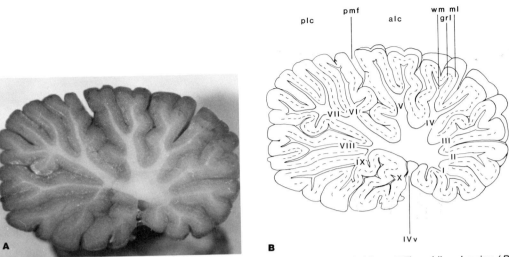

Fig. 3–11. Sagittal section through cerebellar vermis, shown in photograph (*A*, × 5.7) and line drawing (*B*). The Roman numerals refer to the numbered cerebellar lobules. See Table 3–1 for key.

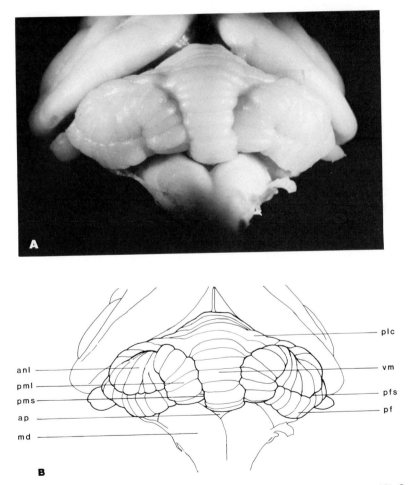

Fig. 3–12. Caudal view of cerebellum in situ, shown in photograph (*A*, × 3.1) and line drawing (*B*). See Table 3–1 for key.

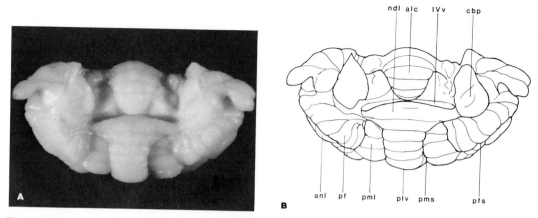

Fig. 3–13. Ventral view of detached cerebellum, shown in photograph (*A*, × 3) and line drawing (*B*). See Table 3–1 for key.

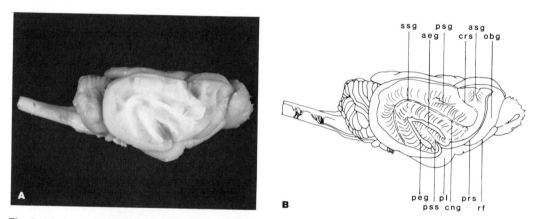

Fig. 3–14. Lateral aspect of forebrain after removal of the cortical gray matter, shown in photograph (*A*, × 1.2) and line drawing (*B*). The ridges of the arcuate fibers are labeled with the names of the gyri under which they normally lie. See Table 3–1 for key.

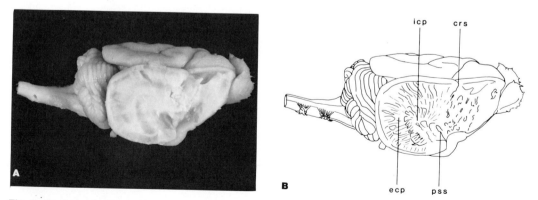

Fig. 3–15. Lateral aspect of forebrain after removal of the arcuate fibers, shown in photograph (*A*, × 1.2) and line drawing (*B*). Caudally, fibers of the "external capsule" can be seen converging on the internal capsule. See Table 3–1 for key.

superficial part of the internal capsule. For simplicity, this fanlike structure will be referred to as the external capsule.

The axons in the external capsule include long association fibers connecting noncontiguous gyri with each other in the same hemisphere, together with commissural fibers that have crossed from one hemisphere to the other in the corpus callosum, and fibers from the internal capsule connecting the cortex to subcortical structures. If the most dorsomedial fibers are removed, a longitudinal bundle of axons can be seen running rostrocaudally above and perpendicular to the corpus callosum (Fig. 3–16). This is the cingulum, which links allocortical structures of the limbic system together. When the cingulum is removed the corpus callosum is seen crossing between the hemispheres, and its contribution to the external capsule is more evident. The corpus callosum is flat in the midline. Its splenium is only 1 mm short of the caudal limit of the cortex, whereas the genu is 7 mm short of the frontal pole. It is

therefore about 70% of the length of the hemisphere at this level, and lies relatively caudally. The forceps frontalis (minor) turns rostrally toward the frontal pole, while the forceps occipitalis (major) sweeps laterally and caudally.

The external capsule forms the roof and lateral wall of the lateral ventricle. Removal of the external capsule exposes the whole extent of the lateral ventricle (Figs. 3–17 and 3–18). Rostral to the interventricular foramen, its anterior horn is bounded dorsally by the corpus callosum, medially by the septal and associated nuclei, laterally by the corpus striatum, and rostrally by the forceps frontalis of the corpus callosum. The body is also roofed over by the corpus callosum. Its floor is formed rostrolaterally by the caudate nucleus and caudomedially by the thalamus, covered by the fornix and choroid plexus. Caudally, the body is limited by the forceps occipitalis of the corpus callosum, and there is no posterior horn. The body of the ventricle sweeps in a wide curve, first ventrolater-

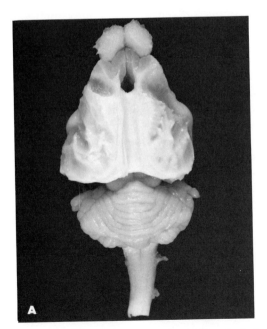
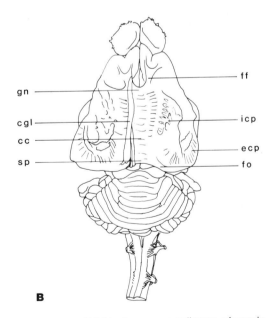

Fig. 3–16. Dorsal aspect of brain after removal of all structures superficial to the corpus callosum, shown in photograph (A, × 1.4) and line drawing (B). See Table 3–1 for key.

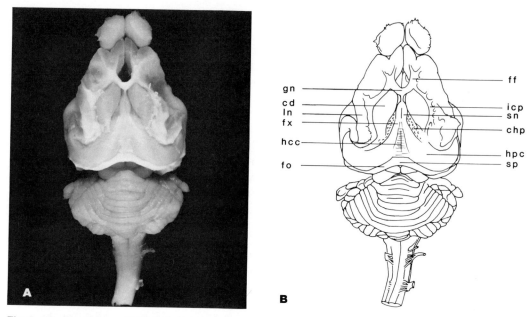

Fig. 3–17. Dorsal view of brain after removal of the corpus callosum, shown in photograph (*A*, × 1.4) and line drawing (*B*). See Table 3–1 for key.

ally, then rostrally, to become the inferior horn. Its lateral wall is formed by fibers in the external capsule and corpus callosum. The inferior horn ends rostrally at the amygdala. Most obvious in its floor is the large hippocampal formation, which is covered by a thin film of axons, the alveus. These axons collect on the inner edge of the hippocampus to form the fimbria prior to becoming the fornix. The fibers of the fornix are predominantly axons of the subiculum and septal nuclei. Dorsocaudally, the hippocampus is enclosed in the fibers of the forceps occipitalis. Medially, the commissural fibers of the fornix can be seen crossing to the other side below the corpus callosum (Fig. 3–17).

The hippocampal complex forms a C-shaped concavity rostrally, with the upper limb dorsomedial and the lower limb ventrolateral. It can be shelled out from the forebrain without damage, making it a very attractive structure to investigate (Fig. 3–19). The inferior surface is the subiculum, which is continuous around

the caudal convex edge of the complex with the hippocampus proper, via the presubiculum, in the depths of the hippocampal fissure. The hippocampus forms the upper surface of the complex and then rolls inward to end in its center, embraced by the dentate gyrus. If the subiculum is peeled off the lower surface, the regularly segmented dentate gyrus, is exposed. It is curved into a C shape, both in the long axis of the complex and in the short axis perpendicular to this. Thus, the blades of the dentate gyrus clasp the recurrent part of the hippocampal complex (field CA3). A blunt instrument can be inserted between the hippocampus and the dentate gyrus, separating them completely and permitting them to be analyzed independently.

Rostromedial to the hippocampal formation is a large oval structure of gray matter, the corpus striatum (Fig. 3–17). The corpus striatum lies immediately ventral to a horizontal plane drawn through the ends of the coronal and pseudosylvian sulci. Its rostral limit is a sharp vertical edge tucked in behind the forceps frontalis (minor) of the

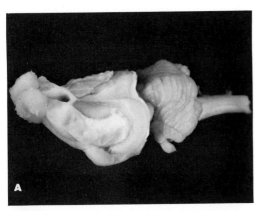

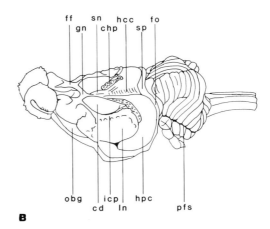

Fig. 3–18. Dorsolateral view of brain after removal of the corpus callosum, shown in photograph (*A*, × 1.2) and line drawing (*B*). See Table 3–1 for key.

corpus callosum, and has a much greater dorsoventral extent than the caudal end. Its caudal limit is almost level with the rostral limit of the hippocampus. The lateral surface of the corpus striatum lies almost directly above and parallel to the lateral olfactory tract. The corpus striatum is divided by the anterior limb of the internal capsule into the caudate nucleus dorsomedially and the lentiform nucleus ventrolaterally (Fig. 3–18). Ventral to the lentiform nucleus, the corpus striatum merges with the amygdala, which, like the lentiform nucleus, was initially covered by the external capsule and claustrum.

The caudate nucleus can be removed as an entity, but this is more difficult than in the case of the hippocampal formation because of the intimate relation of the striatum to the internal capsule (Fig. 3–20). Once it is removed the smooth rounded dorsal surface of the caudate, covered by ependyma, can be seen. The medial surface is also smooth, and its rostral part is flattened by the septal nuclei and by nuclei of the diagonal band, molding it into a sharp vertical edge. The rostral edge terminates ventrally in a point. The most rostro-ventro-, medial part of the structure removed may include part of the nucleus accumbens, lying medial to the groove formed by the anterior commissure. The lateral surface of the striatum is smooth dorsally and rostrally, but is roughened by broken axons and by the internal capsule ventrally. The ventral surface tapers rapidly in a caudal direction, reaching the dorsal surface at its caudal limit. This surface is deeply notched by the broken axons of the internal capsule, through which strands of gray matter previously connected the caudate to the lentiform nucleus (hence the name "corpus striatum").

Removal of the hippocampal formation exposes the deep surface of the entorhinal cortex. When the latter is removed the colliculi on the dorsal surface of the midbrain can be seen, together with the large ovoid thalamus (Fig. 3–21). The thalamus is continuous with the rostrolateral aspect of the superior colliculus. Its dorsal and caudal surfaces are smooth, and covered with pia or ependyma. The medial surface forms part of the lateral wall of the third ventricle, which it partly obliterates as it fuses across the midline to form the massa intermedia. The junction of the medial and dorsal thalamic surfaces is marked by the stria medullaris thalami (see Figs. 3–27 and 3–28), which runs caudally toward the habenula, a slight swelling on the most dorsal caudal part of the thalamus. The habenular com-

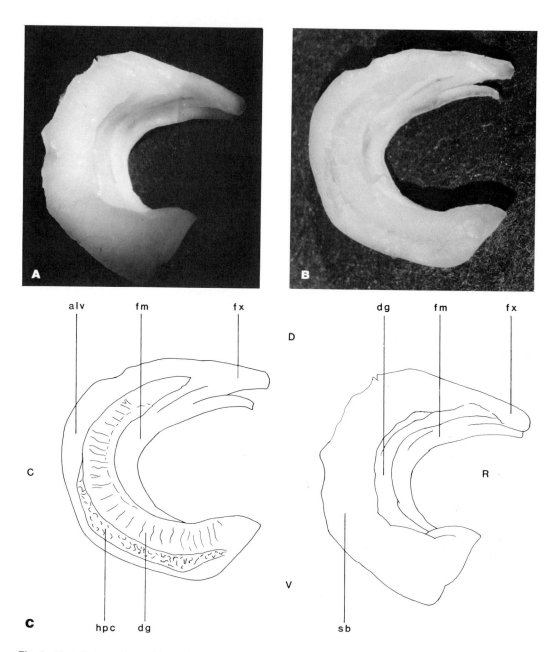

Fig. 3–19. Inferior surface of the isolated left hippocampal complex before and after removal of the subiculum, shown in photographs (*A* and *B*, × 10.5) and line drawing (*C*). See Table 3–1 for key.

missure can be seen crossing to the opposite side just rostral to the superior colliculus (see Figs. 3–27 and 3–29). The midline pineal gland is visible dorsal and caudal to the habenular commissure (Fig.

3–5). The lateral surface of the thalamus is roughened by its contribution to the internal capsule, the posterior limb of which separates it from the lentiform nucleus (Fig. 3–22). The stria terminalis

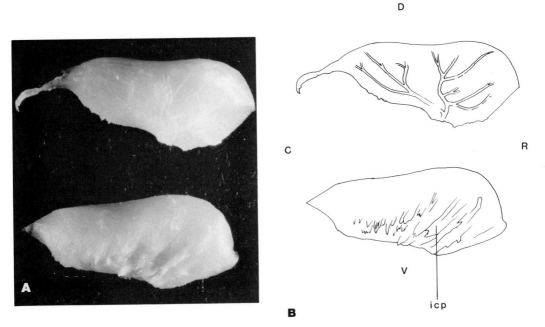

Fig. 3–20. Medial view of the isolated left caudate nucleus and lateral view of the right caudate nucleus, shown in photograph (*A*, × 5.5) and line drawing (*B*). See Table 3–1 for key.

encircles the roughened lateral surface, running first caudally from the amygdala, then dorsally, and finally rostromedially, between the thalamus and the corpus striatum, on its way to the hypothalamus. Ventrally, the optic tracts can be seen entering the ventrolateral part of the thalamus, where the lateral geniculate nucleus, pars ventralis, can be found (Fig. 3–23). The main part of the tract continues dorsally and caudally to reach the pars dorsalis of the lateral geniculate nucleus, situated on the dorsocaudal extremity of the lateral surface of the thalamus. The continuity of the internal capsule and the crus cerebri is evident immediately deep to the entry of the optic tract into the lateral geniculate nucleus. Caudal and medial to the lateral geniculate nucleus, the more prominent medial geniculate body can be seen receiving the brachium of the inferior colliculus (Fig. 3–23).

As the gray matter of the thalamus is scraped away, the axons of the brachium of the superior colliculus are seen running between the superior colliculus and the lateral geniculate body, dorsolateral to the medial geniculate body. The full extent of the internal capsule can be exposed by removal of the thalamus and the corpus striatum. It has an anterior limb intervening between the lentiform nucleus and the caudate, a genu, and a posterior limb separating the lentiform nucleus from the thalamus.

If the remains of the fornix are followed rostrally, it is seen entering a vertical wedge of gray matter directly under the corpus callosum (Figs. 3–5, 3–21, and 3–24). The wedge is comprised of septal and associated nuclei, and is perforated by the anterior commissure (Fig. 3–24). The septal nuclear complex can be removed as an entity (Fig. 3–25). The dorsocaudal part of this wedge is comprised of septal nuclei. The more ventral part of the wedge, adjacent to the anterior commissure includes the bed nuclei of the stria terminalis and of the anterior

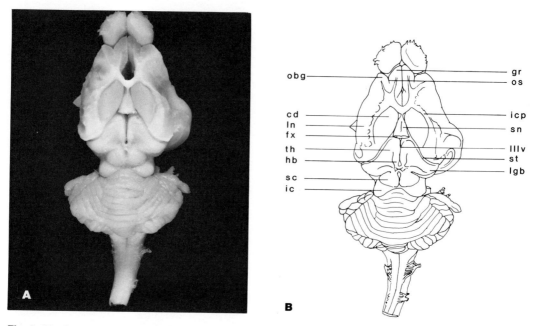

Fig. 3–21. Dorsal view of forebrain after removal of the hippocampal complex, shown in photograph (*A*, × 1.5) and line drawing (*B*). See Table 3–1 for key.

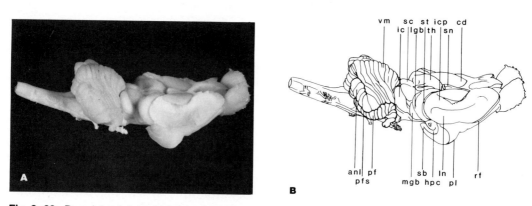

Fig. 3–22. Dorsolateral view of forebrain after removal of the hippocampal complex, shown in photograph (*A*, × 1.2) and line drawing (*B*). See Table 3–1 for key.

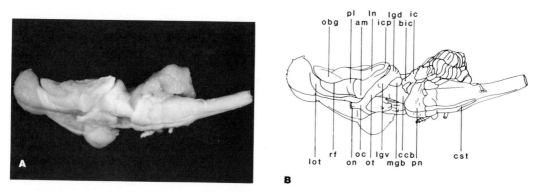

Fig. 3–23. Inferolateral view of brain demonstrating optic tract reaching the thalamus, shown in photograph (*A*, × 1.2) and line drawing (*B*). See Table 3–1 for key.

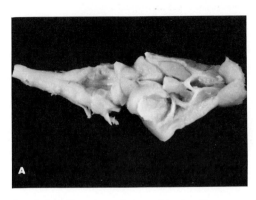

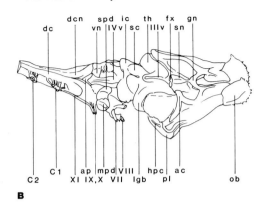

Fig. 3–24. Dorsolateral view of brain after removal of the cerebellum and right caudate nucleus, shown in photograph (*A,* × 1.2) and line drawing (*B*). See Table 3–1 for key.

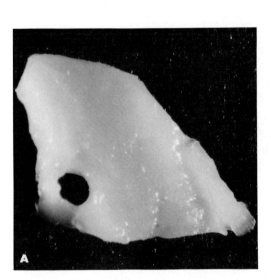

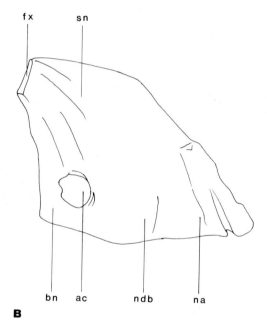

Fig. 3–25. Isolated septal nuclear complex, shown in photograph (*A,* × 7.4) and line drawing (*B*). The foramen was occupied by the anterior commissure prior to its removal. See Table 3–1 for key.

commissure. Rostral to the anterior commissure is the nucleus of the diagonal band ventromedially. The diagonal band can be seen from the medial aspect of a bisected brain (Fig. 3–26), curving dorsally onto the medial surface from the ventral surface and therefore hooking itself inside the concavity of the anterior commissure. Before removal, the nucleus

accumbens was rostrolateral to the diagonal band nuclei. The most rostromedial part of the septal nuclear complex is the lateral septal nucleus. It would be very difficult to differentiate these structures in a macroscopic dissection. When these nuclei are removed, the pillars of the fornix (Fig. 3–27) are seen descending toward the anterior commissure, where

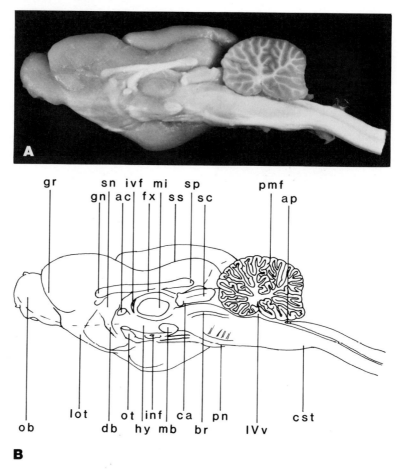

Fig. 3–26. Inferomedial view of sagittally bisected brain after removal of the pineal gland and hypophysis, shown in photograph (*A*, × 1.9) and line drawing (*B*). This is one stage earlier than that represented in Figure 3–6. See Table 3–1 for key.

some fibers pass rostrally, but most continue ventrally and then caudally into the hypothalamus, ending mainly in the mamillary bodies. The pillars of the fornix form the rostral boundary of the interventricular foramen, with the thalamus as the caudal boundary (Fig. 3–5). Ventral and rostral to the anterior commissure is the preoptic region, with the hypothalamus more caudally. The third ventricle extends rostrally into the preoptic region, technically part of the telencephalon but functionally more closely associated with the hypothalamus. In the lateral wall of the third ventricle, a groove running from the interventricular foramen to the cerebral aqueduct demarcates the hypothalamus ventrally from the thalamus dorsally (Fig. 3–6). This is the hypothalamic sulcus.

The hypothalamus is divided into a medial cell-rich zone and a lateral more fiber-rich zone by the fornix coursing toward the mamillary bodies. The hypothalamus extends from the optic chiasma rostrally to the mamillary bodies caudally, with the tuber cinereum in between. Unless great care is taken, the infundibular stem arising from the median eminence of the tuber cinereum will

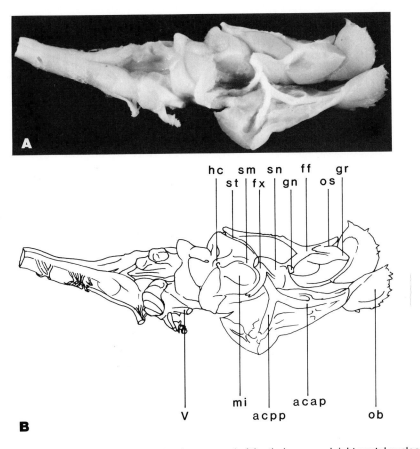

hc   sm   sn   ff   gr
st | fx | gn | o s

V   mi   acap
B   acpp   ob

Fig. 3–27. Fornix and anterior commissure following removal of the thalamus and right septal nuclear complex one stage after that represented in Figure 24, shown in photograph (*A*, × 1.8) and line drawing (*B*).

be severed, because the hypophysis is usually trapped in the hypophyseal fossa by a layer of dura, the diaphragma sella.

Once the thalamus and caudate and septal nuclei have been removed, the lateral olfactory tract can be seen running caudally from the olfactory bulb to the rostroventral aspect of the amygdala. Medial to the lateral olfactory tract, and on a deeper (more dorsal) plane, the thick bundle of fibers forming the rostral part of the anterior commissure travels rostrally toward the olfactory bulbs (Figs. 3–27 and 3–28). A slightly less substantial bundle of axons forms the caudal part of the anterior commissure, traveling laterally and slightly caudally to enter the pyriform lobe. The anterior commissure disappears below the ventral part of the corpus striatum.

BRAIN STEM (MIDBRAIN, PONS, AND MEDULLA)

Whereas gray matter and white matter are distinct from each other in the forebrain, and can therefore be dissected macroscopically, large parts of the brain stem consist of the reticular formation in which, by definition, cell bodies and axons are not segregated. This makes macroscopic dissection unrewarding, and no description is offered. The major tracts of white matter can be displayed and may be of heuristic interest, but it is doubtful if specimens of a quality adequate for research purposes could be prepared reproducibly in this way. It is recommended that researchers who wish to work on the brain stem use thick slices and take biopsies under microscopic guidance. At least one atlas of the ferret brain stem has been prepared.[3]

The cerebellum can be removed, exposing the fourth ventricle (Figs. 3–28 and 3–29). The superior cerebellar peduncle runs rostrally and medially to the midbrain. It is crossed laterally by the inferior cerebellar peduncle coming from the medulla. Both of these peduncles are embraced and hidden by the larger middle cerebellar peduncle coming from the pons. The fibers of the middle peduncle run in a more dorsoventral direction than those in the superior peduncle.

The floor of the fourth ventricle is diamond-shaped. Rostrally, it leads into the cerebral aqueduct and caudally it continues into the central canal. Caudally it is obscured by the choroid plexus (Fig. 3–29), which must be removed to expose its floor (Fig. 3–28). The midline is marked by a deep groove, lateral to which

the white matter of the medial longitudinal fasciculus is visible (Fig. 3–30). There is a deep fossa rostrally, the superior fovea, and a groove, the sulcus limitans, running caudally from this, at first medially and then laterally. Between the sulcus limitans and the midline the floor is raised to form the medial eminence, part of which covers the facial nerve as it curves around the abducens nucleus, thus forming the facial colliculus. Caudally, the medial part of the floor overlies the hypoglossal nucleus. Lateral to the sulcus limitans is the well-marked diamond-shaped gray matter, which constitutes the vestibular nuclei. Caudal to the vestibular nucleus a triangular area marks the vagal nuclei. The most caudal structure of the ventricle is the area postrema, which is a midline U shape in the ferret, with each limb running rostrally in the caudolateral margins of the fourth ventricle. The obex is immediately caudal to the area postrema.

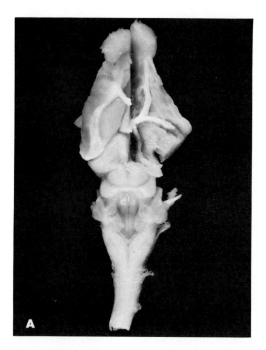
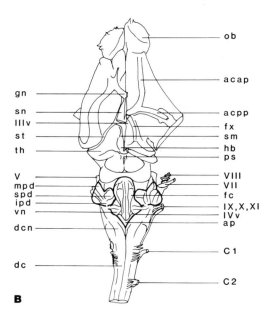

Fig. 3–28. Dorsal view of the same stage as that represented in Figure 3–27, shown in photograph (*A*, × 1.5) and line drawing (*B*). The fourth ventricle and cerebellar peduncles are heavily outlined. See Table 3-1 for key.

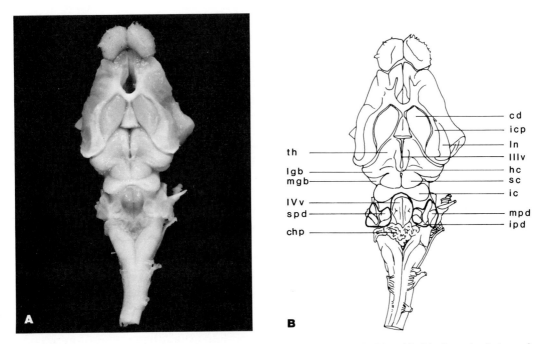

Fig. 3–29. Dorsal view of the stage between those represented in Figures 3–21 and 3–24, shown in photograph (*A*, × 1.5) and line drawing (*B*). The cerebellum has been removed to expose the choroid plexus of the fourth ventricle. See Table 3-1 for key.

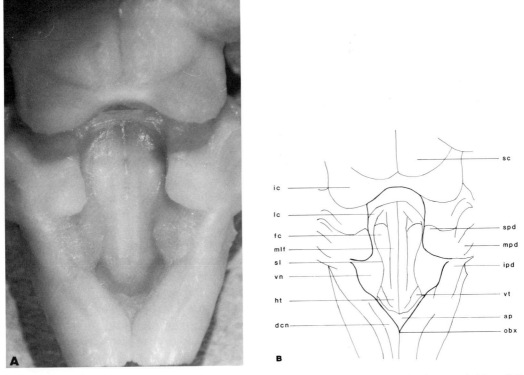

Fig. 3–30. The floor of the fourth ventricle after removal of the choroid plexus, shown in photograph (*A*, × 6.9) and line drawing (*B*). See Table 3-1 for key.

REVIEW OF THE LITERATURE

FOREBRAIN: CEREBRAL HEMISPHERES

Cerebral Cortex

The ferret brain, although gyrencephalic like that of other carnivores, has one of the simplest forebrains in this order. It differs from another carnivore, the cat, in having a relatively narrow forebrain.[4] This reflects a decrease in the diameter of the frontal parts of the hemispheres during development,[1] and relates to the decrease in the diameter of the postorbital constriction of the ferret skull in older animals.[5] There is no ectosylvian sulcus on the dorsolateral surface, nor a suprasplenial sulcus on the medial surface.[4]

It has been presumed[4] that the motor cortex is in the anterior sigmoid gyrus, the sensory cortex in the posterior sigmoid gyrus, the auditory cortex in the ectosylvian gyrus, and the visual cortex in the lateral gyrus. Evoked potentials indicate that olfactory information reaches the pyriform cortex.[2]

The development of the ferret brain has been studied in embryos, ranging from 5.5 to 38 mm in length.[6] The brain of the youngest embryo is divided into telencephalon, diencephalon, mesencephalon, and rhombencephalon by grooves, and the optic primordium and trigeminal and vestibulocochlear nerves are apparent. No cerebral hemisphere, olfactory system, nor cerebellum are evident. The development of the cortex from an original two-layered structure, at 10 mm, to a four-layered structure, at 17 and 38 mm, has been described.[6] Although no cortical grooves are apparent at 17 mm, two grooves are seen extending caudolaterally from the "rhinencephalon," a deep posterior groove delimits the temporal lobe, and a groove is seen on the medial surface,[6] possibly indicating the site of the future crural sulcus.

In contrast to Krabbe's report,[6] postnatally the cerebral cortex is described as smoothly convex at birth,[1] with no more than slight transverse narrowing, but the rudiments of all the adult sulci and gyri develop within 1 week. Prior to weaning growth is symmetric around three relatively stable points, the interventricular foramen and the caudal ends of the ectosylvian and orbital gyri. After weaning, however, the hemispheres increase in length and height but diminish relatively in breadth, particularly rostrally, so that, with the development of the frontal pole, the originally rectangular shape becomes triangular. The floors of sulci are displaced little relative to the underlying white matter. Smart and McSherry have postulated that one system of gyri, comprised of the splenial, posterior and anterior sigmoid, and orbital gyri, folds back on itself because of the constraints imposed on the growth of the frontal pole.[7] A second set of concentric folds is formed by the coronal and ectosylvian gyri, the growth of which is determined by their attachment to the underlying striatum.

Operative interference with the brain of young ferrets has produced corresponding changes in endocranial casts,[8] indicating that the convolutional pattern of the endocranial cast depends on that of the brain. Depressions in the brain produce depressions in the skull. Darlington supposed that the endocranial surface is molded by the arachnoid mater tethered to the brain by arachnoid trabeculae; when the trabeculae are severed, the arachnoid is free to move away from the brain and create a depression in the overlying bone.[8]

Intracortical development has been studied.[7] Cell nuclei grow in radial columns that diverge superficially in gyral crowns but recurve toward each other in sulcal floors, where their deeper parts are eventually replaced through tangential growth and they become shorter. The cortical subplate grows most in the crowns but only minimally in sulcal floors; its neurons disperse and then disappear altogether. Cell nuclei in the cortical plate are initially elongated but become rounder and more dispersed, although new cells migrate from the depths to fill the expanding cortical volume. If cell columns are measured along their length instead of perpendicular to the surface they, and the thickness of cortical layers, are found to be relatively conserved.

Analysis of cell production gradients in the ferret cortex[9, 10] indicates that cortical plate growth depends on an increase in depth by an accumulation of migratory neurons from a subjacent periventricular germinal layer, and on an increase in area resulting from germinal cells being recruited into neuron production at the periphery of the plate. At 29 days postconception there is a laterodorsal gradient of neuron production, which is greater laterally than dorsally, and a rostrocaudal gradient greater rostrally than caudally. Both gradients are therefore the expression of a single rostrolateral focus. By 36 days postconception the laterodorsal gradient persists only in caudal sections, and the rostrocaudal gradient is present only dorsally. This analysis was based on profile counts without stereologic correction, and the change in numbers could be partly due to a change in cell size as well as number, but the results nevertheless indicate a rostrolateral focus of cortical plate formation.

The timing of these production gradients may explain why methylazoxymethanol acetate administered at 32 days postconception causes lissencephaly mainly in the caudal third of the cortex,[11] while at 38 days it produces little disruption, causing the loss of only the ansate sulcus.[12]

Olfactory Bulb and Pyriform Lobe

The development of dendritic and somatic spines of granule cells in the olfactory bulb has been studied in relation to the imprinting of prey odors that occurs between 60 and 90 days postnatally in the ferret.[13] Although somatic spines decrease continuously, dendritic spines show a temporal overshoot.

The accessory olfactory bulb receives the vomeronasal nerve.[4] The anterior olfactory nucleus situated in the olfactory crus contributes to the lateral olfactory tract.[4] The pyramidal cells of the olfactory tubercle form a corrugated sheet.[4]

The pyriform lobe of ferrets is smaller than in other carnivores such as cats and dogs, and the cortical amygdaloid nucleus occupies a relatively greater proportion of it, in the gyrus lunaris.[2] Three layers of neurons have been described in the rostral part of the ferret pyriform cortex and five have been described caudally.[4] The cortex of the pyriform lobe that receives fibers from the lateral olfactory tract is histologically distinct, as described in detail by Dennis and Kerr.[2] The prepyriform cortex of the ferret, and a caudolateral extension (the flatter, rostral part of the pyriform lobe), has been designated as the "anterior olfactory cortex," and most of the periamygdaloid cortex or entorhinal area has been designated as the "posterior olfactory cortex."[2] This area is bounded by the rhinal fissure, the cortical amygdaloid nucleus, the subiculum, and the angular cortex. It is histologically distinct from the "anterior olfactory cortex."[2] The cell-sparse plexiform band, layer IV, is less well developed in ferrets than in other carnivores.

The functionally unbiased terms "prepyriform," "periamygydaloid," and "parahippocampal" would seem preferable to "olfactory cortex," given the problems associated with changing views on function such as occurred with the term "rhinencephalon." Function is determined by what a region does with the information it receives, as well as by the nature of the information itself.

The parts of the pyriform cortex not receiving a direct olfactory input include the angular cortex, a part of the entorhinal cortex at the angle between the temporal and occipital lobes. Based on antidromic stimulation, it has been claimed that the medial part of the olfactory tubercle of the ferret does not receive fibers from the lateral olfactory tract,[2] and its function is unclear.

Subcortical Structures

The nuclei of the ferret amygdala have been divided into a corticomedial group of four nuclei and a basolateral group of five nuclei, together with an undifferentiated anterior amygdaloid area.[4] A morphometric study, however, has indicated the existence of eleven nuclei distributed in five major groups, together with a further four individual nuclei.[14] Physiologic studies have implicated the ferret amygdala in gonadal function,[15] and it is likely to contribute to many other endocrine, autonomic, affective, and mnemonic processes.

The dorsal group of septal nuclei (dorsal septal nucleus and septohippocampal nucleus) is poorly represented in the ferret. A group of cells just caudal to the anterior olfactory nucleus is variously considered to be an anterior hippocampal remnant or part of the septal group of nuclei.[4]

The putamen is fused with the tail of the caudate and the tail is not in continuity with the body. The claustrum is divided into a dorsal insular portion and a ventral prepyriform portion, caudolateral to the amygdala and dorsomedial to the pyriform cortex.[4]

FOREBRAIN: DIENCEPHALON

Thalamus

The thalamus is small in relation to the midbrain.[4,16] Its component nuclei are divided into anterior, medial, lateral, and ventral groups. The following account is

a brief synopsis of a detailed paper by Herbert,[16] unless otherwise specified. The anterior group occupies the rostral pole of the thalamus and consists of anteroventral (actually dorsolateral in the ferret), anteromedial, and anterodorsal nuclei. The anterodorsal nucleus is smaller than in the rat, possibly indicating a gradual phylogenetic regression of the anterodorsal and anteromedial nuclei.

The medial group, dorsomedial to the internal medullary lamina, has been defined by Herbert as the nucleus medialis dorsalis, centrum medianum, midline, and intralaminar nuclei. The dorsomedial nucleus is the largest, and occupies most of the medial thalamus. Its lateral part, projecting to the frontal cortex, is increasing phylogenetically while the medial part is regressing. The medial part of the nucleus paracentralis crosses the midline. The centrum medianum, once denied as a subprimate nucleus, is the second largest of Herbert's medial group of nuclei. The centrum medianum has been described as primordial in another mustelid, the mink,[17] but a large area corresponding to Herbert's centrum medianum is unlabeled. A medial part of this nucleus is sufficiently distinct in the ferret to be discerned as the nucleus parafascicularis, unusual in subprimates. The midline group of nuclei includes the nucleus paraventricularis, nucleus paratenialis, nucleus reuniens, and the nucleus rhomboidalis. Except for the paratenial nucleus, these nuclei all fuse across the midline.

The ventral group is well developed in the ferret and lies ventrolateral to the internal medullary lamina. It includes the nucleus ventralis anterior, medialis, arcuata (the largest of the ventral group), externa, and posteroinferior (which differs in ferrets from that in other carnivores because it lacks a commissural component).

The lateral group lies dorsolaterally, and is best developed caudally. It is comprised of the nucleus lateralis anterior, intermedia, and posterior, and the nucleus posterior. No pulvinar, which is very well developed in primates, has been recognized, although one is described in the mink[17]; the difference may be in terminology. Nevertheless, this region of the thalamus is less developed in the ferret than in species considered to lead to primates.

The nucleus reticularis consists of scattered cells in the external medullary lamina. It blends with the nucleus ventralis anterior in the rostral part of the ferret thalamus, but is more distinct elsewhere.

There has been a substantial amount of work done on the lateral geniculate nucleus (described below, Visual System). The medial geniculate nucleus forms the caudolateral limit of the thalamus. It consists of a pars principalis and a pars magnocellularis, ventromedial to the pars principalis. The nucleus suprageniculatus lies along the dorsomedial border of the medial geniculate nucleus, and the pregeniculate nucleus lies rostral to the lateral geniculate nucleus.

The habenula, properly part of the epithalamus, can be divided into a medial and a lateral nucleus. The habenulopeduncular tract (fasciculus retroflexus) originates more from the lateral than the medial nucleus, and courses ventrally through the thalamus to reach the interpeduncular nucleus.

In a paper published before the advent of modern tract tracing techniques, Herbert pointed out the unsatisfactory nature of subjective interpretations of histologic material.[16] It is now time for a quantitative morphologic study of the thalamus to be combined with these modern techniques.

A mass of small, neuroglial-like cells and larger, mature neurons has been described on the ventricular surface of the ferret thalamus,[4] possibly representing the ganglionic eminence, a developmental defect.

Hypothalamus

As is fitting for an animal that has made such a long and prominent contribution to neuroendocrinology, the hypothalamus of the ferret has been described. It is divided into supraoptic, tuberal, mamillary, and periventricular regions, and the telencephalic preoptic region is described with it. The fiber tracts in the ferret hypothalamus are similar to those in other species. The following account is based on that of Westwood.[18]

The preoptic region lies above the rostral half of the optic chiasma and below the anterior commissure. It is divided into a medial and a lateral area, which is penetrated by the medial forebrain bundle.

The supraoptic region consists of the supraoptic, paraventricular, and suprachiasmatic nuclei, together with the anterior hypothalamic area. The supraoptic nucleus, extensive in the ferret, has rostral and caudal parts, with the latter varying in position in different ferrets. The suprachiasmatic nucleus is better developed in the ferret than in almost any other animal. It is easily recognized as closely packed cells bordering the ventral part of the ventricle, dorsal to the optic chiasma. The anterior hypothalamic area is ill defined in the ferret.

The tuberal region includes ventromedial and dorsomedial nuclei, and posterior, dorsal, and lateral hypothalamic areas. No perifornical nucleus has been identified in the ferret. The ventromedial nucleus is the most prominent structure, larger and better defined than in cats and dogs. Conversely, the dorsomedial nucleus is inconspicuous in the ferret, contrasting with the rat, and in some ferrets it has not been identified. The posterior hypothalamic area is poorly developed with little cellular aggregation into a nucleus, as in other carnivores, but in contrast to its differentiation in primates, particularly humans. Westwood has related this to the visceral expression of emotion. The lateral hypothalamic area is also poorly developed in the ferret. The numerous fiber tracts in this region cast doubt on "centers" identified by electrical stimulation or lesion experiments.

The mamillary region, well marked in the ferret, is comprised of medial and lateral mamillary nuclei, and the intercalated, premamillary, and supramamillary nuclei. The medial mamillary nucleus is the largest nucleus in the hypothalamus, evident as the mamillary body. The fornix, mamillothalamic, and mamillotegmental tracts enter or leave it. Rostrally it can be subdivided into dorsal and ventral zones. The lateral mamillary nucleus lies ventral to the fornix, from which it receives numerous connections. It contributes to mamillothalamic and mamillotegmental tracts, and receives the mamillary peduncle. This nucleus is present in cats, but the nucleus referred to as the "lateral mamillary" in dogs is probably equivalent to the intercalated nucleus. Although more conspicuous in ferrets than in other animals, the intercalated nucleus is subject to terminologic confusion. It is subpial in location, ventrolateral to the lateral mamillary nucleus, and it also receives the mamillary peduncle. The premamillary nucleus is ill defined in the ferret.

The periventricular region includes preoptic, anterior, posterior, and arcuate periventricular nuclei. These are narrow subependymal zones of cells, 3 to 12 layers or more deep, lining the third ventricle. The arcuate periventricular nucleus (or nucleus infundibularis) is well demarcated, but the distinction between anterior and posterior periventricular nuclei is arbitrary.

Like Herbert, Westwood has also warned against the pitfalls in the subjective interpretation of histological sections,[18] and against the pervasive tendency to label some structures (e.g., the preoptic region and the hypothalamus) as "olfactory."

VISUAL SYSTEM

The visual system of the ferret has been studied extensively,[19-27] partly for developmental reasons, partly because of the role of the visual system in photoperiodism, and partly because of peculiarities of this system in the ferret.

Retina

The tapetum and retina of the ferret have been compared to those of other carnivores, and found to resemble those of the dog more closely than the cat.[27] Histochemical localization of cytochrome oxidase has revealed mosaics of differentially stained cells and parts of cells in the retina of four species, including ferrets.[21] The ferret retina contains the same proportion of alphalike cells but fewer betalike cells than the cat retina.[26] Virtually all alphalike cells project contralaterally in pigmented ferrets. The immature retina of the neonatal ferret has been described.[26]

Lateral Geniculate Nucleus

The lateral geniculate nucleus is divided into a much larger dorsal part and a ventral part.[16] The dorsal part is lateral to the midbrain and dorsal to the medial geniculate body. It is concave, with a rostromedial hilum, and is divided into a lamina principalis (corresponding to laminae A and A1 in the dog and cat), a lamina magnocellularis, and a lamina parvocellularis. The ventral part of the lateral geniculate nucleus lies on the ventrolateral aspect of the thalamus, covered by the large lateral part of the optic tract. Although less developed in ferrets than in other carnivores, the lateral geniculate nucleus is larger than in rats, commensurate with a relative increase in geniculate rather than collicular termination of the optic tract.

The lateral geniculate nucleus of the ferret is smaller, the laminae are flatter and less distinct, and the nucleus is less sigmoid sagittally than in the cat. The binocular input is relatively restricted in comparison to the large monocular segment and in comparison to other mammals. There is a well-differentiated laminar pattern in related mustelids, weasels and minks, indicating that ferrets may not have been bred for visual abilities. In the albino ferret, lamina A1, which normally receives an ipsilateral retinal input, is broken up into clusters of cells, and there are fewer retinal fibers projecting to lamina C1.[19]

The development of the dorsal lateral geniculate nucleus has been studied in the ferret because it is born with an unlaminated nucleus comparatively soon after conception, and 30 days before the eyes open.[23] In the adult, lamina A receives crossed and A1 receives uncrossed retinal inputs. Situated between lamina A1 and the optic tract, laminae C and C2 receive crossed, C1 uncrossed, and C3 no retinal inputs. In contrast to the flat laminae of the mink, ferret laminae form a medial transverse (binocular) limb and a lateral (monocular) longitudinal limb. Leaflets within the A and A1 laminae are less well defined than in minks, but no leaflets are seen in other carnivores. The C laminae are better defined than in cats. The medial interlaminar nucleus and geniculate "wing" are innervated, mostly contralaterally, but the perigeniculate nucleus may not be. The perigeniculate nucleus is large in ferrets and minks and traversed by several retinofugal fibers, in contrast with the situation in cats. Uncrossed fibers show some localization within the optic tract.

The postnatal lateral geniculate nucleus is originally innervated binocularly, but the ipsilateral fibers withdraw to a small binocular region, leaving a large monocular region to the contralateral fibers. Soon afterward the contralateral fibers withdraw from this small binocular region. This occurs earlier and more completely in the A layers. Conversely, the C layers attain an adult structure slightly before the A layers, commensurate with their greater development in ferrets than in cats. Segregation of axons begins before cell layers are apparent, but ends after lamination has been completed, indicating that the two processes may be independent. The lateral geniculate nucleus bends posteriorly to form the transverse limb of the adult. These patterns of development appear to be rather general across species.

The distribution of cytochrome oxidase in the lateral geniculate nucleus is different in ferrets, cats, *Macaca*, and *Saimiri*, and suggests that "off-center" cells are more active in carnivores while "on-center" cells are more active in primates.[21]

Accessory Optic System

Older, less reliable techniques have failed to reveal any accessory optic tract in ferrets,[20] and it has been confirmed that there is no anterior accessory optic tract, no fibers in the lateral hypothalamus nor in the cerebral peduncle, and none in the subthalamus.[25] This is typical of carnivores, insectivores, and primates, but contrasts with rodents and lagomorphs.

Crossed fibers of the posterior optic tract, however, have been found leaving the brachium of the superior colliculus caudal to the medial geniculate body, and passing to a small elevation, the lateral terminal nucleus, immediately lateral to the crus cerebri.[25] These fibers continue as the transpeduncular tract to reach the medial terminal nucleus. The lateral and medial terminal nuclei, situated on either side of the crus cerebri, consist mainly of medium-sized round cells and large oval cells.[25] The ferret appears to lack a dorsal terminal nucleus, although this is present in both rats and cats.

The predominantly contralateral retinal projections to the suprachiasmatic nucleus found in most mammals have been confirmed by autoradiographic but not degenerative techniques.[25] This is particularly interesting in view of the marked development of this nucleus in the ferret, and because of the role of photoperiodism in the ferret endocrine and reproductive systems.

Visual Cortex

The laminar distribution and stripelike configuration of the intrinsic connections of ferret striate cortex resemble those in cats but differ from those in primates. Extrinsic ipsilateral and contralateral connections to areas homologous to areas 18 and 19 and to the suprasylvian region have been described.[24]

BRAIN STEM

There has been very little work published on the anatomy of the ferret brain stem. The representation of auditory space has been mapped in the deep layers of the superior colliculus,[28] and it has been found that cells have a preferred direction of sound input that usually corresponds to the preferred direction of visual input to overlying cells in the superficial layers of the colliculus. The anatomic implications of a nucleotopic organization of projections from the superior olivary complex have not yet been investigated. The inferior colliculus has a dominant central nucleus, with a marked rostroventral extension and more diffusely packed external and pericentral nuclei.[29] The ferret inferior colliculus has a tonotopic and binaural organization similar to that found in other species, but has neurons that are particularly active under barbiturate anesthesia.[29]

Vagal afferents to the ferret brain stem have been studied autoradiographically.[30]

Axons from the nodose ganglion terminate in the ipsilateral nucleus of the tractus solitarius. Terminations are greater laterally in rostral parts and medially in caudal parts of the nucleus, but greatest both laterally and medially near the obex. The lateral labeling in the rostral part of the solitary nucleus has not been reported in other species. Only the medial caudal parts of the nucleus have been labeled contralaterally, and the labeling is less intense. Both the area postrema and the area subpostrema are lightly labeled bilaterally. Slight labeling of the dorsal part of the ipsilateral dorsal motor nucleus of the vagus is seen, and this has been tentatively attributed to vagal afferents from the aortic and carotid sinuses. Labeled fibers are seen traversing the commissural nucleus.

No label is seen in the nucleus ambiguus, the external cuneate nuclei, any trigeminal nuclei, the reticular formation, nor cervical segments. Positive reports of labeling in these structures in other species have all involved horseradish peroxidase, which labels fibers of passage presumably originating in cells in the superior vagal ganglion. All autoradiographic studies are reputedly negative for these structures, regardless of species.[30] Major species differences have been found in comparison to the hen, which has a contralaterally labeled tractus solitarius, innervation of the reticular nucleus, and no innervation of the dorsal motor nucleus, area postrema, nor area subpostrema. The ferret vagal afferents therefore resemble those found by using axonal transport techniques in monkeys and cats and, with the exception of the area postrema, also in rats.

Odekunle and Bower have indicated that the ferret dorsal motor vagal nucleus is the principal source of cranial efferents to the subdiaphragmatic gastrointestinal tract.[31] Other sources are the nucleus ambiguus, nucleus retroambiguus, and nucleus dorsomedialis. The nucleus ambiguus is the principal source to the esophagus, which is striated in the ferret and has a myelinated innervation. Varied patterns of efferent projections have been found for different parts of the gut, but the viscerotopic organization is indistinct and requires study by more powerful quantitative techniques.[32, 33]

The spinal cord has been investigated, and reasons have been given for the use of the ferret as a model of spinal cord injury.[34]

CEREBELLUM

Specific points referring to the ferret have been extracted from a chapter on the comparative anatomy of the mammalian cerebellum.[35] As in humans and *Macaca*, lobules IV and V are of relatively greater length in the ferret than in cats, goats, and *Hyrax*. The prepyramidal fissure of the ferret, between lobules VII and VIII, resembles its human counterpart in stopping near the lateral border of the cerebellum, whereas in several other species this fissure reaches the border. The area lacking a cortex in the interparafloccular fossa extends to the paramedian sulcus and isolates the vermal cortex of lobules X, IX, and part of VIII from the hemisphere, with the ferret resembling goats and monkeys in this respect.

Spinocerebellar afferents, revealed by mossy fiber degeneration, are restricted to the crowns of folia in lobules I, II, III, and VIII in the ferret, as in a number of other species.[35] Ferret, goat, hedgehog, and *Macaca* differ from other species in lacking a spinocerebellar input to lobule IX. Use of the Haggqvist stain reveals that the white matter of the ferret cerebellum can be divided into alternating bands of small and large (3 to 4-μm) fibers.[35] There are five such zones on each side of the anterior lobe, and two or three in the caudal part of the posterior lobe. These parasagittal zones are more marked than in the cat. The cerebellar cortex can also be divided into parasagittal zones on the basis of projections to deep nuclei. Zone A, projecting to the fastigial nucleus and zone B, projecting to the lateral vestibular nucleus, have been identified in the anterior lobe of the ferret. Zone C is subdivided in this species into a medial part projecting to the anterior interposed nucleus and a lateral part, absent in lobules I and II, projecting to the posterior interposed nucleus. Fifth and sixth zones project to different parts of the lateral cerebellar nucleus.[35]

Electrophysiologic evidence indicates that there is a monosynaptic mossy fiber input to lobules V and IV in the paravermal zone, 4 mm lateral to the midline, from periodontal receptor afferents traveling in the inferior alveolar nerve.[36] The conduction velocity of these afferents is 49 to 52 m/sec, indicating a myelinated fiber diameter of approximately 8 μm. It is thought that these axons are mossy fiber collaterals of sensory neurons in the caudal part of the mesencephalic nucleus of the trigeminal nerve. Cutaneous afferents in the mental branch of the inferior alveolar nerve do not project directly to the cerebellum, and muscle afferents in the masseter-temporalis nerve do not evoke early cerebellar responses either. These muscle afferents, and periodontal afferents, produce later, large slow waves attributed to a climbing fiber input, implying a route through the olivary complex. The afferents studied probably signal the pressure and direction of force applied to the teeth, together with the end point of jaw closure. This information may be used to recalibrate muscle spindle afferents periodically.[36]

USE OF THE FERRET IN NEUROLOGIC STUDIES

The ferret is an animal of proven value in neuroscientific investigations. One of the earliest consistent uses has been in the study of neuroendocrinology, particularly in relation to the influence of photoperiodism. In this connection the marked development of the suprachiasmatic nucleus, with an accessory optic input, may contribute to the importance of the use of the ferret in the investigation of photoperiodism, endocrinology, and reproduction. The ferret visual system has been studied partly because of its peculiarities in both relatively normal fitches and in less normal albinos; the preponderant contralateral visual input is enhanced in albinos. The lateral geniculate nucleus, although relatively less laminated than in the cat, nevertheless shows greater development of the C layers and a marked indication of leaflets in the A layers, with each leaflet corresponding to either on- or off-center types of receptive fields[37]; the biologic significance of this restricted differentiation of part of the system against the background of an otherwise poor visual differentiation should prove interesting.

Another clear trend is in the use of the ferret for developmental studies. One line of research has exploited the immaturity of the nervous system at birth. Special senses can be investigated before the ferret develops vision and hearing at 4 weeks of age, or smell at 13 weeks when it leaves the nest. Another line of research has concentrated on the convolutional patterns of the ferret cortex. Although gyrencephalic, the cortex is simpler than in many other species; thus, gyri can be readily identified and used as landmarks, but at the same time they are less complex and variable than in more advanced species. This has been exploited in both anatomic and teratologic studies.

A potential problem in the neuroscientific investigation of the developing ferret brain is the fact that body weight is not a good predictor of brain weight.[38] A study of variations in the ferret skull has shown that two landmarks, however, the zygomatic process and the occipital crest, can be used to improve the accuracy of intracranial location.[5] Using these two landmarks, brain sites can be accurately located in adults of all ages, regardless of variation in body weight. This technique could presumably be extended to very young animals.

In conclusion, the ferret is an animal of proven value to neuroscience. Its reputation for viciousness can be shown to be ill founded if proper care and frequent handling are practiced. No doubt this species will be used more often in future neuroscientific investigations.

REFERENCES

1. Smart, I.H.M., and McSherry, G.M.: Gyrus formation in the cerebral cortex in the ferret. I. Description of the external changes. J. Anat., 146:141, 1986.
2. Dennis, B.J., and Kerr, D.I.B.: Olfactory bulb connections with basal rhinencephalon in the ferret: An evoked potential and neuroanatomical study. J. Comp. Neurol., 159:129, 1975.
3. Hawthorn, J.: An atlas of the ferret brain stem. Unpublished observations.
4. Lockard, B.I.: The forebrain of the ferret. Lab. Anim. Sci., 35:216, 1985.
5. Lawes, I.N.C., and Andrews, P.L.R.: Variation in the ferret skull (*Mustela putorius furo* L.) in relation to stereotaxic landmarks. J. Anat., 154:157, 1987.
6. Krabbe, K.H.: Studies on the Morphogenesis of the Brain in Hyracoidea, Ungulata, Carnivora and Pinnipedia, pp. 41–54. Copenhagen, Einar Munksgaard, 1947.
7. Smart, I.H.M., and McSherry, G.M.: Gyrus formation in the cerebral cortex in the ferret. II. Description of the internal histological changes. J. Anat., 147:27, 1986.

8. Darlington, D.: The convolutional pattern of the brain and endocranial cast in the ferret (*Mustela furo* L.) J. Anat., *91*:52, 1957.

9. McSherry, G.M.: Mapping of cortical histogenesis in the ferret. J. Embryol. Exp. Morphol., *81*:239, 1984.

10. McSherry, G.M., and Smart, I.H.M.: Cell production gradients in the developing ferret isocortex. J. Anat., *144*:1, 1986.

11. Haddad, R.K., Dumas, R., and Burgio, P.: Methylazoxymethanol-induced malformations in the ferret. Teratology, 9:118, 1974.

12. Haddad, R.K., and Rabe, A.: Use of the ferret in experimental neuroteratology: Cerebral, cerebellar and retinal dysplasias induced by methylazoxymethanol acetate. *In* Neural and Behavioural Teratology. Edited by T.V.N. Persaud. Lancaster, UK, MTP Press, 1980.

13. Rehn, B., Breipohl, W., Mendoza, A.S., and Apfelbach, R.: Changes in granule cells of the ferret olfactory bulb associated with imprinting on prey odours. Brain Res., *373*:114, 1986.

14. Baleera, L.G., and Lawes, I.N.C.: A morphometric study of the ferret amygdala. Unpublished observations.

15. Baum, M.J., and Goldfoot, D.A.: Effect of amygdaloid lesions on gonadal maturation in male and female ferrets. Am. J. Physiol., *228*:1646, 1975.

16. Herbert, J.: Nuclear structure of the thalamus of the ferret. J. Comp. Neurol., *120*:105, 1963.

17. Sloane, M.W.M.: The diencephalon of the mink. . Comp. Neurol., *95*:463, 1951.

18. Westwood, W.J.A.: Anatomy of the hypothalamus of the ferret. J. Comp. Neurol., *118*:323, 1962.

19. Guillery, R.W.: An abnormal retinogeniculate projection in the albino ferret (*Mustela furo*). Brain Res., *33*:482, 1971.

20. Jefferson, J.M.: A study of the sub-cortical connection of the optic tract system of the ferret with special reference to gonadal activation by retinal stimulation. J. Anat., *75*:106, 1940.

21. Kageyama, G.H., and Wong-Riley, M.T.: The histochemical localization of cytochrome oxidase in the retina and lateral geniculate nucleus of the ferret, cat, and monkey, with particular reference to retinal mosaics and on/off-center-visual channels. J. Neurosci., *4*:2445, 1984.

22. Le Gros Clark, W.E., McKeown, T., and Zuckerman, S.: Visual pathways concerned in gonadal stimulation in ferrets. Proc. R. Soc. Lond. [Biol.], *126*:449, 1939.

23. Linden, D.C., Guillery, R.W., and Cucchiaro, J.: The dorsal lateral geniculate nucleus of the normal ferret and its postnatal development. J. Comp. Neurol., *203*:189, 1981.

24. Rockland, K.S.: Anatomical organization of primary visual cortex (area 17) in the ferret. J. Comp. Neurol., *241*:225, 1985.

25. Thorpe, P.A., and Herbert, J.: The accessory optic system of the ferret. J. Comp. Neurol., *170*: 295, 1976.

26. Vitek, D.J., Schall, J.D., and Leventhal, A.G.: Morphology, central projections, and dendritic field orientation of retinal ganglion cells in the ferret. J. Comp. Neurol., *241*:1, 1985.

27. Wen, G.Y., Sturman, J.A., and Shek, J.W.: A comparative study of the tapetum, retina and skull of the ferret, dog and cat. Lab. Anim. Sci., *35*:200, 1985.

28. Hutchings, M.E., and King, A.J.: A map of auditory space in the ferret superior colliculus. J. Physiol., *358*:31P, 1984.

29. Moore, D.R., Semple, M.N., and Addison, P.D.: Some acoustic properties of neurones in the ferret inferior colliculus. Brain Res., *269*:69, 1983.

30. Odekunle, A., and Bower, A.J.: Brain stem connections of vagal afferent nerves in the ferret: An autoradiographic study. J. Anat., *140*:461, 1985.

31. Odekunle, A., and Bower, A.J.: Brain stem localization of vagal efferents to the gastrointestinal tract. Unpublished observations.

32. Lawes, I.N.C., and Payne, J.N.: Quantification of branched neuronal projections labeled by retrograde fluorescent tracing. J. Neurosci. Methods, *16*:175, 1986.

33. Payne, J.N., Wharton, S.M., and Lawes, I.N.C.: Quantitative analysis of the topographical organization of olivocerebellar projections in the rat. Neuroscience, *15*:403, 1985.

34. Eidelberg, E., et al.: A model of spinal cord injury. Surg. Neurol., *5*:35, 1976.

35. Voogd, J.: Comparative aspects of the structure and fibre connexions of the mammalian cerebellum. *In* The Cerebellum, Progress in Brain Research, Vol. 25, pp. 94–134. Edited by C.A. Fox, and R.S. Snider. Amsterdam, Elsevier, 1967.

36. Taylor, A., and Elias, S.A.: Interaction of periodontal and jaw elevator spindle afferents in the cerebellum—sensory calibration. Brain Behav. Evol., *25*:157, 1984.

37. Stryker, M.P., and Zahs, K.R.: On-and-off sublaminae in the lateral geniculate nucleus of the ferret. J. Neurosci., *3*:1943, 1983.

38. Andrews, P.L.R., and Lawes, I.N.C.: A stereotaxic atlas of the ferret brain: A demonstration of some problems. J. Physiol., *346*:12P, 1983.

chapter 4

THE PHYSIOLOGY
OF THE FERRET

P. L. R. Andrews

This chapter reviews several aspects of the physiology of the ferret. The information presented reflects the interests of investigators in particular areas of physiology. Little, if anything, is known about certain aspects, and this chapter will highlight the need to investigate other physiologic systems before a complete account of the physiology of the ferret can be given. Some systems have been studied fairly thoroughly, illustrating particular aspects of the ferret's physiology that have encouraged its use in biomedical research.

In deciding which experimental animal to use for investigating a particular problem one question often comes to mind; does the model mimic similar systems in humans? To answer this question completely, however, a considerable body of data must already have been accumulated about the physiology of various systems in the animal (and in humans) to allow meaningful comparisons to be made. In addition, physiologists often look for species in which the system of interest is readily manipulated by external cues (e.g., photoperiod) or is adapted to operate in extreme environments (e.g., kidney of the desert rat). Animals may also be selected because certain anatomic features may make the system of interest particularly amenable to study (e.g., squid giant axon).

Such considerations have all played a role in the choice of the ferret for the study of particular systems. Each section of this chapter describes a physiologic system and, although reference is made to relevant anatomic and histologic studies, the reader is referred to Chapters 2 and 3 for a more detailed description of ferret anatomy.

Attention has been focused on some more recently studied aspects of ferret physiology, particularly systems that have not been reviewed previously (e.g., gastrointestinal tract) or have not been discussed in a more appropriate context elsewhere in this volume.

CARDIOVASCULAR SYSTEM

Most studies on the cardiovascular system of the ferret have investigated the biophysics of the cardiac muscle, mainly because the ventricular trabeculae and papillary muscles are a convenient source of a thin homogeneous strip of muscle for in vitro studies. The trabeculae from several species have been investigated, and it has been generally agreed that the ferret provides the most experimentally durable source of this tissue. This is evidenced by the widespread use of ferret cardiac tissue as representative of the carnivore heart. In their study of the anatomy of the ferret heart, Truex and colleagues[1] have reported that the sinoatrial node is discrete (3 × 1 × 1 mm) and easily identifiable, the conduction system is well differentiated, and the left coronary artery is dominant and supplies the left ventricular myocardium and the nodal regions. These anatomic features could certainly be exploited in further investigations. Although the biophysics of

the heart has been extensively studied, a detailed discussion of this aspect is beyond the scope of this book (see Frederick and Babish[2]). Attention will therefore be focused on the more general aspects of the cardiovascular system.

One anatomic feature of the ferret cardiovascular system requires clarification. Several workers have reported a single innominate artery arising from the arch of the aorta, instead of the more usual arrangement of two carotid arteries. It must be emphasized that the innominate artery divides into two carotid arteries within the thorax and these continue on either side of the neck, closely applied to the vagi and internal jugular vein, to supply the brain.[3] The impression given by some authors that the ferret possesses a single direct ascending artery supplying the brain is misleading. It has often been suggested that the presence of an innominate artery would be advantageous in maintaining cerebral perfusion as the animal turns its head while maneuvering in a confined space,[4] but it is difficult to envisage how this would operate because the innominate artery is located entirely within the thorax in its most inflexible region.

HEART RATE AND BLOOD PRESSURE

Heart rate and blood pressure measurements have been made in both anesthetized and conscious animals, although considerably more data are available for the former.

Basal Values

Under barbiturate or urethane anesthesia, mean systolic blood pressure values between 140 and 164 mm Hg have been reported, with diastolic values of 110 to 125 mm Hg.[3,5] The only study of blood pressure in the conscious animal recorded mean systolic values of 161 mm Hg (males) and 133 mm Hg (females).[6] In both conscious and anesthetized animals, individual animals with pressures as high as 190 mm Hg were encountered, but it is not known whether this represents the extreme end of the normal range or animals with a pathologic degree of hypertension.

In contrast to the values for blood pressure a greater discrepancy is found for heart rate measurements. Under urethane anesthesia the heart rate is 387 ± 54 beats/min,[3] whereas under barbiturate anesthesia considerably lower values of 230 ± 26 beats/min are recorded.[6] In the barbiturate-anesthetized mink a heart rate of 324 ± 9 beats/min has been reported, with a blood pressure of 198/143 ± 37/ 26 mm Hg.[7] In the conscious state heart rates of 341 ± 39 beats/min and 200 to 255 beats/min have been reported.[3,6] In assessing the results from conscious animals, one problem is that the heart rate must be influenced by the animal's behavior at the time of measurement. Thornton and associates[6] did not comment on the activity of their animals, but Andrews and co-workers[3] studied freely moving animals that were allowed to feed at will. Monitoring one animal as it went to sleep revealed that the heart rate decreases to 246 ± 15 beats/min, comparable to the barbiturate-anesthetized and "conscious" animal values reported by other workers. Andrews and Illman[8] emphasized the importance of making heart rate measurements under various behavioral conditions. They suggested that the problem of the variations in heart rate described earlier could be resolved by regarding the heart rates under barbiturate and urethane anesthesia as two ends of a spectrum, between which the heart rate in the unanesthetized animal operates according to its activity level.

The electrocardiogram measured from standard limb leads shows the characteristic P, QRS, and T waves, with the QRS complex recorded at 1.84 ± 0.61 mV in lead II and becoming progressively smaller in leads III and I.[3]

In their study of barbiturate-anesthetized ferrets, Kempf and Chang[5] measured a cardiac output of 139 ml/min (range 82–200 ml/min) and circulation times of 6.8 ± 1.2 sec (fluorescein) and 4.5 ± 0.7 sec (cyanide).

Thus, it is apparent that considerably more studies, particularly in conscious animals, are required to characterize the cardiovascular system of the ferret adequately.

Control

The nervous system and humoral agents influence heart rate and blood pressure.

Nerves. In the urethane-anesthetized animal cervical vagotomy has little effect on the heart rate, indicating that little vagal tone is present. Electrical stimulation of the peripheral cut end of the cervical vagus at voltages sufficient to activate small-diameter myelinated fibers produces a profound frequency-related bradycardia blocked by atropine. At 50-Hz stimulation cardiac arrest is produced within a few seconds and with prolonged stimulation (>15 sec) "vagal escape" can be demonstrated.[3]

The effect of sympathetic nerve stimulation on the heart has not been studied, but it would be of great interest to determine whether or not a high tonic sympathetic discharge is responsible for the high heart rate in the urethane-anesthetized animals. Of the rat, guinea pig, rabbit, cat, and ferret, it has been found that the ferret has the highest levels of noradrenalin (11.11 ± 1.43 μg/g) and dopamine (0.222 ± 0.088 μg/g) in the atria.[9]

The reflex control of the circulation in the ferret has seldom been investigated, but the following brief observations are relevant. In the anesthetized animals, distension of the biliary system to noxious levels evokes a reflex increase in blood pressure mediated by the sympathetic nerves,[10] and I have produced similar responses by distension of the duodenum and gastric antrum. It has been suggested that changes in blood pressure may be used to distinguish between innocuous and noxious levels of stimulation of the abdominal viscera[10]; the studies cited earlier indicate that the urethane-anesthetized ferret is a useful model for the investigation of visceral pain mechanisms.

Humoral Agents. This section only describes the effect of humoral agents on the systemic circulation; influences on particular regions are discussed below. Acetylcholine (0.1–1 μg/kg IV) and neostigmine (1 mg/kg IV) produce a bradycardia and concomitant fall in blood pressure. Adrenalin (0.5–50 μg/kg IV), noradrenalin (1–20 μg/kg IV), angiotensin II, and vasopressin produce increases in systemic blood pressure.[3, 11, 12] Atropine has little effect on blood pressure but guanethidine (5 mg/kg IV), propranolol (2 mg/kg IV), and phentolamine (2 mg/kg IV) all cause a decrease in blood pressure, indicating the importance of a tonic sympathetic adrenergic drive in the maintenance of blood pressure in the ferret, as in other species. The nicotinic cholinergic receptor antagonist *d*-tubocurarine produces a biphasic change in blood pressure; at low doses (0.1–1 mg/kg IV) hypotension results whereas higher doses (4 mg/kg IV) produce hypertension. Because ganglionic blockade is not produced by low doses it has been suggested that the characteristic hypotensive response to *d*-tubocurarine is caused by the release of vasodilator agents.[13] More detailed pharmacologic investigations of the cardiovascular system have been undertaken in the mink.[7]

CIRCULATION IN SPECIFIC REGIONS

The vasculature and circulation of several specific areas in the ferret have been the subjects of investigation.

Testes

Seasonal variations in testicular blood flow have been investigated by Joffre and Joffre,[14] who demonstrated that testicular blood flow is at a minimum in July (21.3 ± 1.5 ml/min/100 g), and increases to a maximum of 35.2 ± 1.2 ml/min/100 g between January and March. Spermatozoa are present in the seminiferous tubules between January and June. These changes are presumably regulated by seasonal fluctuations in levels of the reproductive hormones.

Gut

Measurements of systemic blood pressure following administration of drugs into the celiac artery via the abdominal aorta provides insight into some influences on the mesenteric circulation. Vasoactive intestinal polypeptide (1 μg/kg) and substance P (100 ng/kg) produce a fall in blood pressure, bradykinin produces a biphasic change (50 μg/kg), and a delayed increase is noted by high doses of neurotensin (1 μg/kg).[15] Stable analogues of ATP produce a marked vasoconstriction in the ferret gut in contrast to the vasodilator action usually associated with ATP. In my laboratory stimulation of the peripheral cut end of the greater splanchnic nerve has been seen to produce a large increase in blood pressure because of a direct effect on the mesenteric bed and the release of adrenalin from the adrenal glands. Noradrenalin and dopamine have been detected in the mesenteric artery and spleen.[9]

Data are not available on the blood flow to each region of the gut, nor on the relative distribution of blood flow between the gut muscle and mucosa.

Pituitary

Direct measurements of the blood flow to the pituitary have not been made, but the pituitary vasculature has been the subject of detailed anatomic studies. The hypothalamic-pituitary portal system has also been investigated because of its involvement in the endocrine functions of the pituitary.[16]

Pulmonary Vasculature

Several studies have investigated the response of the isolated blood-perfused ferret lung to hypoxia. All agree that, of several species investigated (e.g., rat, rabbit, cat, dog, pig), the ferret has the most marked pulmonary vasoconstriction in response to hypoxia, with a maximum response occurring at about 25 mm Hg.[17–20] Further decreases in Pi_{O_2} result in vasodilatation. The mechanism of this vasoconstriction has not been elucidated but there is evidence to implicate histamine and ATP, although the ferret lung contains relatively little histamine in comparison to that in other laboratory animals.[21,22] Once the vasoconstriction is established it can be reversed by adenosine and dopamine.[23] The extreme sensitivity of the ferret pulmonary vasculature to hypoxia makes it a very useful model for investigating this condition, which is an important component in the development of pulmonary hypertension in humans. It has been suggested that the sensitivity to hypoxia in the ferret may be an adaptation to burrowing.[24]

RESPIRATORY SYSTEM

Studies have focused primarily on the mechanisms and control of tracheal secretion in the ferret, because the trachea is relatively long for its size (10 cm in a 1-kg animal), and a large number of submucosal glands are present. More recently, pulmonary mechanics and airway smooth muscle activity have been investigated (also see earlier discussion on pulmonary vasculature).

PULMONARY MECHANICS

The resting respiratory rate in the conscious ferret is reported to be 33 to 36 breaths/min[25] as compared to values of 31 ± 6 breaths/min in urethane-anesthetized animals[3] and 26.7 ± 3.9 breaths/min or 43.5 ± 4.6 breaths/min in pentobarbital-anesthetized animals.[24,26] The disparity among the results from the latter studies may have been caused by differences in the size of animals used (553–870 g, versus 200–360 g), but also the dose of pentobarbital was 25 mg/kg in one study[26] and 30 to 50 mg/kg (+ 10 mg/kg supplement) in the other[24]; a dose of 25 mg/kg IP served only to sedate the animal. Other differences were observed in the two studies (e.g., compliance), and these also may have been produced by the level of anesthesia or by variations in measurement technique. Both papers contain a wealth of data characterizing the respiratory system.[24] The lung in the ferret is large in relation to body weight, and hence has a total lung capacity 297% of the predicted value. The only comparable animal is the sea otter, an aquatic mustelid, in which the large lung capacity (462% of predicted) has been suggested as an adaptation to diving.[27] In addition, the chest wall of the ferret is very compliant and, along with the large lung capacity, it is argued that these features are adaptations to facilitate subterranean hunting activity.[24]

These studies provide a useful initial guide to lung mechanics but, because the animals used were smaller than those generally used for physiologic studies, a similar study of larger animals is needed. It would be of particular interest to determine whether or not the lung-to-body weight ratio remains constant as the animal grows.

AIRWAY SECRETION

Histologic and histochemical studies of the tracheobronchial tree have been undertaken,[28, 29] and the major findings are as follows.

The epithelium is composed of ciliated cells, nonciliated dark cytoplasmic cells (with or without secretory granules), and a few goblet cells. The number of goblet cells increases toward the bronchus, where about 60 cells/mm are found; many of these contain acidic material (possibly glycosaminoglycans). Submucosal glands are numerous, and extend from the larynx at least to the level of the smaller bronchi. Glands containing acidic material are more numerous in the distal airways. Because of the large number of submucosal glands it is probable that fluid collected from the respiratory tract is mainly of glandular origin, a hypothesis supported by the functional studies described below. In addition, immunohistochemical studies have localized lysozyme in the secretory granules of serous but not mucous cells in the ferret trachea. Thus, by monitoring lysozyme secretion, factors influencing the control of serous cell secretion can be studied.[30]

Various techniques have been used for studying tracheal secretion in the ferret, including the in vivo construction of tracheal pouches,[31] the in vitro collection of secretions from entire tracheas,[32] and studies of ion fluxes from tracheal segments mounted in modified Ussing chambers.[33] The results discussed below are all from in vitro studies.

Fluid Secretion and Ion Fluxes

The volume of fluid appearing on the luminal surface of the trachea depends on the rates of fluid secretion and fluid absorption. Under resting conditions little if any spontaneous secretion is present.[33, 34] Under basal conditions there is a net reabsorption of fluid, which is con-

sistent with ion flux studies that demonstrated a net absorption of sodium with little or no active chloride secretion.[35] The short circuit current is reduced to zero by ouabain, reduced by amiloride, and unaffected by bumetanide.

In the studies described later, the measured volume of tracheal fluid probably represents the secretion of the submucosal glands.[34] Although this fluid undoubtedly contains mucoproteins, the secretions are referred to as fluid secretions rather than mucous secretions because the mucoproteins were not measured directly. The secretion of macromolecules will also be discussed.

Nerve stimulation, phenylephrine, and acetylcholine enhance fluid secretion, and it has been proposed that the autonomic innervation of the submucosal glands regulates fluid secretion via α-adrenergic and muscarinic cholinergic receptors. Ion flux studies demonstrate a stimulation of chloride secretion by isoproterenol and a stimulation of sodium and chloride ion secretion by methacholine.[33]

It is probable that, like other tissues, the movement of these ions provides the mechanism by which the tracheal fluid is secreted, but an involvement of macromolecules cannot be excluded.[36] Using the whole trachea, in vitro basal secretory rates of 0.22 ± 0.03 μl/min were obtained; stimulation with methacholine increased these to 3.9 ± 0.33 μl/min. An increased stimulation of secretion was also produced in this preparation by phenylephrine, and histamine, and a decreased secretion was produced by salbutamol and substance P.[37]

Secretion of Macromolecules

Using $^{35}SO_4$ as a marker, electrical field stimulation, acetylcholine, phenylephrine, terbutaline, and norepinephrine produced an increased in vitro secretion of macromolecules ($>10^6$ molecular weight). It was concluded that tracheal innervation is involved in the secretion of macromolecules by muscarinic cholinergic receptors and by both α- and ß-adrenergic receptors.[38] A nonadrenergic, noncholinergic (nanc) component has also been identified. Because vasoactive intestinal peptide (VIP) has been shown to enhance the output of sulfated macromolecules in the ferret trachea, it is tempting to suggest that it may be responsible for the nanc component of the neural response.[39] VIP does not, however, stimulate ion transport in this tissue.

Studies of lysozyme release in incubated tracheal segments show that cholinergic and α-adrenergic receptor agonists stimulate lysozyme release, whereas ß-adrenergic agonists have only a small effect.[30] Lysozyme is only found in the secretory granules of the serous submucosal gland cells. A morphometric study has demonstrated that serous cell granules are only discharged by α-adrenergic and cholinergic stimuli, an observation consistent with the results of the forementioned studies on lysozyme release.[40]

Autoradiographic studies have demonstrated the presence of α$_1$- and ß-adrenergic receptors on both epithelial and submucosal gland cells.[41,42]

AIRWAY SMOOTH MUSCLE ACTIVITY

Most studies have been performed on the smooth muscle of the trachea. The cells had a resting membrane potential of 58.31 ± 2.10 mV and an input resistance of 21.3 ± 5.31 mV.[43] Control of the tracheal smooth muscle has been investigated in two different preparations, discussed below.

In vitro increases in luminal pressure have been produced in the whole trachea by methacholine, phenylephrine, histamine, bradykinin, and kallidin histamine.[37] The last two substances have no effect on fluid secretion, whereas the remainder stimulate secretion. Autoradi-

ographic studies have revealed a differential distribution of α- and ß-adrenergic receptors and muscarinic cholinergic receptors: α receptors are numerous in small bronchioles but sparse in large airways; ß receptors are present in the highest density in the bronchioles, although their density is relatively high throughout the airway; and cholinergic receptors are most dense in the bronchial muscle and decrease in density toward the distal bronchioles.[41,42,44]

RESPIRATORY REFLEXES

The defensive respiratory reflexes have been studied in the pentobarbital-anesthetized ferret. Coughing is evoked by mechanical stimulation of the bronchi and larynx, but not the trachea. Sulfur dioxide also elicits coughing, but this is weaker than that evoked by mechanical stimulation. Other reflexes elicited were the aspiration, expiration, and sneeze reflexes.[45] The absence of a cough reflex in response to tracheal stimulation may be related to the absence or paucity of epithelial nerves in the trachea.[28] The deflation reflex is present in the urethane-anesthetized ferret, and persists in the presence of vagotomy.[46] The reflex respiratory changes accompanying retching and vomiting are discussed later (see p. 115).

It is apparent that from the brevity of this account that further studies of the reflex control of respiration are required. For instance, nothing is yet known of the reflex control of airway secretion.

GASTROINTESTINAL TRACT

Physiologic studies of the ferret gastrointestinal tract have been undertaken mainly over the past 20 years, although the earliest report was a study of the colon by Elliott and Barclay-Smith in 1904.[47] As with other aspects of its physiology, the gut has been investigated largely to determine the potential of the ferret for use as an alternative carnivore to the cat and dog in laboratory investigations. Most gut regions have been investigated, but the bulk of the studies have concentrated on gastric function.

The gross morphology of the gastrointestinal tract has been described[48] and is detailed elsewhere in the text (see Chap. 2), as have more detailed studies of specific regions.

SALIVARY GLANDS

The gross and microscopic anatomy of the major and minor salivary glands has been described.[49] Ferrets possess parotid, submandibular, sublingual, molar, zygomatic, and lingual glands. Histochemical studies of the glands reveal the presence of several different types of secretory products in the gland cells, with carboxylated and sulfated mucins being the most common.[50] Although the mucous substances in the salivary glands have been relatively well characterized, nothing is known of the types of enzymes secreted by the glands or of the stimuli that induce secretion of mucus- or enzyme-rich saliva.

More information is available about the physiologic processes underlying the aqueous and ionic components of salivary secretion. Micropuncture studies in barbiturate-anesthetized ferrets have examined the secretion of monovalent ions and water and their handling by the salivary duct system.[51,52] These studies have revealed an interesting difference between the parotid and submandibular glands. In the unstimulated state both glands produce a primary secretion in their secretory segment (acinus plus intercalated duct) that is isotonic with plasma and has a similar ionic composition in regard to levels of Na^+, K^+, Cl^-, and HCO_3^-.

When stimulated by pilocarpine (100 μg/kg IV), which evokes secretory rates of up to 600 μl/min/g wet weight gland, the parotid gland secretes a hypertonic fluid whereas the submandibular gland secretion remains isotonic. The increase in osmolarity of the parotid fluid is mainly due to Na^+ and HCO_3^- ions. Although the submandibular fluid remained isotonic, its composition changed: $[HCO_3^-]$ decreased from 24.2 $\pm$ 3.8 to 11.5 $\pm$ 3.3 mEq/L, whereas $[Cl^-]$ increased from 106.1 $\pm$ 6.5 to 134.5 $\pm$ 6.2 mEq/L.

These observations suggest that a chloride-bicarbonate exchange mechanism may be involved, as suggested in other salivary glands. The production of an isotonic primary secretory fluid by one gland and a hypertonic one by another in the same animal may be unique to the ferret; hence, this animal could provide a very useful model for investigating the factors influencing each type of secretion.

The final saliva in the ferret is usually hypotonic relative to plasma, and the role of the duct system in the modification of the primary secretion has therefore been investigated.[51,52] In both the submandibular and parotid glands the duct system is impermeable to water both in the resting and unstimulated states; thus, changes in the composition of the primary secretion must be a result of transductal movements of ions. The ducts involved are striated, and they bring about a net reabsorption of sodium and chloride (lumen to blood) and a net secretion of potassium (blood to lumen) in both glands, although the sodium and chloride fluxes are larger in the submandibular gland. In the parotid gland there is some reabsorption of bicarbonate ions.

The handling of calcium by the parotid gland has also been studied,[53] revealing that most calcium in the saliva is nonionized, and that there is little variation in [Ca] when changes in salivary flow between 17 and 363 μl/min/g wet weight tissue are evoked by pilocarpine (2 mg/kg

IV). In contrast, the ionized calcium concentration is related to flow rate, suggesting that some ionized calcium from the primary secretion is reabsorbed in the duct system.

Although information exists about the secretory processes occurring in the glands, less is known of the control of the secretion. Electrical stimulation of the parasympathetic auriculotemporal nerve in the pentobarbital anesthetized ferret provokes secretion (190 mg/min) in the parotid gland.[54] This secretion is markedly reduced (25 mg/min) but not abolished by atropine (2 mg/kg IV). Secretion is also stimulated by methacholine (0.1–2 μg/kg) and substance P (0.05–0.1 μg/kg), but not by adrenalin (20 μg/kg), phenylephrine (100μg/kg), isoprenaline (100 μg/kg), or VIP polypeptide (100μg/kg). These preliminary studies demonstrate a potent cholinergic stimulation of gland secretion and, in addition, provide preliminary evidence for a noncholinergic stimulation of secretion, similar to that observed in other species. This finding has attracted considerable interest because of the possible involvement of cotransmission.

Based on these few studies, it appears that the control of salivary secretion in the ferret is similar to that in other carnivores, although more studies are needed. Because ferrets tend to ingest their natural food quickly it is unlikely that salivary enzymes play a significant role in digestion, although the lubricant function of saliva may be important (particularly when the animals are receiving a pelleted diet). Mangos and colleagues[51] have noted that "the secretory patterns were similar to those in the man and monkey, thus making the ferret an excellent model for the study of salivary gland function."

ESOPHAGUS

The entire supradiaphragmatic portion of the esophagus is composed of striated muscle, a pattern found in various other species, including the dog. In humans the esophagus is comprised of striated muscle in the upper portion and smooth muscle in the lower portion, and in this respect the ferret is not a suitable model. Nothing is known of the anatomy nor properties of the sphincters at either end of the esophagus.

Preliminary studies of the esophagus have shown that its intrathoracic portion is innervated by the vagus.[55] A single vagal stimulus produces twitchlike contractions of the esophagus and, with increasing frequencies of stimulation (>25 Hz), these contractions fuse to produce a sustained tetanic contraction. The vagal efferent fibers involved are small myelinated axons with a conduction velocity of <20 m/sec. The contractions are blocked by tubocurarine, indicating that they are mediated by activation of nicotinic cholinergic receptors on the muscle; this is also the case in the dog.

The esophageal lining is composed of keratinized stratified squamous epithelium, which is patchy in the lower portion and absent in the subdiaphragmatic continuation.[48] Submucosal glands are present, but their secretion and control, have not been characterized.

STOMACH

The ferret stomach, both in the fasted and fed states, is similar to that of humans in gross morphologic appearance. As in other carnivores the stomach has a considerable storage capacity, as illustrated by the observation that adult ferrets will drink over 100 ml of milk in 10 min. Following a meal about 80% of the food is stored in the proximal stomach, with the circular muscle layer undergoing the largest change in length.

The gastric mucosa has been studied both at light and electron microscopic levels in normal,[56,57] caffeine-,[58] cinchophen-,[59] and glucocorticoid-[60] treated animals. The histochemistry of the glands has also been investigated.[61] A detailed description of the mucosal histology is beyond the scope of this chapter, but the main conclusion relevant to the physiology of gastric secretion is that the structure of the mucosa at the cellular level is remarkably similar to that of humans.

A comparison of the vagal innervation of the stomach in humans and the ferret has been undertaken,[62] demonstrating that the gross innervation of the ferret stomach generally represents a simplified version of that in humans and the fiber composition of the nerve trunks is similar, with unmyelinated nerve fibers predominating.

It is apparent that on anatomic grounds the ferret stomach is similar to that of humans, as evidenced by the physiologic investigations described below.

Gastric Secretion

The gastric secretions of both hydrochloric acid and proteolytic enzymes have been studied, although the control of the former has been studied more extensively.

Hydrochloric Acid. The study of gastric secretion in the ferret was greatly enhanced by the surgical preparation of a ferret with a chronic gastric fistula.[63] Experiments reveal that, in the interdigestive state, the ferret is a spontaneous secretor of hydrochloric acid. The secretory volume is 0.72 ± 0.088 ml/kg body weight/15 min, the pH 3.0 is 0.23, the titratable acidity is 35.6 ± 3.09 meq/l, and the acid output is 17.0 ± 2.33 μEq/15 min. The urethane-anesthetized ferret is also a spontaneous secretor of acid. The magnitude of basal acid secretion is not influenced by the estrous state of the animal.[64]

Acid secretion is stimulated by histamine—an optimal dose of 67.3 μg/kg IP produces an acid output 30 min after administration of 177.0 ± 39.14 μEq/15 min. Histamine has been implicated in the physiologic control of gastric acid secretion, and in this context a biochemical study of histamine metabolism in the ferret is of interest.[22] The stomach contains relatively low concentrations of free histamine (12 μg/g) and lacks the histamine-forming enzyme, specific L-histidine decarboxylase, although histamine-destroying activity is present. I have noted that the histamine H_2 receptor antagonist cimetidine abolishes the acid secretory response to exogenous histamine, and reduces it to pentagastrin. The response to histamine (67.3 μg/kg IP) is reduced by 30% by atropine and abolished by EDTA.[65, 66]

The peptide pentagastrin has its maximal effect on acid secretion after 30 min at a dose of 10 μg/kg, and produces 490 ± 50 μEq/15 min. The response is reduced by atropine and abolished by EDTA. Gastric acid secretion is also stimulated by calcium, a response that is abolished by atropine; this suggests an action via acetylcholine. Because calcium infusion in the ferret stimulates gastrin release,[67] it is unclear whether the effect of atropine blocks the release of gastrin or prevents its action on the secretory cells. Gastrin cryptic peptide B has been identified in extracts of ferret gastric antral and duodenal mucosa, with larger amounts being present in the antral mucosa (708 $\pm$ 278 pmol/g).[68]

The cholinomimetic bethanecol (0.4 mg/kg IP) evokes a stimulation of acid output comparable to that of histamine (67.3 μg/kg) but, in a volume of about 5 ml/15 min, approximately doubles that produced in response to histamine.[65, 66]

The role of the vagus in the control of acid secretion has also been investigated. Hypoglycemia induced by insulin (1.5 units/kg IP) produces a sustained stimulation that is markedly reduced by atropine and vagotomy.[66] Unilateral (dorsal) vagotomy reduces the basal acid secretion by about 60% and also reduces the response to pentagastrin and histamine, with the former being affected to a greater extent.[69] Studies in the urethane-anesthetized ferret have demonstrated that vagal activation by cytoglycopenia (induced by 2-deoxy-D-glucose, 120 mg/kg IV) or electrical stimulation both evoke a significant increase in acid secretion that is markedly reduced by atropine.[70]

Gastric acid secretion has also been studied in vitro in the fundic mucosa of 8 to 15-week-old ferrets.[71,72] The mucosa secretes acid spontaneously (0.6–1.8 μEq/cm^2/hr), and this increases to between 3 and 4.6 μEq/cm^2/hr by acetylcholine (1 $\times$ 10^{-4} M), pentagastrin (6.5 $\times$ 10^{-7} M), and histamine (1.6 $\times$ 10^{-6} M).

Proteolytic Enzymes and Mucus. In addition to being a spontaneous secretor of acid, the ferret stomach also secretes proteolytic enzymes under basal conditions. Histamine produces an increase in the secretion of proteolytic enzymes from a basal value of 757 $\pm$ 274.6 μg/15 min to 1698 $\pm$ 575.3 μg/15 min.[63,65,66] A dose of histamine of 1080 μg/kg, however, is required to produce this doubling of output in contrast to the considerably lower dose (67.3 μg/kg) required to produce a tenfold increase in acid output 30 min after histamine injection. A pentagastrin dose of 2 μg/kg produces a maximal response in protease secretion, in contrast to the 10 μg/kg required to provoke a maximal acid secretory response. Studies in the anesthetized ferret have demonstrated that vagal stimulation also provokes proteolytic enzyme secretion.

The physiology of gastric mucus in the ferret has been described in a study of the effect of carbenoxolone on gastric glycoprotein synthesis.[73] Carbenoxolone promotes the healing of gastric ulcers in humans. The ferret study demonstrated an increased rate of incorporation of N-acetyl glucosamine, glucosamine, galactosamine, and N-acetyl neuraminic acid into glycoproteins. No effect is observed on the incorporation of galactose or of threonine into the acid-precipitable glycoproteins. It was suggested that carbenoxolone may stimulate specific glycosyl transferases, leading to the formation of a modified glycoprotein with superior protective properties.

Although little data are available about the physiology of gastric mucus, surface mucous cells have been studied at the ultrastructural level.[56] Histochemical studies[61] have demonstrated that the surface mucous cells are PAS-positive. In the pyloric region compound tubuloacinar glands are seen with "foaming" cytoplasm, giving PAS- and PAS-AB positive reactions that indicate the presence of neutral mucosubstances. Two features are of particular note: (1) the pyloric and duodenal Brünner's glands are similar, whereas in most other mammals they are markedly different in their mucosubstances; and (2) of the species so far studied, only the glands in humans and ferrets do not contain acid mucosubstances. These observations suggest that the ferret stomach may be a suitable model for the study of pyloric mucous secretion in humans.

Integrity of the Gastric Mucosa. Permeability changes in the gastric mucosa have long been implicated in the etiology of gastric ulceration. Gastric transmural potential differences (pd) decrease following mucosal damage, thus providing a convenient index of mucosal integrity. In the ferret the resting transmural pd is 39 $\pm$ 7 mV (lumen $-$ Ve [negative]), which decreases as the concentration of a damaging solution of acetic acid (50–200 mM) increases.[74] Flux studies reveal that as the permeability of the mucosa increases by the effect of acetic acid, H$^+$ ions are lost from the lumen while Na$^+$ ions enter the lumen. The ferret stomach therefore appears to be a convenient system for the study of substances that influence the permeability of the gastric mucosa, and of its possible involvement in the production of gastric ulcers.

Gastric Motility

The ferret stomach possesses an inner circular smooth muscle layer and an outer logitudinal layer. It has been reported that no oblique muscle layer is present, but this awaits confirmation.[48] Gastric motility to date has only been systematically investigated in anesthetized ferrets, although preliminary studies show that gastric antral contractions can be monitored in the conscious animal with implanted strain gauges.

Studies of gastric motility have concentrated on the role of extrinic autonomic innervation in the regulation of the overall gastric pressure (tone) and of the amplitude of the rhythmic contractions. Two experimental approaches have been used—direct electrical stimulation of the nerves, and the effect of nerve lesions on gastric motor reflexes.

Influence of the Vagus. Electrical stimulation of the peripheral cut end of the cervical or abdominal vagi evokes a frequency-related increase in the amplitude of the gastric contractions, with a maximal response being produced at 10 Hz. Responses are only evoked with stimulus parameters sufficient to activate unmyelinated axons. With stimulation periods >10 sec multiple contractions are produced at a frequency similar to those occurring spontaneously. The excitatory effects of vagal stimulation are mimicked by close intra-arterial injection of acetylcholine (10–100 μg/kg) and are blocked by atropine (1 mg/kg IV), as is the response to acetylcholine.[75] Further studies have revealed that the pattern of vagal stimulation also plays a complex role in determining motility and secretory responses.[76]

In the anesthetized ferret the stomach may be divided into corpus and antral regions while retaining their extrinsic innervation. Using this preparation it was demonstrated that the vagus stimulates activity in both regions; in the presence of atropine, however, differences are observed. In the antrum vagal stimulation inhibits the ongoing spontaneous antral contractions, whereas in the corpus a profound long-lasting decrease in the mean pressure is observed. Following a 10-sec period of stimulation at 10 Hz, it takes longer than 10 min for the corpus pressure to recover. These and other experiments demonstrate that the vagal preganglionic fibers activate both cholinergic, excitatory, and noncholinergic nonadrenergic inhibitory intramural neurons in both regions of the stomach. The nature of the inhibitory transmitter is unknown, but it has been suggested that vasoactive intestinal polypeptide is involved in the corpus and neurotensin in the antrum.[15]

The ease with which the stomach can be divided in the ferret greatly facilitates our understanding of the functions of the two gastric regions by highlighting differences between them in their responses not only to nerve stimulation but also to drugs such as 5-HT[77] and the novel prokinetic Cisapride.[78]

Motor Reflexes. The adaptive motor responses to gastric distension have been most extensively studied, although the role of the chemical environment of the lumen in the regulation of motility has been investigated more recently.

The capacity of the stomach has been measured by monitoring the volume of milk ingested in a single continuous session so that the motor responses observed in response to experimental gastric distension could be related to normal gastric physiology. In ferrets with a mean body weight of 784 ± 60 g (n = 11) 94.5 ± 7.5 ml of milk is ingested at a rate of 13.0 ± 0.7 ml/min.[79]

Two components of gastric motility have been studied, tone and rhythmic contractions.

Tone. Inflation of the stomach with 50 ml of 154 mM Nacl produces a stable tone of

6.3 ± 0.85 cm H_2O (relative to atmospheric pressure).[80] Most (80%) of the fluid is accommodated in the corpus region, and pressure studies in the divided stomach demonstrate that this region is mainly responsible for determining the overall gastric tone in response to physiologic levels of distension. Lesion studies reveal that the major reflex responsible for the relaxation of the corpus muscle in response to distension is a vagovagal reflex, involving vagal afferent activation of the intramural nonadrenergic noncholinergic inhibitory neurons described above.[15] In the absence of the vagus, a splanchnosplanchnic adrenergic reflex is also demonstrated, although its characteristics are markedly different from the vagovagal reflex.[81] More recent studies have shown that this vagovagal inhibitory reflex may be inhibited at a central site by the $GABA_B$ receptor agonist baclofen.[82]

The vagal efferents driving the intramural nonadrenergic, noncholinergic inhibitory neurons can also be activated reflexly by stimulation of gastric mucosa either mechanically or chemically, thus raising the possibility that the gastric motor response to a meal is determined both by the volume and the chemical nature of the food.[83, 84]

Contractile Activity. The reflex control of contractile activity has been studied less thoroughly than the control of tone. One of the most striking features of the ferret stomach is that it is "spontaneously" rhythmically active under urethane anesthesia, as is the rest of the gut immediately following surgery. The overall frequency of contraction is 7.1 ± 0.005 contractions/min, although the antrum and corpus contract at different frequencies when surgically uncoupled.[75] The amplitude of the contractions is reduced but not abolished by vagotomy or atropine, indicating that both cholinergic and noncholinergic systems are involved in their production.

The best-defined reflex involving contraction amplitude is the corpoantral reflex. Using the divided stomach preparation, it has been demonstrated that inflation of the corpus evokes an increase in the amplitude of antral contractions. This reflex is mediated by the vagus, and it may be involved in the initiation of gastric emptying. Distension of the duodenum produces a splanchnosplanchnic adrenergic reflex inhibition of gastric motility by a direct effect on the muscle and by modulation of cholinergic ganglionic transmission.[81] This enterogastric reflex is also implicated in the regulation of gastric emptying.

PANCREAS AND BILIARY SYSTEM

Both the exocrine and endocrine portions of the ferret pancreas have been the subject of preliminary investigations. Under urethane anesthesia the pancreas has a very sparse spontaneous secretion of fluid (0.05 g/10 min), which can be increased by secretin to about 0.5 g/10 min in a dose-related manner. The ferret pancreas has been used for the bioassay of the stability of secretin and its analogues.[85] Vagal stimulation and pancreozymin-cholecystokinin stimulate the secretion of amylase in animals receiving a submaximal infusion of secretin.

A comparative study of the islets of Langerhans, including those of the ferret, revealed capillary connections between the islets and exocrine tissue.[86] The direction of blood flow appears to be from the islets to the exocrine tissue, thus supporting the hypothesis that the endocrine pancreas influences the exocrine portion, possibly in a trophic manner via this vascular link.[87]

A glycogenolytic factor has been extracted from the ferret pancreas,[88] but studies have not been undertaken to identify the hormones present in the islets. A small quantity of gastrin cryptic peptide B has been identified in pancreatic extracts.[68]

The gross and microscopic anatomy of the biliary system has been described,[89] but nothing is known of the composition of the bile, its rate of secretion, nor the enterohepatic circulation. In a study concerned with biliary tract pain,[10] it was noted that the resting biliary pressure is 1.5 to 4 mm Hg, and increasing the pressure by 5 to 7 mm Hg evokes a reflex opening of the sphincter of Oddi.

It is apparent that considerable further work needs to be done on the pancreatic and biliary systems in the ferret.

SMALL INTESTINE

The gross morphology of the small intestine has been described in Chapter 2. In their histologic study, Poddar and Murgatroyd[48] identified villi and goblet cells in all regions of the small intestine. Brunner's glands are found in the submucosa of the duodenum proximal to the opening of the bile duct, and these contain only neutral mucosubstances, as in humans.[61] The physiology of the small intestine has been less extensively investigated than the stomach, but a number of interesting features are present.

Hormone Release

The mucosa of the upper part of the small intestine contains a number of gastrointestinal hormones, in particular those involved in the control of pancreatic function—secretin and pancreozymin-cholecystokinin (PZ-CCK). Although the mechanisms underlying the release of antral gastrin are relatively well defined, this is not the case for PZ-CCK.[90] This problem has been the subject of an in vitro study of segments of ferret jejunum[90] and the PZ-CCK released was assayed in the isolated perfused cat pancreas. The released PZ-CCK is stimulated by 30 mM tryptophan or phenylalanine, 7.5 mM Ca^{2+}, or 50 mM K^+. The response to phenylalanine is reduced by the removal of Ca^{2+} but is unaffected by atropine (10^{-6} M) or theophylline (10^{-3} M). Interestingly, an unidentified vasoconstrictor substance (probably not 5-HT) is also released from the mucosa by phenylalanine. These data demonstrate that this preparation has the potential for use in the study of the factors influencing the release of substances from the intestinal mucosa.

Secretion and Absorption

Using changes in transmural potential difference (pd) as an index of electrogenic intestinal secretion, the relationship between jejunal motility and pd in the urethane-anesthetized ferret has been studied.[91] These studies reveal that spontaneous bursts of jejunal motility (see later discussion) are associated with increases in the pd, with the lumen becoming more negative, and that vagotomy, atropine, or tetrodotoxin abolish both responses.

Motor and pd changes are evoked by stimulation of the peripheral end of the cervical vagus. These results suggest that the spontaneous bursts of motor activity and pd changes are closely linked, but whether the two events are produced by the vagus influencing both the mucosa and muscle or whether the vagus evokes the motor changes, which in turn stimulates secretion, is unknown. Other studies provide some evidence that the vagus can influence secretion directly in this tissue by both cholinergic and noncholinergic mechanisms. This linkage between motor and secretory events in the intestine has been reported in humans, and thus the ferret appears to be a useful animal model for the study of this interaction.

Very little is known of the absorptive processes in the ferret gut. "Closure" of the gut occurs relatively late, with values from 28 to 42 days having been reported.[92,93] Corticosteroids cause premature gut closure in the rat but not in the ferret, suggesting different mechanisms of closure in rodents and carnivores.[93]

Phenylalanine (1.5–12 mM) produces a dose-related increase in the in vitro jejunum preparation in the transmural pd, indicating an electrogenic (probably sodium-dependent) transport mechanism of this amino acid.[90] This preliminary experiment demonstrates that the transport characteristics of the ferret intestine can be investigated using the Wilson and Wiseman technique that is so widely employed for such studies in the rat. In addition to an understanding of these transport processes, a full description of intestinal absorption in the ferret requires information on the mucosal enzymes responsible for digestion at the brush border. Disaccharidase activity (e.g., maltose, sucrose, lactose, and trehalose) is present in extracts of ferret jejunal mucosa.[94]

Motility

Under urethane anesthesia the ferret jejunum is spontaneously active, with characteristic bursts of contractions that last about 1 min each.[95] This activity is abolished by atropine or vagotomy and mimicked to a large extent by vagal stimulation. In the presence of atropine the immediate response to vagal stimulation is converted to a small, amplitude-delayed response. These observations indicate that the vagus influences jejunal motility mainly by a cholinergic pathway, although there is also some suggestion of a noncholinergic vagal excitatory pathway. The periodicity of the bursts is probably organized within the myenteric plexus, with the tonic vagal activity having a permissive role.

COLON

A major problem in studying the physiology of the colon in the ferret involves delineation of its limits. No external division is visible between the ileum and colon, but it is possible to identify the approximate site of this junction by the vascular anatomy (see Chap. 2). Histologic studies have identified subserosal lymphoid formations that mark the most rostral limit of the colon, and electromyographic studies (see later discussion) confirm this as the region of the ileocolic junction. Also at this point, which coincides with the splenic flexure, villi are no longer present. Tubular glands with goblet cells containing predominantly or exclusively sulfated mucosubstances are found in the colon.[96] The wall of the colon is formed from circular and longitudinal muscle layers but, in contrast to several other species (e.g., guinea pig), taenia coli are not present. The only aspect of colonic physiology studied to date is motility.

Motility

Using conscious ferrets[97] electrical activity of the intestine has been used to identify the location of the colon. In the electrodes anterior to the subserosal lymphoid tissue, activity is characterized by continuous slow wave activity (3.06 ± 0.6 cycles/min). Irregular and regular spiking activities of 37.2 ± 6.7 min and 5.9 ± 0.4 min, respectively, have also been recorded, resembling that seen in the dog ileum. Tissue activity typical of that recorded in the colon of related species is observed at recording sites in the 8 to 10 cm of intestine caudal to the subserosal lymphoid tissue; slow wave activity with a frequency of 9 to 13 cycles/min is present only 7% of the time. Long and short spike bursts have been recorded; the former had a duration of 21.3 ± 7.8 sec and the latter 4.6 ± 2.5 sec. Long spike bursts are propagated aborally, whereas short bursts are not. Histologic studies reveal a strip of fibrous connective tissue that disrupts the continuity of the muscle layers between the intestinal region with "ileal" electrical activity and with "colonic" electrical activity. This strip of connective tissue prevents the electrotonic spread of the migrating myoelectric complex from the ileum to the colon, a function subserved by the ileocolonic sphincter in the dog.

Under urethane anesthesia, colonic pressure activity changes with a similar temporal pattern to the electrical activity recorded in the conscious animal have been observed.[98, 99] This "spontaneous" activity is markedly reduced by atropine (1 mg/kg IV) or by vagal cooling, suggesting that much (but not all) of the colonic contractile activity is due to a vagal-cholinergic pathway. Electrical stimulation of the peripheral cut end of the cervical or abdominal vagus evokes a frequency-related increase in colonic motility, with a peak response occurring at 10 Hz. This response is markedly decreased by atropine, and is replaced by a delayed noncholinergic nonadrenergic excitatory response. Similar colonic responses are observed when the vagal efferents supplying the colon are activated reflexly by vagal afferent stimulation. These results demonstrate that the motor activity of the ferret colon is largely vagus-dependent, mediated by both cholinergic and noncholinergic transmitter systems, with the former predominating.[98, 99] The vagal noncholinergic excitation of colonic motility is of particular interest in view of the increasing importance attached to this type of control system.

The influence of sacral innervation on the colon has been the subject of preliminary investigation.[47] The colonic excitatory fibers are confined to the first sacral segment, and the excitatory effect is mainly the result of an effect on the longitudinal muscle coat. Two aspects are of interest in this paper: (1) the importance of lymphoid tissue for distinguishing the ileum from the colon was recognized; and (2) retroperistalsis was evoked in the colon.[47] Such activity has been observed in other gut regions prior to vomiting, and a study of the mechanisms underlying this

phenomenon in the ferret colon would be of interest, because such disordered motility has been implicated in the genesis of vomiting.

Gut transit time was only measured in one study, and values between 148 and 219 min were reported for animals fed a meat-based diet.[100] Further studies are required using different diets and markers to confirm these rather rapid times.

VOMITING

The study of the physiology of emesis is an area in which use of the ferret has become firmly established as an alternative animal model to the cat and dog. The ferret exhibits all three phases of emesis. Prior to retching or vomiting the animal displays characteristic behavior, including licking, chin rubbing, walking backward, and slit eyes, which are regarded as equating with the subjective sensation of nausea in humans. Further studies are needed to quantify these correlates of nausea before the ferret can be used to investigate antinausea drugs. As in the cat and dog, retching is characterized by large (>50 mm Hg) negative oscillations (1/sec) in intrathoracic pressure, with concomitant increases in intra-abdominal pressure but no ejection of stomach contents. During vomiting both the intrathoracic and intra-abdominal pressure oscillations become positive, and this is associated with the expulsion of the upper gastrointestinal contents. I have recorded the intrathoracic pressure changes during retching and vomiting in both conscious and urethane-anesthetized animals.

In the 5 years that the ferret has been more widely used for emetic studies, it has been shown to respond to various stimuli, including the following: cytotoxic agents used in chemotherapy (cisplatin,[101, 102] cyclophosphamide[103]; radiation x-rays, 200–800 rad); vagal afferent stimulation under urethane anesthesia[105];

and intragastric irritants (e.g., $CuSO_4$, NaCl) (results from our laboratory).

Studies of the mechanisms by which these stimuli evoke vomiting have concentrated on the role of the area postrema, the "chemoreceptor trigger zone" for vomiting located in the fourth ventricle. Recent studies, however, have demonstrated that abdominal vagotomy produces a marked reduction in the vomiting evoked by high doses of radiation and by the cytotoxic drugs cyclophosphamide and cisplatin,[103,104] suggesting an important role for abdominal innervation in triggering vomiting by these two stimuli.

Because of its sensitivity to a number of clinically important emetic stimuli, the ferret is now being used routinely for testing novel antiemetic agents. These studies reveal that 5-HT M-receptor antagonists are particularly effective against radiation and cytotoxin-induced vomiting.[103,106,107] The site of action of these new antiemetics is not known precisely, but our preliminary studies suggest that they may prevent activation of the abdominal vagal afferent pathway to the vomiting center.

BLOOD

Hematologic and serum chemistry data for the ferret have been reported by Thornton and colleagues.[6] Similar results have been reported by Lee and associates,[108] who studied fitch ferrets in contrast to the albino animals investigated in the study by Thornton and associates. Hematologic data are also available for the mink,[109] polecat,[110] and Siberian ferret[11] (also see Chap. 7).

HEMATOCRIT AND ERYTHROCYTE PHYSIOLOGY

The hematocrit is in general higher than in other common laboratory species, as is the erythrocyte count itself. For practical purposes we have found it necessary to take a blood sample three times the volume of the desired plasma sample. In addition, Thornton and co-workers reported that ferret blood must be spun for about 20% longer than that of other species.

Membranes

Red blood cells have been used as a convenient and plentiful source of cell membranes for the investigation of the transport and permeability characteristics of biologic membranes in general. Preliminary studies have been performed on ferret red cells to determine its potential as an alternative source to the cat and dog for carnivore red cells. The concentrations of cations inside the cells is as follows, given as the mean ± standard error per liter of original cells: Na^+, 95.7 ± 1.1 mmol/L; K^+, 3.9 ± 0.2 mmol/L; Mg^{2+}, 3.01 ± 0.12 mmol/L; Ca^{2+}, 8 to 10 μmol/L.[112] The ATP concentration was also measured, and found to be 0.60 ± 0.04 mmol/L original cells, sufficient to drive sodium or calcium pumps although the ferret red cell does not appear to have an active sodium pump.[112] Ionic flux studies[113] reveal that the red cell membranes are highly permeable to potassium, in contrast to cat and dog red cells, and this can be resolved into a rapid component that accounts for 70 to 90% of the movement and a slow component that accounts for the remainder. The high-ceiling loop diuretic bumetanide (0.1 mM) inhibits potassium influx by 80 to 90% and sodium by 60 to 70%, suggesting that these ions move into the cell using a sodium-potassium cotransport system. There is evidence that the red cells may be divisible into two populations based on potassium transport characteristics. The ferret red cell membrane has a number of transport characteristics not found in other carnivores, which makes further studies of these cells of great interest.

Hemoglobin

A sexual dimorphism has been observed in the red cell content of hemoglobin, and the values in both sexes are higher than those in the dog and rat.[6] No data are available on the oxygen transport characteristics of ferret hemoglobin, although measurements of the blood oxygen content indicate that they are likely to be similar to those of other species. An electrophoretic mobility study of carnivore hemoglobin[114] revealed that five species of the genus *Mustela*, including *M. putorius*, have two major hemoglobins, with mobilities of 0.85 and 0.65. The functional significance of these observations awaits further studies.

BLOOD GASES AND pH

These parameters have only been measured in urethane-anesthetized animals, and the following values therefore serve only as a guide to those that would be expected in the conscious animal. The arterial blood pH is 7.283 ± 0.025, with a bicarbonate concentration of 15.7 ± 0.7 mM.[95] In a different study we found that the arterial blood pH is 7.218 ± 0.014, Pa_{CO_2} is 30.4 ± 0.6 mm Hg and Pa_{O_2} is 95.0 ± 1.4 mm Hg. These observations demonstrate the stability of the urethane-anesthetized ferret.

In the barbiturate-anesthetized animal, Kempf and Chang[5] reported that the oxygen content of arterial blood is 15.7 ± 2.6 ml/100 ml blood and that of venous blood is 10.2 ± 1.8 ml/100 ml blood, giving an arteriovenous difference of 5.5 ± 1.7 ml/100 mL blood and an oxygen consumption of 7.2 ± 2.5 ml/min (body weight, 823 ± 114 g; surface area, 0.51–0.67 m^2).

SERUM CHEMISTRY

Several parameters have been measured in ferret serum, including serum glucose, a serum ammonia, and plasma protein levels, as well as osmolarity.

Glucose

In one study the blood glucose level was 131 mg/dl,[25] a value remarkably close to those obtained by others in a more recent study, who reported mean values of 126 (94–169) mg/dl in males and 145 (100–207) mg/dl in females.[6] In the fasting state the ferret has a relatively high blood glucose level, and this has led to some difficulties in adapting the 2-deoxy-D-glucose autoradiographic technique to the ferret.[115] Further studies are required to identify the reason for such a high glucose level, and in particular to investigate whether these values are a consequence of a pelleted laboratory diet.

Osmolarity

In the conscious ferret, plasma osmolarity is 328 ± 1 mOsm/kg and, following water deprivation for 24 hr, this increases to 366 ± 11 mOsm/kg.[116]

Plasma Proteins

In the ferret the total serum lipoprotein concentration is as high as in humans and dogs.[117] The major lipoprotein fraction is of high density (1.063–1.21 g/ml). The very low-density lipoprotein contains proportionately less triglyceride and more phospholipid than in humans, and the low-density lipoprotein contains proportionately more triglyceride and less cholesterol than in humans. Marked similarities have been observed in the gel electrophoretic pattern of human and ferret lipoprotein apoproteins, and in the solubility of apoproteins in tetramethylurea. These similarities between human and ferret lipoproteins may make it a useful animal model for the study of lipid metabolism.

In Aleutian disease, hypergammaglobulinemia is seen both in the ferret and the mink[118] (see Chap. 17).

Ammonia

The resting serum ammonia level in the ferret is 200 to 400 μg/dl, and is therefore considerably higher than in humans (17–80 μg/dl).[119] Hyperammonemia (2000–7000 μg/dl) is produced 2 to 3 hr after feeding a diet containing less than 0.3% arginine, or by an intraperitoneal injection of jack bean urease. These results are important for several reasons. First, ferrets appear to tolerate very high levels of ammonia, and remove ammonia from their system rapidly. Second, the ease with which hyperammonemia can be induced makes the ferret an ideal animal model for the study of ammonia metabolism, which is of particular relevance because of the association between hyperammonemia and Reye's syndrome (see later discussion and Chap. 5).

NERVOUS SYSTEM

The role of the nervous system in general and of the hypothalamus in particular in the regulation of reproduction in the ferret has been the subject of study for over 50 years, and is certainly the best characterized CNS function in this animal. Use of the ferret in the study of reproductive neuroendocrinology is reviewed elsewhere in this book, as is the influence of sex hormones on behavior (see Chaps. 18 and 19). The general anatomy of the ferret brain has been reviewed by Lockard[120] and in Chapter 3 of this volume. The hypothalamic-pituitary relationship in the ferret and other animals has been described in detail.[16] This section will concentrate on some more recent neurophysiologic studies, and highlights areas of research for which the ferret, with its relatively large gyrencephalic brain, may be of particular use.

CENTRAL NERVOUS SYSTEM

For convenience the central and autonomic components of the nervous system are discussed separately, and subdivisions made on both functional and anatomic grounds.

SPECIAL SENSES

The neurophysiology of the special senses is the major area of study. These investigations originally began because of the influence of photoperiod on reproduction. More recent studies, however, have shown that at birth the ferret nervous system is relatively immature, particularly when compared with the cat, and thus provides a system in which the development of the CNS can be studied postnatally at stages that occur in the cat in utero.

Visual System. Behavioral studies have demonstrated that at 50 cm from a target the visual resolution in ferrets trained to distinguish gray and striped patterns the ferret is 8′24″ at 220 lux, and 17′24″ at 0.01 lux; the absolute visual threshold is between 8.6×10^{-5} and 8.6×10^{-6} cd/m^2.[121] Ferrets preferentially follow and attack "prey targets" moving at 25 to 45 cm/sec, close to the escape speed of a mouse.[122]

It has been reported that the Mustelidae in general and the ferret in particular have a retina rich in cones and ganglion cells[123]; this observation awaits present quantitative confirmation. The possession of cones does not provide evidence for color vision, although simple behavioral studies provide some evidence that red may be distinguished but not blue, yellow, or green.[124] Further studies are needed to determine the presence of color vision in the ferret.

The morphology of the retina and its connections with the lateral geniculate nucleus have been the subject of several studies, but there are relatively little physiologic data available to complement these anatomic investigations. Nevertheless, anatomic studies will be briefly outlined because they provide an insight into the physiologic processes of the nervous system.

Retina. The retina is about 12.5 mm diameter in an adult. Its structure has been the subject of studies examining photoreceptors,[125] vasculature,[126] and development.[127]

Three types of ganglion cells are found in the retina, and are classified based on cell body size (range, 8–28 μm) and dendritic morphology: (1) ganglia with large cell bodies, coarse axons (1 μm), and large dendritic fields; (2) ganglia with medium-sized cell bodies and small dendritic fields; and (3) ganglia with medium-sized cell bodies and large dendritic fields. These three cell types resemble the alpha, beta, and epsilon ganglion cells described in the cat retina. In addition, a large number of cells in the retina, with cell bodies ranging in size from 8 to 20 μm, do not fall into any of the above categories, and were therefore described as unclassified. Each ganglion cell type was found in the following proportions: alphalike, 3 to 4%, betalike, 25%, and unclassified, 72%; in the cat, the corresponding percentages were 5, 40, and 55%, respectively.[128] The peak density of ganglion cells of 5200 cells/mm^2 occurs in the area centralis, 2.7 mm from the temporal margin and 2.6 mm from the center of the optic disc. A horizontal visual streak with an average density of >3000 cells/mm^2 is found throughout. This is consistent with the presence of a horizontal slit pupil described in the ferret.

Using cytochrome oxidase (CO) stain as a marker for cells with high levels of physiologic activity and oxidative metabolism, Kageyama and Wong-Riley[129] have revealed further details of the func-tional anatomy of the ferret retina. The inner segments of the rods and cones have an intense affinity for CO, with the cones staining more heavily than the rods, although this difference is not as marked as in primates. Medium to dark staining occurs in the ganglion cell dendrites in the inner plexiform layer, and two types of ganglion cell are distinguishable—large (20–26 μm) and medium to small (12–16 μm). Eighty-four percent of the large ganglion cells and 98% of the small ganglion cells have moderate to darkly staining dendrites projecting into sublamina A. This finding suggests a high level of activity in the off channel, known to be highly active under conditions of low light intensity. In addition, differences in CO staining are observed in the ganglion cells; alphalike cells show both dark and moderate staining, and it was proposed that these could represent off- and on-center cells, respectively. Dark staining is seen in beta-like cells, proposed to be off-center cells, but a functional correlate was not proposed for the medium-staining small cells.

Studies on the retina have shown many broad similarities to the cat retina. The CO staining of cells suggests functional division of on and off channels; confirmation of this awaits further neurophysiologic studies of the ganglion cells.

Retinogeniculate Projections. Two aspects of this projection are of interest, the degree of crossing of optic nerve fibers from nasal and temporal visual fields, and the organization of the retinal projection to the lateral geniculate nucleus (LGN).

Albino and pigmented ferrets, like many other animal species, differ in the degree of crossing of optic nerve fibers from the retina to the LGN. The major difference is the number of optic nerves projecting to the ipsilateral LGN from the temporal retina, being considerably reduced in the albino ferret. This is supported by recordings from the LGN.[130, 131] The functional implications are not clear, but perhaps this variation could be exploited in investigations of genetic influences on the development of the nervous system.

The structure and development of the LGN in the ferret has been described in detail.[132] Similar to other species the LGN has a laminar structure, with laminae A and C receiving inputs from the contralateral eye and lamina A1 inputs from the ipsilateral eye. In contrast to the cat, laminae A and A1 are divided into sublaminae A (inner), A' (outer), and A1 (inner), A1' (outer). Recordings of activity from these laminae demonstrate a clear segregation of off- and on-center retinal projections, with sublaminae A' and A1' containing cells responding only to off-center stimuli and those in A and A1 responding only to on-center stimuli.[133] Cytochrome oxidase reveals darker staining in the large cells in sublaminae A' and A1', providing further support for a high resting level of activity in the off channel.[129] Interestingly, in the mink, no cells in laminae A and A1 respond to color-coded stimuli.[133] In the C sublamina of both the ferret and mink,[133, 134] cells with responses to on- and off-center stimuli given to the contralateral eye were reported. The parvocellular C lamina is particularly well developed in the ferret, and this may be associated with the large proportion of small ganglion cells that are thought to be involved in the W visual system.[128, 133]

Considering these observations on the retina and the LGN together, it appears that on and off channels are segregated at the level of the retina and the LGN. Also, the segregation at the LGN is more distinct than in the cat. In addition, as in other species, the laminar organization of the LGN serves to segregate information from the two eyes. The function of this finding and the segregation of on-off information is unclear. One particularly interesting feature is that virtually all the alphalike large retinal ganglion cells in

the temporal retina project to the contralateral LGN. It was suggested that there may be no uncrossed alphalike ganglion cell projections,[128] which is noteworthy for two reasons: first, this organization would facilitate experimental investigations of the central projections of the alpha cells; and second, data from the cat associate the alpha cells with the Y visual system. This system appears to be especially involved in signaling the presence of moving objects in the visual field. Information processing of this type is of particular use to a predatory carnivore such as the ferret. It would be of interest to investigate whether these cells discharge to visual stimuli moving at speeds preferentially attacked by the ferret.

Nothing is known of the projections from the LGN to the visual cortex. The strict segregation of laminae and on-off information in the LGN suggests that such information may remain segregated at the cortical level; confirmation awaits further neurophysiologic studies.

Accessory Optic System. Because of the role of the prevailing photoperiod and of the pineal gland in the onset of estrous, the pathway linking the retina with the pineal gland has been the subject of several investigations. Lesions in the major visual pathways have no effect on the reproductive response to light, and it was therefore proposed that the accessory optic system is involved.[135, 136] In contrast to the rat, the ferret has only a posterior (superior) accessory optic tract. This tract contains only crossed fibers and terminates in two nuclei, the lateral and medial terminal nuclei located on either side of the cerebral peduncle.[136] In view of the differences in the degree of crossing of optic nerve fibers between pigmented and albino ferrets, it would be of interest to know whether this tract is completely crossed in both pigmented and nonpigmented ferrets. Lesions of these terminal nuclei do not modify the estrous response to light, and another pathway must therefore be involved.[137] The retinal projection to the hypothalamic suprachiasmatic nucleus may be involved.[137] Because recordings have not been made from the accessory optic pathways, the components of the visual input projecting to these areas are unknown.

Development. A preliminary account of the development of the retina reveals that 4 days after birth the retinal area is 25% the size of that in the adult. The ganglion cell layer resembles that of the cat at 3 weeks before birth, and the area centralis and visual streak are not visible.[128] The development of the LGN has also been described. Further studies[138] have shown that binocular enucleation in the neonate disrupts the laminar organization of the LGN. This suggests that the retinal afferents are involved in determining or maintaining this organization, particularly in laminae A and A1. Because the eyes in the ferret do not open until about 28 days after birth, the ferret provides an ideal animal model for studying not only the general development of the visual system, but also how it is influenced by usage of the eyes. In addition to the advantage of an immature visual system at birth, there are differences in the visual system between albino and pigmented ferrets. The ferret therefore provides an experimental system in which both the genetic and developmental influences on the visual system can be investigated separately and in combination.

Olfactory System. The olfactory epithelium has not been studied histologically, although the morphology of the nasal chambers has been the subject of a comparative study. The ferret, like many other carnivores, has an extensive turbinate system.[139] A detailed description of the olfactory cortex noted that the lateral olfactory tract (LOT) projects to most of the pyriform cortex.[140] The posterior olfactory cortex receives fine LOT collaterals with a conduction velocity of about 0.6 m/sec, and the anterior olfactory cortex larger diameter fibers have a conduction velocity of about 6.0 m/sec.

Electrophysiologic studies have not been performed to characterize the olfactory information projected to the CNS, but activity in the olfactory bulb has been recorded. These studies are technically feasible.[140] A series of behavioral studies demonstrated a sensitive phase for the development of olfactory preference,[141] which occurred at about 3 months. This coincides with the time at which ferrets would normally begin to live independently.

Auditory System. Recordings have been made from the superior and inferior colliculi, the subcortical regions involved in the processing of auditory information.

The inferior colliculus is histologically similar to that of the cat, although it is more compressed rostrocaudally and the central nucleus has a prominent rostroventral extension.[142] Under barbiturate anesthesia many of the neurons in the central nucleus are active, making the ferret particularly useful for the study of inhibitory mechanisms. The neurons in the central nucleus are sharply tuned (comparable to those of the cat), and a large proportion are inhibited by a band of frequencies on either side of the maximally effective frequency. The most sensitive units had the best frequencies in the range of 4 to 15 kHz, and most (80%) units had inputs from both ears. As in other animals the central nucleus is tonotopically organized, with units with "low" best frequencies located dorsally and those with "high" best frequencies located ventrally. A preliminary study of the superior colliculus has revealed that many of the cells respond preferentially to sound from a particular direction, suggesting that the superior colliculi may contain a map of auditory space in both the vertical and horizontal dimensions.[143] The auditory system in the ferret offers a suitable alternative to the cat for studies of auditory physiology, and the developmental study described below suggests a number of advantages over use of the cat.

Behavior studies have revealed that a startle response to a loud clap is only present 32 days after birth, which coincides with the time at which the ear canals[144] and the eyes open. Prior to this time ferrets exhibit a range of behavior, including defecation, vocalization, exploration, sucking, and withdrawal from a noxious stimulus. Electrophysiologic studies on the midbrain of animals before 32 days of age reveal that, although there is spontaneous activity, it is unaltered by auditory stimuli. At 32 days after birth auditory evoked responses are recorded but their threshold is higher than in the adult, and the frequency range is narrow (1–6 kHz) compared to that of the adult (at least 4–15 kHz). The frequency sensitivity and threshold change rapidly toward adult values, and recordings from two ferrets aged 39 and 42 days showed the adult pattern. These results demonstrate that the ferret auditory system is primitive at birth as compared to that of the cat, thus offering an opportunity to investigate the development of the auditory system during stages that would occur in the cat in utero. The visual and auditory systems both appear to become functional at about the same time (30 days); because the two systems are known to interact, it would be of interest to investigate their developmental interactions in this model.

The adult auditory system appears to undergo functional changes following pregnancy. Neonatal animals emit distress calls with frequency components of up to 100 kHz, and these elicit searching behavior in lactating females who will preferentially orient themselves toward frequencies >16 kHz. Responses to these stimuli, however, are not evoked in non-lactating females.[145] Although the mechanism is unclear it would be of interest to know the time course of the change, and to determine whether or not it could be produced in males by suitable manipulation of sex hormones.

Hypothalamus

The vast majority of studies on the hypothalamus have investigated its interactions with the pineal gland and the pituitary, and their roles in reproduction. These aspects are discussed elsewhere (see Chap. 19), and this section will briefly discuss the levels of neurotransmitters in the hypothalamus.

5-HT was detected by radioenzymatic assay in the septum, preoptic area, suprachiasmatic area, medial forebrain bundle, pineal and lateral (LHA) and anterior hypothalamic (AHA) areas; the pineal has the highest levels.[146] The levels of 5-HT in the pineal region and of the LHA and AHA, vary slightly with time of day. Only the LHA and pineal levels are influenced by the prevailing photoperiod. Differential rhythms in pineal and anterior hypothalamic 5-HT levels reported by Yates and Herbert[147] were not found.[146] Although 5-HT is probably a neurotransmitter in the ferret hypothalamus, the proposal that the pineal influences the hypothalamic-pituitary axis via 5-HT requires further studies before definitive answers can be given regarding its role in the modulation of reproduction.

In homogenates of the entire hypothalamus, activities of adrenalin (163 ± 11 pmol/g), noradrenalin (3912 ± 330 pmol/g), dopamine (701 ± 99 pmol/g), and noradrenalin N-methyl transferase (NMT; 246 ± 30 pmol/hr/g) have been identified. The levels of noradrenalin, dopamine, and NMT are closer to those for the dog than the cat, but the adrenalin level is substantially lower than either the dog or cat.[148]

Cerebellum

Two types of study on the physiology of the ferret's cerebellum have been undertaken, one type directed toward understanding its role in jaw reflexes[149, 150] and the other toward elucidation of its role in locomotion.

Field potentials were evoked in lobules 4 and 5 (ipsilateral > contralateral) in response to stimulation of the inferior alveolar nerve. The conduction velocity of the inferior alveolar axons in their peripheral course was 52 m/sec, and further calculations of conduction time within the CNS indicated that the projection to the granular layer is direct. The function of such a rapid direct first-order projection needs further evaluation.

In decerebrate ferrets recordings have been made from cerebellar Purkinje cells in lobules 5 and 6 during treadmill walking.[151] A complete description of this study is beyond the scope of this chapter, but it was shown that during locomotion the Purkinje cell discharge is not very well modulated. If locomotion is suddenly perturbed, however, the discharge is clearly modulated, and this is particularly associated with an increase in complex spikes. This report suggests that the ferret may be a suitable alternative to the cat for this type of locomotor research. In addition, the ferret has been used for investigation of the effects of spinal compression injuries on locomotion.[152] A combination of these two types of locomotor studies may provide insight into the problems of locomotion in persons with selective cord lesions.

Brain Stem

The brain stem has been investigated in the ferret mainly to determine the location and characteristics of the cells of origin of the abdominal vagus. The anatomy of the vagal brain stem connections have been described in Chapter 3, and the vagal afferents were the subject of a more detailed study.[153] Recordings from the dorsal medulla in the region of the obex reveal respiratory or cardiovascular phased multiunit activity. Ventral to this layer, in the region of the dorsal motor vagal nucleus, single units have been identified and demonstrated by collision to project axons to the abdomen.[154] The conduction velocity of the axons is in the range for that of unmyelinated fibers. Indirect evidence suggests that some of the abdominal vagal efferents may be reflexly activated by vagal afferents via monosynaptic or polysynaptic pathways.[155] Electrophysiologic studies of brain stem auditory evoked responses are discussed later (see Reye's syndrome).

The levels of various neurotransmitters have been measured in homogenates of whole brain stem: adrenalin 45 ± 5 pmol/g; noradrenalin, 2125 ± 109 pmol/g; and dopamine, 174 ± 19 pmol/g. These values lie midway between those for the cat and dog measured in the same study.[148] The levels of noradrenalin N-methyl transferase (191 ± 37 pmol/hr/g tissue) are comparable to those in the dog but very low in comparison to those in the cat (895 ± 53 pmol/hr/g tissue).

Stimulation of abdominal vagal afferents produces an increase in the uptake of [^{3}H]-2-deoxyglucose by the area postrema.[156] This provides evidence that vagal afferents may evoke vomiting by direct activation of the vomiting chemoreceptor trigger zone located within the area postrema (see earlier discussion on vomiting).

Disease Models

The ferret has been used in neurophysiologic studies to elucidate the mechanisms of several neurologic disorders.

Lissencephaly. Although lissencephaly is a rare syndrome in humans, the importance of an animal model in which this syndrome can be readily produced lies in two areas. First, in humans, lissencephaly is associated with epileptic seizures. Thus, a study of the lissencephalic cortex may provide insight into the genesis of such seizures in patients with far less extensive lesions. Second, an understanding of how lissenchephaly may be induced experimentally will yield important information about the mechanisms of normal cortical histogenesis, and reveal how this may become disordered to produce various disturbing CNS birth defects.

Treatment of pregnant ferrets with the alkylating agent methylazoxymethanol acetate on gestation day 32 or 33 leads to the production of offspring with lissencephalic hydrocephalic cerebral hemispheres and a brain weight 28% less than normal.[157] Behaviorally, the animals have a markedly impaired learning ability when tested in several types of maze.[157] The spectrum of EEG activity is modified, particularly during sleep. Although the stimulation current required to evoke an epileptiform afterdischarge is no different from that for control animals, the duration of afterdischarges and seizures is longer. This effect indicates a generally enhanced sensitivity in the lissencephalic animals. Also, these animals respond to treatment with antiepileptic drugs, although less well than gyrencephalic animals.[157] Neurochemical studies have revealed an increase in indices of cholinergic and catecholaminergic nerve terminals and little if any change in GABAergic systems.[158] Further studies are required to determine whether neurochemical changes can be related to the EEG changes, which would suggest new approaches for the design of antiepileptic drugs.

Reye's Syndrome. This often fatal childhood syndrome of unknown etiology is characterized by a number of CNS problems, including coma, seizures, cerebral edema, and raised intracranial pressure. Although the cause is unknown its appearance has been associated with hyperammonemia, salicylates, and viruses, particularly influenza. Ferrets are particularly susceptible to influenza B, and hyperammonemia may be readily induced by an arginine-deficient diet.[119] Combining these treatments with acetylsalicylic acid administration results in animals with several of the symptoms of Reye's syndrome. Electrophysiologic studies have revealed that wave 1 (eighth nerve generator potential) of the auditory brain stem evoked response is delayed in latency compared with that of controls, and wave 4 (brain stem nuclei response potential) is initially delayed. By 10 days after treatment, however, the latency returns to near normal values.[159] It was suggested that the central components of the auditory system recover more quickly than the peripheral components. Because of its sensitivity to all three of the factors predisposing to Reye's syndrome, the ferret is an excellent model for the study of its etiology and possible treatments (see Chap. 5 for further discussion).

High-Pressure Neurologic Syndrome (HPNS). The profound neurologic effects (e.g., convulsions) of exposure to high hydrostatic pressures have attracted interest in connection with deep sea diving and as a research method for producing reversible changes in the excitability of the nervous system. In a comparative study of HPNS, the ferret had a high susceptibility to HPNS comparable to that of the mouse, guinea pig, squirrel, and rhesus monkey.[160] These preliminary observations indicate that the ferret may be a useful animal model for the study of HPNS.

AUTONOMIC NERVOUS SYSTEM

A complete anatomic description of the autonomic nervous system in the ferret has not been published, but the innervation of several organs has been reported: trachea[28,161,162]; heart[14]; stomach[62]; kidney[163,164]; and bladder and colon.[47,165]

The influence of the autonomic innervation on a number of visceral functions is discussed in the cardiovascular, respiratory, gastrointestinal, and urogenital sections of this chapter, so this section will describe electrophysiologic studies of the autonomic nervous system that were concerned with the trachea and gut.

TRACHEAL INNERVATION

Because of its length and the large number of submucosal glands, the ferret trachea is popular for use in studies of the neural control of airway secretion. In addition, the parasympathetic nerves contract the tracheal smooth muscle, and the neural control of secretion and motility can thus be investigated in the same tissue. Associated with the ferret trachea are two chains of paratracheal ganglia separated by interganglionic nerve trunks.[161,162] The extrinsic innervation is from the laryngeal nerve. The ganglia each contain 10 to 20 cells, with cell body diameters ranging from 15 to 40 μm. Based on electrical characteristics two cell types may be distinguished—AH cells with a resting membrane potential of -37 ± 7 mV, which have a marked hyperpolarization following an action potential, and nonspiking B cells with a resting potential of -52 ± 11 mV. Stimulation of the nerve trunks evokes fast excitatory and inhibitory postsynaptic potentials in the AH cells and in some of the B cells. The inputs to the ganglia appear to be both cholinergic and noncholinergic. The interganglionic nerve trunks are composed mainly of unmyelinated nerves, as are the postganglionic axons supplying the smooth muscle cells (calculated conduction velocity, 0.1–0.2 m/sec). The interganglionic nerve trunks are

important not only in distributing the extrinsic input to separated ganglion cells but also in the dissemination of postganglionic fibers to the smooth muscle cells.[43,161] The paratracheal ganglia may not act solely as simple relay stations, but may also play a role as peripheral integrators of respiratory reflexes.

Using the above preparation, it was demonstrated that transmission between the pre- and postganglionic nerves could be modulated by norepinephrine acting on presynaptic α-adrenergic receptors. It was concluded that the sympathetic nerves influence tracheal function not only by direct action on the muscle and submucosal glands but also by modulating the effects of the extrinsic parasympathetic drive.[166] A similar mechanism has been proposed for the influence of the greater splanchnic (sympathetic) nerves on gastric motility.[81] Ganglionic transmission in the trachea is also reduced by barbiturates at doses comparable to those producing general anesthesia.[167] This observation suggests that barbiturates may not be the best anesthetics for use in studies of the respiratory system in the ferret; unfortunately, the only reports of pulmonary mechanics in this species used a barbiturate.[24,26]

GASTROINTESTINAL INNERVATION

Afferent activity has been recorded in vagal fibers supplying the esophagus and stomach,[55,79] and in greater splanchnic nerves innervating the gallbladder and biliary tree.[10] Recordings have been made from vagal afferent mechanoreceptors supplying the midthoracic striated muscle portion of the esophagus. The discharge rate is related to the degree of esophageal distention, and stretch of the circular muscle produces a more marked response than longitudinal distention, although the discharge is relatively slow-adapting in both cases. The afferent axons are small diameter myelinated fibers, with conduction velocities between 7.5 and 15 m/sec.[55]

In contrast to the esophageal mechanoreceptors, the vagal afferents innervating the gastric smooth muscle are unmyelinated, with a mean conduction velocity of 0.91 ± 0.21 m/sec.[79] The most interesting feature of the gastric mechanoreceptors is that their precise response to gastric distention depends on their location in the stomach. During gastric filling most fluid is accommodated in the gastric body, and the discharge in the mechanoreceptors with receptive fields in this region gradually increases with increasing volume. The antrum is little distended but an increase in the level of contractile activity is reflexly evoked,[84] and this is signaled by the antral mechanoreceptors. The receptors in both regions are "in series" tension receptors. The nature of their response is largely determined by differences in the properties of the muscle in the two gastric regions. The "in series" nature of the corpus mechanoreceptors has recently been confirmed.[168]

The only study of visceral afferents traveling with the abdominal sympathetic nerves investigated the role of biliary system afferents in the production of visceral pain.[10] In response to distension of the gallbladder and biliary ducts, two types of afferent activity were evoked: (1) low-threshold afferents activated by levels of distension but not producing reflex increases in blood pressure (innocuous stimulation); and (2) high-threshold afferents activated by degrees of distension that evoked changes in blood pressure (noxious stimulation). The latter type was most commonly found in the biliary tree. These results indicate that specific nociceptors may exist in the gallbladder, and the ferret may thus provide a suitable animal model for the investigation of visceral nociception.

ENDOCRINE SYSTEM

Most studies of ferret endocrinology have investigated aspects of the reproductive system; these are reviewed in Chapters 18 and 19 and therefore will not be discussed here. For convenience, references are given to studies in which the levels of reproductive hormones were measured. Apart from these investigations there is sparse information on the endocrine system. Preliminary studies have been performed and will be briefly described.

REPRODUCTIVE ENDOCRINOLOGY

Testis. The effect of luteinizing hormone (LH), hypothalamic lesions, the amygdala, development, season, and time of day on testosterone secretion have all been investigated,[169–172] and in addition the influence of LH-RH (releasing hormone) has also been studied. Testosterone has been detected in plasma from spayed and intact females.[172]

Ovary. Progesterone levels in plasma have been measured before and during implantation, and in pregnant and pseudopregnant animals.[173, 174] The influence of day length on the secretion of progesterone, estradiol, and estrone has also been studied.[175] In the ferret progesterone has been shown to increase the level of glycogen in the liver (but not in muscle), and a more marked response is observed in pseudopregnant animals.[176]

Anterior Pituitary. The influence of LH-RH, day length, estrus and anestrus, ovariectomy, the hypothalamus, and development on the secretion of LH have been investigated.[177, 178] Follicle stimulating hormone (FSH) secretion has been studied in relation to development, hypothalamic stimulation, LH-RH, day length, and ovariectomy.[177–179] The half-life of FSH and LH in estrus, anestrus, and ovariectomized animals has been measured by Donovan and Gledhill.[180]

ADRENAL GLANDS

The gross morphology, histology, and vasculature of the adrenal glands have been described by Holmes.[181] The adrenal cortex has three main zones usually encountered in other mammals (glomerulosa, fasciculata, and reticularis) and, in addition, a zona intermedia and juxtamedullaris are also found. One of the most interesting findings was that the adrenal weight is higher in animals in late proestrus or estrus than in animals in anestrus or early proestrus. There is also some indication that the stainable lipid in the cortex increases in estrus, but this finding varies.[181] The functional significance of these observations is unclear, and is unlikely to be resolved until measurements of ferret adreno cortical hormones have been made. These studies are facilitated by the presence of relatively large veins that drain the gland (see Chap. 2).

POSTERIOR PITUITARY

Preliminary studies have demonstrated the presence of bioactive antidiuretic hormone (ADH) in the plasma of anesthetized and conscious ferrets, and the level increases by water deprivation. The control of ADH secretion has not been studied in detail, but large increases in its output are produced by the D_2 receptor agonist apomorphine, and by electrical stimulation of the central cut end of the abdominal vagus.[116]

GASTROINTESTINAL TRACT

Although the gut is usually regarded as the largest endocrine gland, this area has seldom been investigated in the ferret. The features studied have been previously discussed in this chapter (see Gastrointestinal Tract: Gastric Secretion, Small Intestine, and Pancreas and Biliary System).

URINARY SYSTEM

KIDNEYS

Morphologically the kidneys are similar to those in other species, but histologic studies have revealed two interesting features—first, that ectopic glomeruli are present,[182] and second, that the intrarenal arteries have relatively thicker walls than in other laboratory animals.[6] The functional significance of these observations is unclear.

The autonomic innervation of the kidney is more complex than that reported for other species. In summary, the innervation is from two main sources; the aorticorenal ganglion in the region of the adrenal gland gives rise to two to four fine branches. These course into the kidney in proximity to the renal artery and, in addition, the lower lumbar sympathetic chain gives rise to a single nerve that runs directly to the kidney, termed the "direct" renal nerve. No ganglion was observed along the course of the nerve.[163, 164] Reports of such a direct renal nerve in other species have not been found. Electron microscopic studies of the "direct" and "indirect" renal nerves reveal that they both contain small myelinated and unmyelinated axons, with the latter predominating.

Physiologic studies have demonstrated the presence of efferent activity in both nerves. Of particular interest is the finding that in response to hemorrhage some nerves decrease their discharge rather than the increase reported in other species. It has been speculated that these units may represent sympathetic dopaminergic vasodilator nerves known to supply the kidney in some species, although the dopamine levels in the ferret renal cortex (0.014 ± 0.004 µg/g) are low.[9] Of the rat, guinea pig, cat, and rabbit only the guinea pig has a higher level of noradrenalin (1.44 ± 0.154 µg/g), than the ferret suggesting a predominant role for noradrenalin in the regulation of renal function in these species.

Under Inactin (120 mg/kg IP) anesthesia the ferret kidney produces urine, and lesion of the renal nerves leads to a "denervation natriuresis," as observed in other species. This demonstrates a tonic sympathetically driven reabsorption of sodium ions.[16]

Although nothing is known of the details of urine production, bladder urine osmolarity may reach 2000 mOsm/L, indicating a considerable concentrating ability and supporting the hypothesis that the ferret may have originated from a desert-dwelling animal. Conscious animals fed a commercial dog diet with water ad libitum had a urine output of 8 to 140 ml/24 hr, containing sodium, 0.2 to 6.7 mmol/24 hr, potassium, 0.9 to 9.6 mmol/24 hr and chloride, 0.3 to 8.5 mmol/24 hr.[6] These values depend on the nature of the diet and, in particular, we have found that on a pelleted diet water intake is directly related to the salt content of the diet. In view of the effect of high levels of sodium intake on the development of hypertension, it is possible that some of the high blood pressure values reported in this species were produced by excess dietary sodium. In this study most animals were proteinuric, with urine values for protein of up to 33 mg/dl, but the reason for this is unknown.[6]

BLADDER AND URETERS

Under anesthesia the ureters show spontaneous rhythmic contractions propagating toward the bladder, but nothing is known of the control of this activity.

The bladder in a large ferret (2 kg) can accommodate about 10 ml of urine at a relatively low pressure (5 cm H_2O). The control of the bladder is of particular interest, because both the hypogastric (sympathetic) and sacral (parasympathetic) nerves *both* cause contraction of the entire bladder, whereas in other animals (e.g., cat) the sympathetic nerves usually produce relaxation. The bladder also contracts in response to adrenalin, and the contractions to sympathetic stimulation and adrenalin are converted to a relaxation state by chrysotoxin (an ergot derivative). This experiment was performed in 1905, and it is important because it was one of the first studies to demonstrate that the effects of sympathetic nerve stimulation are mimicked by adrenalin, and more significantly that both responses are similarly modified by an antagonist (chrysotoxin).[12, 164] These experiments on the ferret were undertaken jointly by Elliott and Dale,[183] with Dale winning the Nobel Prize for Physiology and Medicine along with Loewi in 1934 for studies on the mechanism of neurotransmission. Those readers familiar with this topic will recognize these observations as constituting two of "Dale's criteria" for the demonstration of neurotransmission. Thus, the unusual response of the ferret bladder played an important role in the elucidation of neurotransmission mechanisms. Interestingly, the pharmacologic basis of the dual effects of adrenalin and sympathetic stimulation on the bladder has not yet been established, although recent studies have demonstrated contractile responses to cholinergic and purinergic agonists in vitro.[184]

REFERENCES

1. Truex, R.C., Belej, R., Ginsberg, L.M., and Hartman, R.L.: Anatomy of the ferret: An animal model for cardiac research. Anat. Rec., 179:411, 1974.
2. Frederick, K.A., and Babish, J.G.: Compendium of recent literature on the ferret. Lab. Anim. Sci., 35:298, 1985.
3. Andrews, P.L.R., Bower, A.J., and Illman, O.: Some aspects of the physiology and anatomy of the cardiovascular system of the ferret. Lab. Anim., 13:215, 1979.
4. Willis, L.S., and Barrow, M.V.: The ferret (*Mustela putorius furo L.*) as a laboratory animal. Lab. Anim. Sci., 21:712, 1971.
5. Kempf, J.E., and Chang, H.T.: The cardiac output and circulation time of ferrets. Proc. Soc. Exp. Biol. Med., 72:711, 1949.
6. Thornton, P.C., Wright, P.A., Sacra, P.J., and Goodier, T.E.W.: The ferret, *Mustela putorius furo*, as a new species in toxicology. Lab. Anim., 13:119, 1979.
7. Kohler, E., and Bieniek, H.: Pharmacological investigations on the cardiovascular system of the anesthetized mink. Z. Versuchstierkd., 17:145, 1975.
8. Andrews, P.L.R., and Illman, O.: The ferret. *In* Universities Federation for Animal Welfare Handbook, Chap. 25. Edited by T. Poole. Edinburgh, Churchill Livingstone, 1987.
9. Bell, C., and Gillespie, J.S.: Dopamine and noradrenalin levels in peripheral tissues of several mammalian species. J. Neurochem., 36:703, 1981.
10. Cervero, F.: Afferent activity evoked by natural stimulation of the biliary system in the ferret. Pain, 13:137, 1982.
11. Andrews, P.L.R.: Dutia, M.B., and Harris, P.J.: Angiotensin II does not inhibit vagally induced bradycardia or gastric contractions in the anesthetized ferret. Br. J. Pharmacol., 82: 833, 1984.
12. Elliott, T.R.: The action of adrenalin. J. Physiol., 32:401, 1905.
13. Evans, C.A., and Wand, D.R.: A pressor effect of high doses of tubocurarine in the ferret. Pharmacology, 10:32, 1973.
14. Joffre, J., and Joffre, M.: Seasonal changes in the testicular blood flow of seasonally breeding mammals: Doormouse, ferret and fox. J. Reprod. Fertil., 34:227, 1973.
15. Andrews, P.L.R., and Lawes, I.N.C.: Characteristics of the vagally driven non-adrenergic, non-cholinergic inhibitory innervation of the ferret gastric corpus. J. Physiol., 363:1, 1985.
16. Daniel, P.M., and Pritchard, M.M.L.: Studies of the hypothalamus and the pituitary gland. Acta Endocrinol. [Suppl.] (Copenh.), 201, 1975.
17. Barber, G.R., Mohammed, F., Suggett, A., and Twelves, C.L.: Hypoxic pulmonary vasoconstriction in the ferret. J. Physiol., 281:40p, 1978.
18. Peake, M.D., Harabin, A.L., Brennan, N.J., and Sylvester, J.T.: Steady-state vascular responses to graded hypoxia in isolated lungs of five species. Am. J. Physiol., 51:1214, 1981.
19. Emery, C.J., Sloan, P.J.M., Mohammed F.H., and Barber, G.R.: The action of hypercapnia during hypoxia on pulmonary vessels. Bull. Physiol. Pathol. Respir., 13:763, 1977.
20. Suggett, A.J., Mohammed, F.H., and Barber, G.R.: Angiotensin, hypoxia, verapamil and pulmonary vessels. Ann. Exp. Pharmacol., 7:263, 1980.
21. Barber, C.R., Emery, C.J., Mohammed, F.H., and Mongall, I.P.F.: H_1 and H_2 histamine actions on lung vessels; their relevance to hypoxic vasoconstriction. Q. J. Exp. Physiol., 63:157, 1978.
22. Cowan, A., and Watson, N.G.: Distribution of free histamine and histamine-destroying and -forming activities in animal tissues. Comp. Gen. Pharmacol., 3:75, 1972.
23. Bee, D., Day, J.J., and Mona Ghan, C.: Reversal of hypoxic pulmonary vasoconstriction by adenosine and dopamine in the ferret. J. Physiol., 316:24P, 1981.
24. Vinegar, A., Sinnet, E.E., and Kosch, P.C.: Respiratory mechanics of a small carnivore: The ferret. J. Appl. Physiol., 52:832, 1982.
25. Pyle, N.J.: The use of ferrets in laboratory and research investigations. Am. J. Pub. Health, 30:787, 1940.
26. Boyd, R.L., and Mangos, J.A.: Pulmonary mechanics of the normal ferret. J. Appl. Physiol., 50:799, 1981.
27. Stahl, W.R.: Scaling of respiratory variables in mammals. J. Appl. Physiol., 22:453, 1967.
28. Robinson, N.P., Venning, L., Kyle, H., and Widdicombe, J.G.: Quantitation of the secretory cells of the ferret tracheobronchial tree. J. Anat., 145:173, 1986.
29. Jacob, S., and Podder, S.: Mucous cells of the tracheobronchial tree in the ferret. Histochemistry, 73:599, 1982.
30. Tom-Moy, M., Basbaum, C.B., and Nadel, J.A.: Localization and release of lysozyme from ferret trachea—effects of adrenergic and cholinergic drugs. Cell Tissue Res., 228:549, 1983.
31. Barber, W.H., and Small, P.A.: Construction of an improved tracheal pouch in the ferret. Am. Rev. Resp. Dis., 115:165, 1977.
32. Robinson, N., Widdicombe, J.G., and Xie, C.C.: In vitro collection of mucus from the ferret trachea. J. Physiol., 340:7P, 1984.

33. Borson, D.B., Chinn, R.A., Davis, B., and Nadel, J.A.: Adrenergic and cholinergic nerves mediate fluid secretion from tracheal glands of ferrets. J. Appl. Physiol., 49:1027, 1980.

34. Kyle, H., Robinson, N.P., and Widdicombe, J.G.: Mucus secretion by tracheas of ferret and dog. Eur. J. Resp. Dis. (in press).

35. Louchlin, G.M., et al.: Fluid fluxes in ferret trachea. Experientia, 38:1451, 1982.

36. Corrales, R.J., Nadel, J.A., and Widdicombe, J.G.: Sources of fluid component of secretions from tracheal submucosal glands in cats. J. Appl. Physiol., 56:1076, 1986.

37. Kyle, H., Robinson, N.P., Robinson, N.R., and Widdicombe, J.G.: Simultaneous measurement of airway mucus secretion and smooth muscle tone in ferret trachea in vitro. J. Physiol., 327:38P, 1986.

38. Borson, D.B., Charlin, M., Gold, D.B., and Nadel, J.A.: Neural regulations of $^{35}SO_4$ macromolecule secretion from tracheal glands of ferrets. J. Appl. Physiol., 57:457, 1984.

39. Peatfield, A.C., et al.: Vasoactive intestinal peptide stimulates tracheal submucosal gland secretion in ferret. Am. Rev. Respir. Dis., 128:89, 1983.

40. Basbaum, C.B., Ueki, I., Brezina, L., and Nadel, J.: Tracheal submucosal serous cells stimulated in vitro with adrenergic and cholinergic agonists: A morphometric study. Cell Tissue Res., 220:481, 1981.

41. Barnes, P.S., Basbaum, C.B., Nadel, J.A., and Roberts, J.M.: Localization of adrenoreceptors in mammalian lung by light microscopic autoradiography. Nature, 299:444, 1982.

42. Barnes, P.J., Basbaum, C.B., Nadel, J.A., and Roberts, J.M.: Pulmonary α-adrenoreceptors. Autoradiographic localization using tritium-labelled prazosin. Eur. J. Pharmacol., 88:57, 1983.

43. Coburn, R.F.: Neural coordination of excitation of ferret trachealis muscle. Am. J. Physiol., 246:C459, 1984.

44. Barnes, P.J., Basbaum, C.B., and Nadel, J.A.: Autoradiographic localization of autonomic receptors in airway smooth muscle. Am. Rev. Resp. Dis., 127:758, 1983.

45. Korpas, J., and Widdicombe, J.G.: Defensive respiratory reflexes in ferrets. Respiration, 44:128, 1983.

46. Young, S.: The effect of vagotomy on the deflation reflex, tracheal occlusion and the pattern of breathing in the rat and the ferret. J. Physiol., 310:62P, 1981.

47. Elliott, T.R., and Barclay-Smith, E.: Antiperistalsis and other muscular activities of the colon. J. Physiol., 31:272, 1904.

48. Poddar, S., and Murgatroyd, L.: Morphological and histological study of the gastrointestinal tract of the ferret. Acta Anat., 96:321, 1977.

49. Poddar, S., and Jacob, S.: Gross and microscopic anatomy of the major salivary glands of the ferrets. Acta Anat., 98:434, 1977.

50. Jacob, S., and Poddar, S.: The histochemistry of mucosubstances in ferret and salivary glands. Acta Histochem., 61:142, 1978.

51. Mangos, J.A., et al.: Secretion of monovalent ions and water in ferret salivary glands—a micropuncture study. Dent. Res., 60:733, 1981.

52. Mangos, J.A., et al.: Transductal fluxes of water and manovalent ions in ferret salivary glands. J. Dent., 60:86, 1981.

53. Mangos, J.A., et al.: Handling of calcium by the ferret submandibular gland. J. Dent. Res., 60:91, 1981.

54. Ekstrom, J., and Olgart, L.: Substance P-evoked salivary secretion in the ferret. J. Physiol., 372:41P, 1986.

55. Andrews, P.L.R., and Lang, K.: Vagal afferent discharge from mechanoreceptors in the lower oesophagus of the ferret. J. Physiol., 332:29P, 1983.

56. Stephens, R., and Pfeiffer, C.J.: Ultrastructure of the gastric mucosa of normal laboratory ferrets. J. Ultrastruct. Res., 22:45, 1968.

57. Pfeiffer, C.J.: Surface topology of the stomach in man and the laboratory ferret. J. Ultrastruct. Res., 33:252, 1970.

58. Pfeiffer, C.J., and Roth, J.L.A.: Studies on the secretory and cytotoxic actions of caffeine on the ferret gastric mucosa. Exper. Mol. Pathol., 13:66, 1970.

59. Umeda, N., Roth, J.L.A., and Pfeiffer, C.J.: Gastric lesions produced by cinchophen in the ferret. Toxicol. Appl. Pharmacol., 18:102, 1971.

60. Pfeiffer, C.J., and Stephens, R.J.: Ultrastructural changes of the parietal cell in the ferret gastric mucosa induced by pylorus ligation and glucocorticoid administration. J. Ultrastruct. Res., 21:524, 1968.

61. Poddar, S., and Jacob, S.: Mucosubstance histochemistry of Brunner's glands, pyloric glands and duodenal goblet cells in the ferret. Histochemistry, 65:67, 1979.

62. Mackay, T.W., and Andrews, P.L.R.: A comparative study of the vagal innervation of the stomach in man and the ferret. J. Anat., 136:449, 1983.

63. Pfeiffer, C.J., and Peters, C.M.: Gastric secretion in the chronic fistula ferret. Gastroenterology, 57:518, 1969.

64. Pfeiffer, C.J., and Peters, C.M.: Gastric acid secretion in the ferret during estrus and anestrus. Digestion, 5:129, 1972.

65. Basso, N., Roth, J.L.A., and Pfeiffer, C.J.: Gastric secretion after pentagastrin and histamine in the basal secreting ferret. J. Surg. Res., 10:111, 1970.

66. Basso, B., and Passaro, E.: The effect of calcium on pentagastrin, histamine, bethanecol and insulin-stimulated gastric secretion in the ferret. J. Surg. Res., *13*:32, 1972.

67. Watson, L.C., Reeder, D.D., and Thompson, J.C.: Effects of hypercalcemia on serum gastrin and gastric secretion in awake ferrets. Tex. Rep. Biol. Med., *31*:605, 1973.

68. Desmond, H.P., Dockray, G.J., Gregory, R.A., and Spurdens, M.D.: Identification and characterization of a novel peptide generated during gastrin biosynthesis in the pig and ferret. J. Physiol., *354*:P4, 1984.

69. Basso, N., et al.: Effect of unilateral vagotomy on gastric secretion in the ferret. Gastroenterology, 61:207, 1977.

70. Andrews, P.L.R.: The vagal control of the gastrointestinal tract. Ph.D. thesis, University of Sheffield, 1979.

71. Roth, S.H., Schofield, B., and Yates, J.C.: Effects of atropine on secretion and motility in isolated gastric mucosa and attached muscularis externa from the ferret and cat. J. Physiol., *292*:357, 1979.

72. Yates, J.C., Schofield, B., and Roth, S.H.: Acid secretion and motility of isolated mammalian gastric mucosa and attached muscularis externa. Am. J. Physiol., *234*:319, 1978.

73. Shillingford, J.S., Lindup, W.E., and Parke, D.V.: The effects of carbenoxolone on the biosynthesis of gastric glycoproteins in the rat and ferret. Biochem. Soc. Trans., *2*:1104, 1974.

74. Edwards, L., and Aubrey, A.: Relation between transmucosal potential difference, ionic flux and the intraluminal supply of H$^+$ in the ferret stomach. Am. J. Surg., *137*:585, 1979.

75. Andrews, P.L.R., and Scratcherd, T.: The gastric motility patterns induced by direct and reflex excitation of the vagus nerves in the ferret. J. Physiol., *302*:363, 1980.

76. Grundy, D., and Scratcherd, T.: Effect of stimulation of the vagus nerve in bursts on gastric acid secretion and motility in the anesthetized ferret. J. Physiol., *333*:451, 1982.

77. Bingham, S.: A comparison of the effects of 5-HT and vagal stimulation on antral motility in the anesthetized ferret. J. Physiol., *382*:187P, 1987.

78. Bingham, S., and Andrews, P.L.R.: Preliminary studies on the mechanism of action of cisapride. Digestion, *34*:138, 1986.

79. Andrews, P.L.R., Grundy, D., and Scratcherd, T.: Vagal afferent discharge from mechanoreceptors in different regions of the ferret stomach. J. Physiol., *298*:513, 1980.

80. Andrews, P.L.R., Grundy, D., and Lawes, I.N.C.: The role of the vagus and splanchnic nerves in the regulation of intragastric pressure in the ferret. J. Physiol., *307*:401, 1980.

81. Andrews, P.L.R., and Lawes, I.N.C.: Interactions between splanchnic and vagus nerves in the control of mean intragastric pressure in the ferret. J. Physiol., *351*:473, 1984.

82. Andrews, P.L.R., Bingham, S., and Wood, K.L.: A comparison of the effects of vagotomy and GABA$_B$ receptor agonist on gastric corpus pressure in the ferret. J. Physiol., *378*:18P, 1986.

83. Andrews, P.L.R., and Wood, K.L.: The effects of chemical and mechanical stimuli applied to the gastric antral mucosa on corpus motility in the anesthetized ferret. J. Physiol., *348*:63, 1984.

84. Andrews, P.L.R., Grundy, D., and Scratcherd, T.: Reflex excitation of antral motility induced by gastric distension in the ferret. J. Physiol., *298*: 79, 1980.

85. Beyerman, H.C., et al.: On the instability of secretin. Life Sci., *29*:885, 1981.

86. Daniel, P.M., and Henderson, J.R.: Circulation in the islets of Langerhans. J. Physiol., *275*: 10P, 1978.

87. Henderson, J.R.: Why the islets of Langerhans? Lancet, *2*:469, 1969.

88. Audy, G., and Kerly, M.: The content of glycogenolytic factor in pancreas from different species. Biochem. J., *52*:77, 1952.

89. Poddar, S.: Gross and microscopic anatomy of the biliary tract of the ferret. Acta Anat. (Basel), *97*:121, 1977.

90. Scratcherd, T., Syme, G., and Wynne, R.D.A.: The release of cholecystokinin-pancreozymin from the isolated jejunum of the ferret. *In* Stimulus-Secretion Coupling in the GI Tract, p. 341. Edited by R.M. Case, and H. Goebell. MTP Press, 1976.

91. Greenwood, B., and Davison, J.S.: Role of extrinsic and intrinsic nerves in the relationship between intestinal motility and transmural potential difference in the anaesthetized ferret. Gastroenterology, *89*:1286, 1985.

92. Clarke, R.M., and Hardy, R.N.: Structural changes in the small intestine associated with the uptake of polyvinyl pyrrolidine by the young ferret, rabbit, guinea-pig, cat and chicken. J. Physiol., *209*:669, 1970.

93. Carlile, A.E., and Beck, F.: The effect of cortisone acetate on the structure and function of the ileum in the ferret. J. Anat., *129*:879, 1979.

94. Hoare, P., and Messer, M.: Studies on disaccharidase activities of the small intestine of the domestic cat and other carnivorous mammals. Comp. Biochem. Physiol., *24*:717, 1968.

95. Collman, P.I., Grundy, D., and Scratcherd, T.: Vagal influences on the jejunal "minute rhythm" in the anaesthetised ferret. J. Physiol., *345*:65, 1983.

96. Poddar, S., and Jacob, S.: Mucosubstances in the colonic goblet cells of the ferret. Acta Histochem. (Jena), 68:279, 1981.

97. Bueno, L., Fioramonti, J., and More, J.: Is there a functional large intestine in the ferret? Experientia, 27:275, 1981.

98. Collman, P.I., Grundy, D., and Scratcherd, T.: Vagal control of colonic motility in the anesthetized ferret: Evidence for a non-cholinergic excitatory innervation. J. Physiol., 348:35, 1984.

99. Scratcherd, T., Grundy, D., and Collman, P.I.: Evidence for a non-cholinergic excitatory innervation in the control of colonic motility. Arch. Int. Pharmacodyn. Ther., 280:164, 1986.

100. Bleavins, M.R., and Aulerich, R.J.: Feed consumption and food passage time in mink (*Mustela vison*) and European ferrets (*Mustela putorius furo*). Lab. Anim. Sci., 31:268, 1981.

101. Florczyk, A.P., Schurig, J.E., and Bradner, W.T.: Cisplatin-induced emesis in the ferret: A new animal model. Cancer Treat. Rep., 66:187, 1982.

102. Schurig, J.E., Florczyk, A.P., Rose, W.C., and Bradner, W.T.: Antiemetic activity of butorphanol against cisplatin-induced emesis in ferrets and dogs. Cancer Treat. Rep., 66:1831, 1982.

103. Andrews, P.L.R., Hawthorn, N.J., and Sanger, G.J.: The effect of abdominal visceral nerve lesions and a novel 5-HT M-receptor antagonist on cytotoxic- and radiation-induced emesis in the ferret. J. Physiol., 382:48P, 1987.

104. Andrews, P.L.R., Davis, C.J., and Hawthorn, J.: Abdominal vagotomy modifies the emetic response to radiation in the ferret. J. Physiol., 378:16P, 1986.

105. Andrews, P.L.R., Bingham, S., and Davis, C.J.: Retching evoked by stimulation of abdominal vagal afferents in the anesthetized ferret. J. Physiol., 358:103P, 1985.

106. Miner, W.D., and Sanger, G.J.: Inhibition of cisplatin-induced vomiting by selective 5-hydroxytryptamine M-receptor antagonism. Br. J. Pharmacol., 88:497, 1986.

107. Costall, B., et al.: 5-Hydroxytryptamine M-receptor antagonism to prevent cisplatin-induced emesis. Neuropharmacology, 25:959, 1986.

108. Lee, E.J., Moore, W.E., Fryer, H.C., and Minocha, H.C.: Hematological and serum chemistry profiles of ferrets (*Mustela putorius furo*). Lab. Anim., 16:133, 1982.

109. Rotenberg, S., and Jorgensen, G. Some hematological indices in mink. Nord. Vet. Med., 23:361, 1971.

110. Fox, H.: Disease in Captured Wild Mammals and Birds. Philadelphia, J.B. Lippincott, 1923.

111. Carpenter, J.W., and Hill, E.F.: Hematological values for the Siberian ferret (*Mustela eversmanni*). J. Zool. Exp. Med., 10:126, 1979.

112. Flatman, P.W., and Andrews, P.L.R.: Cation and ATP content of ferret red cells. Comp. Biochem. Physiol., 74A:939, 1983.

113. Flatman, P.W.: Sodium and potassium transport in ferret red cells. J. Physiol., 341:545, 1983.

114. Seal, U.S.: Carnivora systematics: A study of hemoglobins. Comp. Biochem. Physiol., 31:799, 1969.

115. Davis: Personal communication.

116. Hawthorn: Personal communication.

117. Cryer, A., and Sawyer, A.M.: A comparison of the composition and apolipoprotein content of the lipoproteins isolated from human and ferret (*Mustela putorius furo L.*) serum. Comp. Biochem. Physiol., 61B:151, 1978.

118. Kenyon, A.J., Howard, E., and Buko, L.: Hypergammaglobulinemia in ferrets with lympoproliferative lesions (Aleutian disease). Am. J. Vet. Res., 28:1167, 1967.

119. Desmukh, D.R., and Shope, T.C.: Arginine requirements and ammonia toxicity in ferrets. J. Nutr., 113:1664, 1983.

120. Lockard, B.I.: The forebrain of the ferret. Lab. Anim. Sci., 35:216, 1985.

121. Pontenagel, V.T., and Schmidt, U.: Untersuchungen zur Leistungsfahigkeit des Gesichtssinnes beim Frettchen. Z. Sauget., 45:376, 1980.

122. Apfelbach, R., and Wester, U.: The quantitative effect of visual and tactile stimuli on prey-catching behavior of ferrets. Behav. Proc., 2:187, 1977.

123. Thompson, A.P.D.: Relation of retinal stimulation to estrus in the ferret. J. Physiol., 113:425, 1951.

124. Gewalt, W.: Beitrage zur Kenntnis des Optischen differenzierungsvermogens einiger Musteliden mit besonderer Berucksightigung des Farbensehens. Zool. Beitr., 5:117, 1959.

125. Braekevelt, C.R.: Photoreceptor fine structure in the domestic ferret. Anat. Anz., 153:33, 1983.

126. Braekevelt, C.R.: Fine structure of the retinal epithelium, Bruch's membrane and choriocapillaris in the domestic ferret. Acta Anat., 113:117, 1982.

127. Greiner, J.V., and Weidman, T.A.: Histogenesis of the ferret retina. Exp. Eye Res., 33:315, 1983.

128. Vitek, D.J., Schall, J.D., and Leventhal, A.G.: Morphology, central projections and dendritic field orientation of retinal ganglion cells in the ferret. J. Comp. Neurol., 241:1, 1985.

129. Kageyama, G.H., and Wong-Riley, M.T.T.: The histochemical localization of cytochrome oxidase in the retina, and lateral geniculate nucleus of the ferret, cat and monkey with particular reference to retinal mosaics and on/off center visual channels. J. Neurosci., 41:2445, 1984.

130. Henderson, Z., Morgan, J., and Thompson, I.D.: Retinal projections to the lateral geniculate nucleus in the albino and pigmented ferret: An anatomical and physiological study. J. Physiol., 345:119P, 1983.

131. Guillery, R.W.: An abnormal retinogeniculate projection in the albino ferret. Brain Res., 33:482, 1971.

132. Linden, D.C., Guillery, R.W., and Cucchiaro, J.: The dorsal lateral geniculate nucleus of the normal ferret and its postnatal development. J. Comp. Neurol., 203:189, 1980.

133. Stryker, M.P., and Zahs, K.R.: On-and-off sublaminae in the lateral geniculate nucleus of the ferret. J. Comp. Neurol., 10:1943, 1983.

134. Le Vay, S., and McConnell, S.K.: On-and-off layers in the lateral geniculate nucleus of the mink. Nature, 300:350, 1982.

135. Le Gros Clark, W.E., McKeown, T., and Zuckerman, S.: Visual pathways concerned in gonadal stimulation in ferrets. Proc. R. Soc. Lond. [Biol.], 126:449, 1939.

136. Thorpe, P.A., and Herbert, J.: The accessory optic system of the ferret. J. Comp. Neurol., 170:295, 1976.

137. Thorpe, P.A., and Herbert, J.: The effect of lesions of the accessory optic tract terminal nuclei on the gonadal response to light in ferrets. Neuroendocrinology, 22:250, 1976.

138. LaMantia, A.S., and Guillery, R.W.: The effects of binocular enucleation on the development of the dorsal lateral geniculate nucleus of the ferret. Soc. Neurosci. Abstr., 8:814, 1982.

139. Bang, B.G., and Bang, F.B.: A comparative study of the vertebrate nasal chamber in relation to upper respiratory infections. Comparative morphology of the nasal chambers of three commonly used laboratory animals: Chicken, rat and ferret. Bull. Johns Hopkins Hosp., 104:107, 1959.

140. Dennis, B.J., and Kerr, D.I.: Olfactory bulb connections with the basal rhinencephalon in the ferret: An evoked potential and neuroanatomical study. J. Comp. Neurol., 159:129, 1975.

141. Apfelbach, R.: A sensitive phase for the development of olfactory preference in ferrets. Z. Sauget., 43:289, 1978.

142. Moore, D.R., Semple, M.N., and Addison, P.D.: Some acoustic properties of neurons in the ferret inferior colliculus. Brain Res., 269:69, 1983.

143. Hutchings, M.E., and King, A.J.: A map of auditory space in the ferret superior colliculus. J. Physiol., 358:31P, 1985.

144. Moore, D.R.: Late onset of hearing in the ferret. Brain Res., 253:309, 1982.

145. Von Solmsen, E., and Apfelbach, R.: Brutpflegewirksame Komponenten im Weinen neonater Frettchen. Z. Tierphysiol. Tiernahr. Futtermittelkd., 50:337, 1979.

146. Carter, D.S.: Studies of pineal and hypothalamic 5-HT in the ferret. Brain Res., 224:95, 1981.

147. Yates, C.A., and Herbert, J.: The effect of different photoperiods on circadian 5-hydroxytryptaminergic rhythms in regional brain areas and their modulation by pinealectomy, melatonin or estradiol. Brain Res., 176:311, 1979.

148. Fuller, R.W., and Hemrick-Luecke, S.K.: Species differences in epinephrine concentration and norepinephrine N-methyltransferase activity in hypothalamus and brain stem. Comp. Biochem. Physiol., 74C:47, 1983.

149. Elias, S.A., and Taylor, A.: Direct projections of jaw proprioceptor first-order afferents to the cerebellar cortex in the ferret. J. Physiol., 353:42P, 1984.

150. Taylor, A., and Elias, S.A.: Interaction of periodontal and jaw elevator spindle afferents in the cerebellum—sensory calibration. Brain Behav. Evol., 25:157, 1984.

151. Lou, J.S., and Bloedel, J.R.: The responses of simultaneously recorded Purkinje cells to perturbations of the step cycle in the walking ferret: A study using a new analytical method—the real time postsynaptic response. Brain Res., 365:340, 1986.

152. Eidelberg, E., Straehley, D., Erspamer, R., and Watkins, C.J.: Relationship between residual hindlimb-assisted locomotion and surviving axons after incomplete spinal cord injuries. Exp. Neurol., 56:312, 1977.

153. Odekunle, A., and Bower, A.J.: Brain stem connections of vagal afferent nerves in the ferret: An autoradiographic study. J. Anat., 140:461, 1985.

154. Andrews, P.L.R., Fussey, I.V., and Scratcherd, T.: The spontaneous discharge in abdominal vagal efferents in the dog and ferret. Pflugers Arch., 387:55, 1980.

155. Blackshaw, L.A., Grundy, D., and Scratcherd, T.: Responses of vagal efferent units modulated by gastrointestinal stimuli to central vagal stimulation. J. Physiol., 378:15P, 1986.

156. Andrews, P.L.R., Davis, C.J., Grahame-Smith, D.G., and Leslie, R.: Increase in [^{3}H]-2-deoxyglucose uptake in the ferret area postrema produced by apomorphine administration or electrical stimulation of the abdominal vagus. J. Physiol., 382:187P, 1987.

157. Majkowski, J., Lee, M.H., Kozlowski, P.B., and Haddard, R.: EEG and seizure threshold in normal and lissencephalic ferrets. Brain Res., 307:29, 1984.

158. Johnson, M.V., Haddad, R., Carman-Young, A., and Coyle, J.T.: Neurotransmitter chemistry of lissencephalic cortex in ferrets by fetal treatment with methylazoxymethanol acetate. Dev. Brain Res., 4:285, 1982.

159. Rarey, K.E., Rush, N.L., Davis, J.A., and Desmukh, D.R.: Altered auditory brain stem-evoked responses in the ferret model for Reye's syndrome. Int. J. Pediatr. Otorhinolaryngol., 7: 221, 1984.

160. Braver, R.W., et al.: Comparative physiology of high pressure neurological syndrome—compression rate effects. J. Appl. Physiol., 46:128, 1979.

161. Cameron, A.R., and Coburn, R.F.: Electrical and anatomic characteristics of cell of ferret paratracheal ganglion. Am. J. Physiol., 246: C450, 1984.

162. Baker, D.G., McDonald, D.M., Basbaum, C.B., and Mitchell, R.A.: The architecture of nerves and ganglia of the ferret trachea as revealed by acetylcholinesterase histochemistry. J. Comp. Neurol., 246:513, 1986.

163. Andrews, P.L.R., Harris, P.J., and Mackay, T.W.: Recordings of neural activity in the direct renal nerve of the anesthetized ferret. J. Physiol., 346:11P, 1984.

164. Andrews, P.L.R., Harris, P.J., and Mackay, T.W.: Physiological and anatomical studies of the innervation of the ferret kidney. J. Physiol., 330:90P, 1982.

165. Elliott, T.R.: The innervation of the bladder and urethra. J. Physiol., 35:367, 1906.

166. Baker, D.G., Basbaum, C.B., Herbert, D.A., and Mitchell, R.A.: Transmission in airway ganglia of ferrets: Inhibition by norepinephrine. Neurosci. Lett., 41:139, 1983.

167. Skoogh, B.E., Holtzman, M.J., Sheller, J.R., and Nadel, J.A.: Barbiturates depress the vagal motor pathway to ferret trachea at the ganglia. J. Appl. Physiol., 53:253 1982.

168. Blackshaw, L.A., Grundy, D., and Scratcherd T.: Discharge characteristics of gastric mechanoreceptors during contraction and relaxation of the ferret corpus. J. Physiol., 378:17P, 1986.

169. Rieger, D., and Murphy, B.D.: Episodic fluctuation in plasma testosterone and dihydrotestosterone in male ferrets during the breeding season. J. Reprod. Fertil., 51:511, 1977.

170. Baum, M.J., and Goldfoot, D.A.: Effect of amygdaloid lesions on gonadal maturation in male and female ferrets. Am. J. Physiol., 228:1646, 1975.

171. Neal, J., Murphy, B.D., and Monger, W.H.: Reproduction in the male ferret. Gonadal activity during the annual cycle, recrudescence and maturation. Biol. Reprod., 17:380, 1977.

172. Erskine, M.S., and Baum, M.J.: Plasma concentrations of testosterone and dihydrotestosterone during perinatal development in male and female ferrets. Endocrinology, 111:762, 1982.

173. Heap, R.B., and Hammond, J.: Plasma progesterone levels in pregnant and pseudopregnant ferrets. J. Reprod. Fertil., 39:149, 1974.

174. Daniel, J.C.: Plasma progesterone levels before and at the time of implantation in the ferret. J. Reprod. Fertil., 48:437, 1976.

175. Donovan, B.T., Matson, L.C., and Kilpatrick, M.J.: Effect of exposure to long days on the secretion of estradiol, estrone, progesterone, testosterone, androstenedione, cortisol, and follicle stimulating hormone in intact and spayed ferrets. J. Endocrinol., 99:369, 1983.

176. Gaunt, R., Remington, J.W., and Edelmann, A.: Effect of progesterone and other hormones on liver glycogen. Proc. Soc. Exp. Biol. Med., 41:429, 1939.

177. Donovan, B.T., and Ter Haar, M.B.: Effects of luteinizing hormone and releasing hormone on plasma follicle stimulating hormone and luteinizing hormone levels in the ferret. J. Endocrinol., 73:37, 1977.

178. Ryan, K.D., Sieger, S.F., and Robinson, S.L.: Influence of day length and endocrine status on luteinizng hormone secretion in intact and ovariectomized adult ferrets. Biol. Reprod., 33:690, 1985.

179. Donovan, B.T., and Ter Haar, M.B.: Stimulation of the hypothalamus and FSH and LH secretion in the ferret. Neuroendocrinology, 23:268, 1977.

180. Donovan, B.T., and Gledhill, B.: Half-life of FSH and LH in the ferret. Acta Endocrinol., 105:14, 1984.

181. Holmes, R.L.: The adrenal glands of the ferret. J. Anat., 95:325, 1961.

182. Moffat, D.B., and Fourman, J.: Ectopic glomeruli in the human and animal kidney. Anat. Rec., 149:1, 1964.

183. Andrews, P.L.R., and Tansey, E.M.: The reaction of the ferret bladder to adrenalin: A modern demonstration of an experiment by T.R. Elliott and H.H. Dale. J. Physiol., 382:5P, 1987.

184. Moss, H.E., and Burnstock, G.: A comparative study of electrical field stimulation of the guinea pig, ferret and marmoset urinary bladder. Eur. J. Pharmacol., 114:311, 1985.

chapter 5

NUTRITION

D. E. McLain

J. A. Thomas

J. G. Fox

As a contemporary laboratory carnivore, the ferret (*Mustela putorius furo*) has found increasing application in such diverse biomedical research areas as cardiology,[1–3] ophthalmology,[4–6] pulmonary physiology and pathology,[7–9] virology,[10–12] bacteriology,[13–15] toxicology,[16–18] and teratology.[19–22] An extensive literature review,[23] however, indicates a paucity of controlled research for establishing nutrient requirements for this species. Experiments designed to establish the minimum nutrient requirements for the ferret are needed to increase the efficiency and validity of using this animal as a model for diverse biomedical applications. The inadvertent use of nutritionally deficient animals or improperly formulated diets with nutrient concentrations that are too high (or too low) may result in erroneous findings. Moreover, the extrapolation of such findings to other animals or humans could have dire consequences.

Some information concerning ferret nutrition and nutrition practices useful to biomedical research can be obtained from commercial formulations and from natural ingredient and purified (open formula) ferret diets.[24] Although nutrient concentrations of these dietary formulations are based on data from relatively small numbers of studies designed to determine nutrient requirements of the mink (*Mustela vison*) or related carnivora, most are patterned after apparently successful natural ingredient ferret diets or estimated from studies in which dietary nutrient concentrations produced acceptable animal performance. Regardless of the method used for formulation, nutrient levels contained in commercially available ferret diets are probably excessive, and can only be viewed as apparent requirements for normal animals maintained in conventional environments. Specific nutrient requirements for growth, maintenance, or reproduction cannot be expressed because no data are available. Nutrient analyses of diets that promote optimal growth and reproductive function are necessary.

For certain nutrients, clinically observable conditions have been shown to be related to the chronic ingestion of either a deficient diet or excessive amounts of the substituents. Unfortunately, the overall incidence of nutrient deficiencies or toxicities in the ferret is also largely unknown, and few syndromes or constellation of indicators of susceptibility have been identified. Several of these dietary imbalances will be briefly reviewed; for other nutritional imbalances it may be assumed that the ferret responds to nutri-

TABLE 5–1. COMPOSITION OF NATURAL INGREDIENT FERRET DIET*

Ingredient	Approximate Weight per Batch (lb)†
Wayne dog food cereal	100
Agway dog food cereal	50
Beef tripe	100
Beef lung	50
Beef liver	10
Cod liver oil (fortified)	1
Water	(varies)

* Courtesy of Gilman Marshall, Marshall Research Animals, North Rose, NY.

† Total batch weight is approximately 1000 lbs. Dry ingredients are added to a mechanical mixer from bags or cans; water is added until desired consistency is achieved.

TABLE 5–2. NUTRIENT ANALYSIS OF NATURAL INGREDIENT FERRET DIET*

Nutrient	Analysis	Units†
Protein (N $\times$ 6.25)	9.50	%
Moisture	73.90	%
Fat	7.40	%
Ash	2.00	%
Crude fiber	0.60	%
Carbohydrates	6.60	%
Calories	131.00	calories/100 g
Vitamins		
Vitamin A	2190.00	IU/100 g
Vitamin C, total	1.00	mg/100 g
Vitamin D	150.00	IU/100 g
Vitamin E	1.43	IU/100 g
Thiamin	0.22	mg/100 g
Riboflavin (B_2)	0.25	mg/100 g
Pyridoxine HCl (B_6)	0.20	mg/100 g
Niacin	2.10	mg/100 g
Vitamin B_{12}	6.40	µg/100 g
Folic acid	36.00	µg/100 g
Minerals		
Calcium	0.35	%
Phosphorus	0.29	%
Potassium	0.15	%
Magnesium	0.55	%
Sodium	0.12	%
Aluminum	16.41	ppm
Barium	2.00	ppm
Iron	69.97	ppm
Strontium	3.12	ppm
Boron	1.15	ppm
Copper	3.15	ppm
Zinc	27.39	ppm
Manganese	14.13	ppm
Chromium	0.44	ppm

* McLain, D.E., and Roe, D.A.: Nutrient composition of a natural ferret diet and the reproductive response to several purified diet formulations. Fed. Proc., *43A*:1318, 1983.

† Units are expressed in wet weight of diet.

TABLE 5–3. AMINO ACID COMPOSITION OF CRUDE PROTEIN FROM A NATURAL INGREDIENT FERRET DIET COMPARED TO VARIOUS SOURCES OF REFINED PROTEIN (mg Amino Acid/g Nitrogen)*

Amino Acid	Crude Protein	Casein	Lactalbumin	Wheat Gluten
Aspartic acid	470	531	792	192†
Threonine	190	340	390	167†
Serine	277	408	331	286
Glutamic acid	944	1730	1197	2452
Proline	445	812	340†	865
Glycine	556	137†	154†	205†
Alanine	435	223†	349†	149†
Valine	298	442	335	226
Cystine	53	79	178	163
Methionine	92	206	188	122
Isoleucine	226	374	363	219†
Leucine	473	651	838	409†
Tyrosine	155	445	260	215
Phenylalanine	231	376	258	331
Lysine	354	585	682	93†
Histidine	144	179	117†	115†
Arginine	396	242†	213†	215†
Ornithine	23			
NH$_3$	53	121	97	238
Kjeldahl N (%)	5.82	13.50	12.70	13.66

* McLain, D.E., and Roe, D.A.: Nutrient composition of a natural ferret diet and the reproductive response to several purified diet formulations. Fed. Proc., *43A*:1318, 1983.

† Deficient amount relative to the reference natural ingredient diet amino acid level.

ent deficiencies and toxicities in a manner analogous to that of other species.

AVAILABLE DIETS

Various types of dietary formulations are commercially available for the ferret.

NATURAL INGREDIENT FORMULATIONS

The greatest economic gain for commercial ferret breeders is realized by maximizing the reproductive performance of the colony while minimizing incapacitating disease processes. Astute animal husbandry may include the implementation of health maintenance programs to control epizootic and other communica-ble diseases, but a sound nutritional program is essential. In this respect, one of the nation's largest ferret breeding facilities, Marshall Farms (MF) USA,* has applied over 50 years experience in natural ingredient dietary formulation toward the optimization of reproductive performance. Their success is measured by the fact that primiparous females in their colony whelp an average 10.3 ± 0.2 kits per litter, successfully wean 80% of these, and produce 3 or 4 litters per year.[19] Because natural ingredient diets are more palatable to the ferret than purified or other commercial formulations,[21] this superior efficacy may be a result of increased consumption patterns. Typical diets (Table 5–1) are high in moisture and derive substantial protein from raw meat. Exclusion of cere-

---

* North Rose, N.Y.

als from natural ingredient diets may make it necessary to fortify the ration with a vitamin and mineral supplement.

PURIFIED FORMULATIONS

Ferret requirements for specific nutrients can eventually be determined by depletion-repletion studies using purified or chemically defined diets. To facilitate these investigations, a detailed analysis of the MF natural ingredient diet has been performed.[21] Table 5–2 lists the reported concentrations of 31 macro- and micronutrients as determined by current analytic methods[25] to be contained in the MF diet. The amino acid profile of MF crude protein (Table 5–3) has also been

determined analytically,[21] and levels of saturated and unsaturated fats and essential fatty acids were calculated[21] from food composition tables.[26] Micronutrient levels not determined in this analytic study were extrapolated from a literature review of the nutrient requirements for other carnivora (Table 5–4).[27–30] Requirements determined by extrapolation were selected primarily at levels representing the geometric mean (GM = antilog $\times$ Σ log n/n) for other species while ensuring optimum balance within the total mixture. Nutrient data compiled in this way are presented below (see Table 5–5). Controlled feeding experiments with this purified ferret diet have not yet been performed, but preliminary findings suggest that flavoring agents may be needed to increase diet palatability.

TABLE 5–4. NUTRIENT REQUIREMENTS OF DIFFERENT CARNIVORES USED FOR EXTRAPOLATION AND COMPARISON OF DIETARY NUTRIENT LEVELS FOR THE FERRET (per 1000 kcal)

Nutrient	Cat*	Dog	Fox	Mink	Mink	Geometric Mean	Ferret
Vitamin A (IU $\times$ 10^3)	2.50	1.25	0.60	0.66	3.00	1.30	16.72
Vitamin D (IU $\times$ 10^3)	0.25	0.13	—†	—	0.30	0.21	1.15
Vitamin E (IU)	20.00	12.50	—	6.25	10.00	11.18	10.92
Thiamin (mg)	1.25	0.25	0.25	0.30	0.50	0.41	1.67
Riboflavin (mg)	1.25	0.55	0.65	0.38	1.00	0.70	1.91
Pantothenate (mg)	2.50	2.50	2.00	1.50	2.00	2.06	—
Niacin (mg)	11.25	2.85	2.50	5.00	10.00	5.26	16.04
Pyridoxine (mg)	1.00	0.25	0.50	0.28	0.50	0.44	1.53
Folate (mg)	0.25	0.05	0.05	0.13	0.25	0.11	0.27
Biotin (μg)	12.50	2.50	—	—	6.30	6.82	—
B$_{12}$ (μg)	5.00	6.00	—	—	10.00	7.00	48.84
Choline (g)	0.50	0.30	—	—	0.25	0.34	—
Calcium (g)	2.50	2.75	1.50	1.00	1.40	1.70	2.65
Phosphorus (g)	2.00	2.25	1.50	1.00	0.75	1.40	2.19
Potassium (g)	0.75	1.50	—	—	1.45	1.20	1.14
Sodium (g)	0.49	1.08	0.49	0.49	0.66	0.61	0.92
Chloride (g)	0.76	1.67	0.76	0.76	1.02	0.94	—
Magnesium (g)	0.13	0.10	—	—	0.10	0.11	4.20
Iron (mg)	25.00	15.00	—	—	51.75	26.90	53.40
Copper (mg)	1.25	1.83	—	—	0.75	1.20	2.40
Manganese (mg)	2.50	1.25	—	—	14.23	3.54	10.78
Zinc (mg)	7.50	12.50	—	—	1.15	4.76	20.90
Iodine (mg)	0.25	0.39	—	—	6.13	0.84	—
Selenium (μg)	25.00	28.00	—	—	—	26.50	—

* Data presented here were obtained and calculated from various sources: cat, National Research Council[29]; dog, National Research Council[27]; fox and mink, Warner, et al.[30] and National Research Council[29]; and ferret, Table 5–2.

† Dashed lines indicate undetermined or unreported requirements or dietary levels.

TABLE 5–5. NUTRIENT COMPOSITION OF DIETS THAT APPEAR ADEQUATE FOR FERRETS*

Nutrient	Unit	Unrefined Natural Ingredient†	McLain-Marshall Purified‡	Ralston Purina 5280§	Agway Feed‖	Ralston Purina Cat Chow#
Protein	%	36.40	36.40	47.20	35.00	34.10
Fat, total, including linoleate	%	28.40	28.40	15.70	18.20	10.50
Linoleic acid	%				1.40	1.40
Carbohydrate	%	25.30	22.10	22.70	35.70	41.80
Fiber	%	2.30	3.00	4.30	2.90	5.10
Ash	%	7.66	10.10	10.10	8.20	8.50
Energy	kcal/g	5.02	4.90	4.25	4.47	3.98
L-Amino acids						
Arginine	%	2.30	3.47	2.44	2.23	—
Glycine	%	3.24	1.85	2.08	3.21	—
Histidine	%	0.84	2.42	1.04	0.63	—
Isoleucine	%	0.84	2.42	1.04	0.63	—
Leucine	%	2.75	8.79	4.09	2.34	—
Lysine	%	2.06	7.90	2.76	1.87	—
Methionine	%	0.54	3.08	0.91	0.47	—
Cystine	%	0.31	1.07	0.78	0.49	—
Phenylalanine	%	1.34	5.08	2.00	1.34	—
Serine	%	1.61	5.51	—	1.67	—
Tyrosine	%	0.90	6.01	1.30	0.98	—
Threonine	%	1.11	4.59	1.67	1.30	—
Tryptophan	%	—	—	0.40	0.32	—
Valine	%	1.73	5.97	2.39	1.22	—
Minerals						
Calcium	%	1.34	1.59	2.02	1.44	1.14
Chloride	%	—	0.89	0.72	—	-0.74
Magnesium	%	2.11	0.17	0.17	0.28	0.16
Phosphorus	%	1.11	1.23	1.19	1.11	0.91
Potassium	%	0.57	0.72	0.67	0.83	0.74
Sodium	%	0.46	0.57	0.72	0.39	0.57
Sulfur	%	—	—	—	—	—
Chromium	mg/kg	1.69	0.16	—	—	—
Cobalt	mg/kg	—	—	1.35	0.80	—
Copper	mg/kg	12.07	15.10	27.64	17.78	13.64
Fluoride	mg/kg	—	—	—	—	—
Iodine	mg/kg	—	3.26	5.06	2.67	1.70
Iron	mg/kg	268.00	338.56	382.02	289.00	284.10
Manganese	mg/kg	54.00	67.67	51.69	45.33	51.14
Molybdenum	mg/kg	—	—	—	—	—
Selenium	mg/kg	—	0.30	—	0.20	—
Vanadium	mg/kg	—	—	—	—	—
Zinc	mg/kg	105.00	131.20	214.61	116.67	102.27
Vitamins						
A	IU/kg	83910.00	20000.00	34830.00	18164.44	11364.00
D	IU/kg	5750.00	2018.75	7530.00	1222.22	1818.00
E	IU/kg	54.80	200.00	247.19	110.56	11.36
K_1 equiv.	mg/kg	—	6.25	3.37	0.98	0.57
Biotin	mg/kg	—	0.20	0.22	0.24	0.09
Choline	mg/kg	—	2500.00	2697.00	2444.44	2500.00
Folacin	mg/kg	1.38	2.50	13.48	1.11	1.14
Niacin	mg/kg	80.50	80.50	71.91	65.16	85.23
Calcium pantothenate	mg/kg	—	18.75	23.60	14.94	22.73
Riboflavin	mg/kg	9.60	12.50	18.76	8.33	5.68
Thiamin	mg/kg	8.40	16.80	97.75	21.59	5.68
Vitamin B6	mg/kg	7.70	7.65	7.87	8.21	5.68
Vitamin B12	mg/kg	0.25	0.14	0.13	0.04	0.02

* All diets expressed as 100% dry matter basis. Dashes indicate undetermined or unreported levels.

† Courtesy of Gilman Marshall, Marshall Farms, North Rose, NY.

‡ ICN Nutritional Biochemicals, Cleveland, OH.

§ Ralston Purina, St. Louis, MO.

‖ Courtesy of Dr. Merle Stillions, Agway, Inc., Ithaca, NY.

Ralston Purina, St. Louis, MO. Carbohydrate calculated by difference.

COMMERCIAL FORMULATIONS

Commercial ferret diets are available that include least cost ration formulations marketed by at least two leading animal feed suppliers (Table 5–5), including the Ralston Purina Ferret Chow 5280, which was developed by Dr. Damon Shelton* in collaboration with several investigators maintaining in-house colonies of ferrets. Although growth, maintenance, and reproduction data have not been published with respect to the nutritional adequacy of Ralston's 5280, the ration appears to be adequate for maintenance of adult animals.

Agway's Marshall Ferret Diet (Table 5–5) was formulated by Dr. Merle Stillions† in collaboration with Marshall Farms USA. Although MF has realized considerable success with their natural ingredient formulations, they have recently elected to feed the Agway diet for maintenance of their colony. The MF natural ingredient diet (or variations), however, is still fed to pregnant and lactating jills as well as to kits up to the age of 12 weeks. Controlled feeding studies using the Agway Ferret Diet are unavailable, but the diet appears to be adequate for maintenance of juvenile and adult animals.

Cat chows are frequently used as ferret chow. Table 5–5 contrasts a typical cat chow (Ralston Purina) with the other more species-specific formulations. The efficacy of cat chows in promoting optimum nutrition in the ferret has not been studied systematically.

DIETARY NUTRIENTS

Delineation of the ferrets' requirements for adequate nutrition has not kept pace with its increasing number of scientific applications. The following general

---

* Ralston Purina, St. Louis, MO.
† Agway, Inc., Ithaca, NY.

guidelines, however, enumerate the nutrients and approximate amounts necessary to promote satisfactory growth and well-being in this species. Because manipulations in nutrition (exogenous or endogenous) may be involved in the pathogenesis of many disease states, the need to update and refine these recommendations constantly is especially apparent.

PROTEIN

In establishing the ferret's protein requirements for the different phases of the life cycle (i.e., growth, maintenance, and reproduction), three factors must be considered: (1) energy concentration of the diet; (2) amino acid composition of the protein; and, (3) digestibility of the protein. Because food intake is related to the energy content of the diet, protein is most properly expressed as the amount of protein with the proper amino acid balance used per unit of diet net energy, or as a calorie-to-protein ratio.

Allen and colleagues[31] and Sinclair and associates[32] have studied the protein and energy requirements of mink (*Mustela vison*) in terms of calorie-to-protein ratios (kcal/% protein) and caloric density. They found that the optimum for growth of male kits up to 16 weeks of age was a calorie-to-protein ratio of approximately 13 and a caloric density of approximately 550 kcal/100 g feed (42% protein). After 16 weeks they suggested that the calorie-to-protein ratio can increase to 17 (36% protein) and possibly to 21 (26% protein). With growing puppies, Ontko and co-workers[33] also concluded that (based on weight gain, feed efficiency, and physical condition) protein requirements increased with increasing caloric density of the diet, and that adequate growth was apparent with a calorie-to-protein ratio of approximately 16.

Commercially available ferret diets listed in Table 5–5 offer calorie-to-protein ratios ranging from 9 (Purina 5280) to 14 (MF Diet). Based on the foregoing discussion, these diets would appear adequate for growth, but nutritional requirements for reproduction (i.e., gestation, lactation) cannot be discerned. In addition, the effect of high-protein (and high-fat) diets on the longevity of ferrets has not been examined.

FAT

Fat has been considered as an optional component of most animal diets, except as a source of essential fatty acids and for its facilitative role in the absorption of fat-soluble vitamins. Limited purified diet feeding trials with ferrets, however,[21] have identified other more subtle functions of this dietary macronutrient that may be especially applicable to carnivora. For example, most food fat occurs in the form of triglycerides. Although pure triglycerides are relatively tasteless, they absorb and retain flavors. In combination with other nutrients, the triglycerides also provide a diet texture that enhances palatability and delays gastric emptying, which may contribute to a feeling of satiety.

Dietary fat may also serve as a concentrated source of energy for the ferret. Because the energy concentration of digestible fat is 2.25 times the energy concentration of digestible carbohydrate or protein, however, substitution of fat for these other macronutrients may increase the energy density of the diet. Ferrets may respond by eating less of this high-energy diet (as compared to a lower energy diet), but the energy intake will be about the same. If the percentages of other macro- and micronutrients in the high-energy diet are not increased appropriately, the daily intake of energy may be sufficient but the intake of protein, minerals, and vitamins may be inadequate.

The minimum level of dietary fat depends on its fatty acid composition. Because fatty acids cannot be synthesized from other dietary components, linoleic, linolenic, and arachidonic acid are considered to be essential fatty acids and have a high propensity for growth.[34] Because arachidonic acid and γ-linolenic are not major components of natural fats, the effectiveness of dietary fat in preventing or reversing a fatty acid deficiency is usually related to its linoleic acid content.

Ferrets appear to be maintained successfully on commercially available diets ranging from 9 to 28% fat (Table 5–5), or 7 to 15% linoleic acid (relative to total fat). It should be noted, though, that the use of high concentrations of unsaturated fats may lead to rancidity and to destruction of other nutrients, such as vitamin E. In view of this, Harris and Embree[35] have recommended that the tocopherol:polyunsaturated fatty acid ratio (mg/g) be at least 0.6 (for all species). The National Research Council Committee on Animal Nutrition[27] has suggested a ratio of at least 0.5 to ensure that the needs for vitamin E are met.

Signs of a dietary fatty acid deficiency are difficult to detect in adult animals, but ferret kits would probably manifest skin lesions similar to those reported for young dogs.[36] Lesions include coarse, dry hair and desquamation. The epidermis may be edematous, with deranged keratinization; parakeratosis may become manifest with advanced deficiency. Resulting skin ulcerations are susceptible to infection.

CARBOHYDRATES

Although no critical studies have been made on the carbohydrate requirements of ferrets, it is probable that they can be maintained without carbohydrates as long as the diet furnishes adequate fat (and thus glycerol) or protein (containing glucogenic amino acids). It should be noted, however, that Naismith and Cursiter[37] found that weanling rats grew more slowly on a carbohydrate-free diet, and there was more carcass fat and less protein compared to rats consuming isocaloric amounts of a carbohydrate-containing diet.

Adult ferrets can efficiently utilize dextrin, maltose and glucose. Large amounts (>50% of diet calories) of sucrose may, however, result in measurable urinary sucrose and fructose levels. Poor reproductive performance has been demonstrated in female ferrets previously intubated with approximately 175 kcal sucrose/kg body weight/day from gestation day 15 through 35, suggesting that there may be low intestinal levels of sucrase and a limited ability to convert fructose to glucose in this species.[20] Carbohydrate composition of commercially available ferret diets ranges from 22 to 44% of total dry matter.

ENERGY

For maintenance, ferrets may consume between 200 to 300 kcal/kg body weight daily. Assuming a mean body weight of 1500 g, daily dry feed intake of diets listed in Table 5–5 may range from 40 to 60 g (MF Natural Ingredient) to 50 to 70 g (Ralston Purina 5280). For growth and reproduction, a ration with a caloric density close to 5000 kcal/kg diet may be necessary, and it is suggested that levels of protein and other essential nutrients be adjusted accordingly.

Depending on the degree of energy deficiency, retardation or cessation of growth may be accompanied by varying stages of emaciation. The fur may be dull and lack sheen, and the animals may appear lethargic. Milk yield may be reduced in lactating females. Conversely, excessive energy intake may lead to obesity in the ferret.

VITAMINS

No data are available concerning the vitamin requirements of ferrets. Common vitamin deficiency and toxicity signs observed with other species are outlined below, and the levels of individual vitamins contained in commercially available ferret diets are discussed.

Vitamin A

Assuming a caloric requirement of 250 kcal/kg body weight daily for maintenance, ferrets fed diets listed in Table 5–5 may consume 1000 (Agway Marshall Ferret Feed and Purified Diet) to 4200 (Natural Ingredient Diet) IU of vitamin A/kg body weight daily (Ralston 5280 Ferret Diet would deliver 2050 IU vitamin A). Plasma and liver vitamin A levels have not been determined in animals consuming these rations, but these dietary concentrations probably provide an excess of the daily requirement. Toxicity (hypervitaminosis A), however, was not observed in pregnant females consuming up to 4200 IU vitamin A/kg body weight daily.[21]

Feeding diets devoid of vitamin A may result in growth failure, night blindness, and muscular incoordination (particularly in the rear quarters). Eyes may be affected, with lenses becoming opaque and the conjunctivae encrusted. Metaplasia of epithelial tissues and fatty infiltration of the liver may also occur. It is not known if ferrets can convert carotene to vitamin A efficiently.

Vitamin D

Commercially available ferret diets may provide between 65 (Agway Marshall Ferret Feed) to 325 (Ralston 5280) IU vitamin D/kg body weight daily. As with other species, the ferret's requirement for vitamin D may depend on dietary concentrations of calcium and phosphorus or on the duration of exposure to ultraviolet light. Other factors include dietary calcium: phosphorus ratio, physiologic stage of development, and sex. Rachitic changes and abnormal bone development may occur when the diet is deficient in vitamin D, calcium, or phosphorus, especially when exposure to ultraviolet light is minimized.

Vitamin E

Yellow fat disease, fatty degeneration of the liver, or steatitis is a frequent complication of feeding diets containing rancid fat or high levels of unsaturated fatty acids. A tocopherol:polyunsaturated fatty acid ratio (mg:g) of at least 0.5 has been recommended[27] in most species to ensure that the needs for vitamin E are met. Commercial ferret diets exceed this ratio, and may provide between 3 (MF Natural Ingredient Diet) and 15 (Ralston 5280) IU vitamin E/kg body weight daily.

Vitamin E deficiency may result in a yellow discoloration of body fat, hemolytic anemia, anorexia, and a progressively impaired gait leading to paralysis.

Vitamin K

The metabolic need for vitamin K has not been established in the ferret, but it is likely that a dry diet concentration of 1.0 mg menadione/kg would sustain normal plasma prothrombin levels. A deficiency may result in hypoprothrombinemia and hemorrhage. Kernicterus and hemolytic anemia may be a manifestation of vitamin K toxicity.

Thiamin

Thiamin concentrations (mg/kg dry diet) of commercially available ferret diets (Table 5-5) range from 8.4 (MF Natural Ingredient Diet) to 97.8 (Ralston 5280). Signs of deficiency may include anorexia, vomiting, impaired locomotion, and cardiac hypertrophy with subsequent failure (see later discussion on dietary imbalances or toxicities). Death caused by depression of the respiratory center may occur with toxic doses, probably in excess of 200 mg/kg body weight.

Riboflavin

Riboflavin requirements for growth and fur production in mink are about 1.5 mg/kg of dry feed.[38] The needs for most other species are met with less than 3 mg/kg. Commercial ferret diets contain in excess of this amount, so signs of deficiency would not be anticipated. When manifested, however, acute deficiency may result in decreased respiratory rate, hypothermia, weakness, and coma. Chronic riboflavin deficiency may result in anorexia, muscular weakness, dermatitis, microcytic-hypochromic anemia, corneal vascularization-opacification, and reduced erythrocyte and urine riboflavin concentration.

Pyridoxine

Testes of mink fed diets devoid of vitamin B_6 become atrophic, aspermatic, and degenerative, while absorption sterility occurs in females.[39] One mg of vitamin B_6/kg dry matter may be sufficient to prevent deficiency signs, and commercially available ferret diets contain eight times this level.

Vitamin B_{12}

Uncomplicated vitamin B_{12} deficiency has not been described in the ferret, but a macrocytic hypochromic, macrocytic normochromic, normocytic hypochromic, or normocytic normochromic anemia might be manifested with deficient vitamin B_{12} intake. Commercially available ferret diets provide between 2 (Agway Marshall Ferret Feed) and 13 (MF Natural-Ingredient Diet) mg vitamin B_{12}/kg body weight daily.

Folacin

Intestinal bacterial synthesis of folic acid has not been studied in the ferret; commercially available rations range from 1 (Agway Marshall Ferret Feed) to 13 (Ralston 5280) mg/kg dry matter (Table 5–5). Folic acid at a level of 0.5 mg/kg of dry feed causes a remission of deficiency symptoms in mink, but levels below this amount have not been tested.[38] Folacin deficiency may result in erratic appetite, poor weight gain, glossitis, leukopenia, and hypochromic anemia with a tendency to microcytosis.

Biotin

Commercially available ferret diets provide approximately 200 μg biotin/kg dry matter, which may supply up to 10 μg/kg of body weight daily. This level is approximately twice the level required for optimum growth in dogs.[27] A deficiency may result in alopecia, hyperkeratosis, graying of fur, conjunctivitis, and fatty liver.

Niacin

The mink, like the cat, requires dietary niacin because it cannot metabolize sufficient precursor tryptophan to meet its niacin requirement.[40] The metabolic conversion of tryptophan to niacin has not been systematically studied in the ferret. Commercially available ferret diets provide 65 to 85 mg/kg dry diet, while 20 mg is tentatively stated as the requirement for mink. Signs of deficiency may include anorexia, profuse salivation, diarrhea, gastrointestinal inflammation, hemorrhagic necrosis, dehydration, and emaciation. High doses of nicotinic acid may produce vasodilation, pruritus, and cutaneous desquamation.

Pantothenic Acid

Calcium pantothenate is present at levels ranging from 15 (Agway Marshall Ferret Feed) to 24 (Ralston 5280) mg/kg dry diet. Requirements for the ferret are probably about 500 to 750 μg/kg body weight, based on the absence of deficiency signs in animals consuming the Agway Marshall Ferret Feed. Pantothenic acid deficiency in ferrets may result in poor appetite, slow growth, reduced blood cholesterol and total lipid levels, loss of conditioned reflexes, alopecia, vomiting, intermittent diarrhea, gastrointestinal disorders, convulsions, and coma.

Choline

In most species, the dietary requirement for choline is markedly affected by dietary protein concentration—more specifically, by the dietary concentration of methionine. Because both choline and methionine may serve as labile methyl donors in metabolism, the dietary supply of one tends to spare the need for the other. Unfortunately, this interaction has not been systematically studied in ferrets, so commercial diets are supplemented with approximately 2500 mg choline/kg dry matter. Plasma phosphatase activity and blood prothrombin times may be elevated following deficiency. There may be an increased alkalinization of urine and decreased ammonia excretion following toxicity.

Vitamin C

Ferrets are likely not to require an exogenous supply of vitamin C, and commercial feed suppliers do not supplement their formulations with this vitamin. Analysis of the MF natural ingredient diet (Table 7–2) indicated approximately 4 mg vitamin C/100 g dry diet.

MINERALS

No data are available concerning the mineral requirements of ferrets. Common mineral deficiency and toxicity signs observed with other species are outlined below. In addition, the levels of individual minerals contained in commercially available ferret diets are discussed.

Calcium and Phosphorus

Calcium and phosphorus requirements are closely related, and must be considered together. A calcium:phosphorus ratio of 1:2 (Agway Marshall Ferret Feed) to 1:7 (Ralston 5280) is found in commercial formulations. The minimum calcium and phosphorus levels may be on the order of 0.4 to 1.0% calcium and 0.4 to 0.8% phosphorus, respectively, as long as the proper ratio is maintained and adequate vitamin D is present. Diets high in calcium and low in vitamin D and phosphorus may produce difficulty in walking and enlargement of the bones. In addition, diets high in calcium and vitamin D may be associated with signs of renal impairment. Calcium deficiency may result in tetany and convulsion. In addition, hemorrhage, reproductive and lactation failures, spontaneous fractures, and altered requirements for other nutrients such as magnesium may occur. Low phosphorus intake may result in slowed growth, poor appetite, and osteomalacia in adult animals.

Iron and Copper

Severe emaciation, growth retardation, microcytic-hypochromic anemia, roughened fur, and lack of underfur pigmentation (achromotrichia) have been linked to an iron deficiency in mink.[41] This deficiency syndrome can presumably occur in ferrets consuming inadequate dietary levels of iron. Without copper, iron absorption may not be impaired, but hemoglobin cannot be formed efficiently. Excessive iron can result in anorexia, weight loss, and a decreased serum albumin level. Fortunately, commercially available ferret diets appear to contain iron and copper in amounts sufficient to prevent a deficiency.

Sodium and Chlorine

Sodium and chlorine are essential for normal physiologic performance, and must be provided by ingredients of the diet or by sodium chloride supplements. In mink, the requirements for sodium and chlorine are met by fortifying the ration with 0.5% salt. A dry diet containing 1% sodium chloride will supply normal needs, and is not excessive for normal dogs. This amount, equivalent to about 242 mg of sodium chloride (or 95 mg of sodium and 147 mg of chlorine)/kg of body weight daily has been designated as a daily allowance, but probably exceeds the minimum requirements for dogs. Commercially available ferret diets provide between 195 (Agway Marshall Ferret Feed) and 360 (Ralston 5280) to 445 (Purified Diet) mg chloride/kg body weight daily. Signs of deficiency include fatigue, exhaustion, inability to maintain water balance, decreased water intake, retarded growth, dryness of skin, and loss of hair.

Zinc

Commercially available ferret diets contain between 105 (MF Natural Ingredient Diet) and 215 (Ralston 5280) ppm zinc. These amounts are apparently adequate in preventing deficiency signs of alopecia, hyperkeratinization and acanthosis, disturbance in growth, anorexia, and emaciation. Diffuse necrosis has recently been attributed to zinc toxicity (1500–3000 ppm) in the ferret (see later discussion on dietary imbalances or toxicities).

Magnesium

Several investigators[42,43] have obtained evidence that the magnesium requirement of dogs varies with the dietary level of phosphorus. Using a 0.6% calcium-

and 0.4% phosphorous-containing diet, the magnesium requirement of mature dogs was estimated at between 80 and 180 mg/kg dry diet.[42] The recommended daily magnesium allowance for dogs, based on the above research and on studies of other species, is 0.04% of the diet on a dry basis. Commercially available ferret diets provide between four (Ralston 5280 and Purified Diet) and seven (Agway Marshall Ferret Feed) times this level. The high level of magnesium contained in the MF Natural Ingredient Diet is probably a result of the mixing apparatus used for grinding the chow.

Magnesium deficiency may be manifest clinically as an alteration in sodium and potassium transport, anorexia, decreased weight gain, irritability, and muscular weakness. Serum magnesium and calcium concentrations may be depressed; inorganic phosphorus levels may be elevated.

Iodine

Ferrets may require a small amount of iodine for prevention of goiter. Other signs of deficiency can include myxedema, skeletal deformity, delayed shedding of deciduous teeth, alopecia, dullness, apathy, drowsiness, and timidity. Commercially available diets provide approximately 3 to 5 ppm iodine, which appears to be adequate for preventing hypothyroidism.

Potassium

A daily allowance for growth of 264 mg potassium/kg of body weight is suggested as a minimum requirement for dogs.[44] Ferrets consuming the commercially available diets listed in Table 5–5 (under Minerals)[44] may consume between 285 (MF Natural Ingredient Diet) and 490 (Agway Marshall Ferret Feed) mg potassium/kg of body weight per day. Signs of deficiency include growth retardation, restlessness, muscular paralysis, dehydration, and lesions of the heart and kidney.

DIETARY IMBALANCES OR TOXICITIES

Several dietary imbalances, produced either experimentally or naturally occurring, have been documented in the literature, and are discussed below.

NUTRITIONAL STEATITIS

Nutritional steatitis, or yellow fat disease, has been described in ferrets fed a high level of dietary polyunsaturated fat (PUFA).[45] In all species in which the disease has been reported (the mink being particularly sensitive), the disease is caused by feeding a diet high in polyunsaturated fats and/or deficient in vitamin E.

Epizootiology and Control. In carnivores, including mustelids, this disease if often associated with feeding excessive quantities of oily marine fish.[46,47] Polyunsaturated fats are highly susceptible to oxidation within the food source as well as within the host's tissue, and vitamin E is a critical nutritional component in protecting tissue lipids from oxidative injury.[45] In an outbreak of steatitis in New Zealand ferrets, the PUFA concentration of the ferrets' diet, 7.7%, was considered excessive, although vitamin E levels of 13 mg/ferret/day would be considered adequate for low-PUFA diet of mink.[48] The squid in the ferrets' diet consisted of 17.9% PUFA, and is not recommended in any diet formulation for ferrets or mink. Young growing ferrets are more susceptible to the disease, and dietary management is particularly important for this age group. The toxic effects of PUFA are prevented or modified by vitamin E, which acts as an electron donor to prevent oxidation and scavenges free radicals within fat tissue. In the New Zealand outbreak of steatitis, a daily vitamin E intake of 13 mg/animal did not protect the ferret, and a dietary supplement of 75 to 150 mg/ferret/day (similar to mink recommendation) is advised when feeding ferrets a high-PUFA diet.[45] The high level of selenium found in the liver of ferrets with steatitis does not reduce the toxicity of the high-PUFA content of the feed, even though selenium does protect tissue against lipoperioxidases.

Clinical Signs and Diagnosis. Young growing kits are found dead or affected kits are depressed, cry out when handled, and are reluctant to move. Affected kits have diffuse firm swellings under the skin, and prominent subcutaneous lumps in the inguinal areas. Hematologic studies reveal a marked neutrophilia with a left shift, and a mild microcytic normochromic anemia.[45] Clinical diagnosis is based on clinical signs and on a history of feeding a high-PUFA diet.

Pathologic Findings. Fat in the subcutaneous and abdominal areas is yellow-brown and of a coarse and granular texture. Histologically, fat is infiltrated with large macrophages, mononuclear cells, and fibroblasts. Focal neutrophilic infiltrates are also noted.[45] Dense deposits of PAS-positive fluorescent lipopigment within macrophages is also prominent in affected tissue.

Treatment. Immediate removal of the offending diet is recommended clinically, and affected animals should be injected with 10 IU vitamin E daily for 2 days.[45] Vitamin E is added to the feed at 30 mg (30 IU)/ferret/day for 10 days, 15 mg for another 5 days, and 10 mg/ferret/day as a maintenance diet.

OSTEODYSTROPHIA FIBROSA (NUTRITIONAL HYPERPARATHYROIDISM)

Although ferrets may be susceptible to true rickets (hypophosphorosis and/or hypovitaminosis), the condition evidently has not been reported in this species. Hyperphosphorosis, associated with feeding an all-meat diet, with no calcium supplementation, has been documented in ferrets.[49]

Epizootiology and Control. The prevalence and susceptibility of the ferret to this nutritional deficiency is unknown; it has, however, been diagnosed in two ferret farms in New Zealand. The disease can be prevented by ensuring adequate calcium intake and a proper calcium:phosphorus (1:1). Natural product diets should be supplemented with 5 to 10% ground bone or an all-meat diet fortified with 2% bone meal or 2% dicalcium phosphate should be given.[49]

Clinical Signs. All ages are susceptible, but rapid growth predisposes ferrets to the disease. Despite an adequate diet, animals will lose weight. Affected ferrets are reluctant to move and support their weight; typical posture is abduction of the forelegs. The bones are soft and pliable, and fractures may be present.

Pathologic Findings. Grossly, bones are soft and rubberlike, and fractures of bones may be noted. Parathyroid glands are hyperplastic. Microscopically, bones are osteoporotic with typical lesions of osteodystrophia fibrosa.

THIAMINE DEFICIENCY

The disease is caused by ingestion of a diet, usually fish, that contains excess thiaminase. Feeding of raw eggs may also predispose ferrets to the disease.

Epizootiology and Control. The prevalence is unknown, but is related to dietary management. The disease has been reported on ferret farms in New Zealand where the diet consisted of fish containing thiaminase: paddle crabs, grey mullet, and dogfish.[49]

Clinical Signs and Diagnosis. The disease is seen in weanling growing animals or adults. Anorexia is marked, with accompanying lethargy. Advanced cases have marked dypsnea, prostration, and convulsions. Signs regress and disappear after parenteral injection of vitamin B complex (5 mg daily for 3 days); this occurs within 1 to 4 hours in mild cases, and usually within 8 hours in ferrets presenting with CNS symptoms.[49]

Pathology. The classic lesion noted in thiaminase deficiency is laminar necrosis in the brain cortex.

ZINC TOXICITY

The condition has been reported in ferrets exposed to excessive levels of zinc in the diet, leached from galvanized feeding pans and water dishes.[49–51]

Epizootiology and Control. Exposure to excess zinc must be avoided. Experimental evidence indicates that ferrets are particularly susceptible to zinc toxicity. Steam sterilization of zinc feed and water dishes has been shown to promote the leaching of zinc into feed and water from the surface of these containers.[51]

Clinical Signs and Diagnosis. Presumptive zinc toxicity is based on clinical signs, and pathologic confirmation is made by analyses of liver and kidney and on demonstration of elevated levels of zinc in the tissue. In proven cases of zinc toxicity, liver levels were 203 to 881 ppm in livers (dry weight) and 785 to 943 ppm in kidneys (dry weight).

All ages are susceptible to the toxicity. Affected animals have pale mucous membranes caused by anemia. Posterior weakness and lethargy are present. The disease was reported on two ferret farms in New Zealand; all animals were affected on one farm.[49]

Pathology. Lesions are primarily restricted to the kidney; grossly, the kidneys are enlarged, pale, and soft. In some cases there are small depressions on the capsular surface.[50] Livers are orange in color, and the stomach has erosions with digested blood on the gastric mucosa surface. Histologically, the kidneys have collapsed glomeruli and dilated tubules, with some tubules containing proteinaceous material and cellular debris. Focal cortical interstitial fibrosis is also seen. Histologically, the liver has periacinar fatty infiltration. Hemorrhage is present in the gastric pits, as well as mucosal erosions, and blood loss occurs into the gastric lumen. Bone marrow analysis shows depression of the erythroid series.

MERCURY TOXICITY

Experimentally, the ferret is susceptible to overt mercury poisoning by ingestion of tissues from chickens.[52] Methyl mercury-dressed wheat (used in crop production) was fed to chickens, and tissues of chicken carcasses, primarily muscles (10 mg/kg) and liver (40 mg/kg), were ingested by adult female ferrets. The total intake of muscle and liver/animal during the experiment was 2500 and 200 g/per ferret, respectively.

Prevalence and Epizootiology. To our knowledge the disease has not been reported under natural conditions. If natural product diets are used, care should be taken to ensure that meats, including fish products, are not contaminated with mercury.[53, 54]

Clinical Signs. Anorexia and weight loss are noted during the clinical course of the disease. Weakness, trembling, and muscle twitching are followed by ataxia, paralysis, and generalized apathy. Periodic episodes of excitation and circling have also been observed.[52]

Pathologic Findings. Muscle atrophy is generalized. All experimental ferrets had subacute ventricular dilatation. Slight to marked fatty degeneration is observed in skeletal and cardiac muscle, hepatic cells, and renal proximal tubular epithelium.[52] The most suspicious histologic changes are confined to the central and peripheral nervous systems. Focal myelin degeneration, with enlarged (focally disintegrated) axon cylinders, are consistently seen in peripheral nerves. Neuronal demyelinization and vacuolization are present in the cerebellar medulla and pons. High levels of mercury are found in the liver, kidneys, and central nervous system. Significant levels are also present in muscle tissue.

Treatment. Other than supportive therapy, there is no effective treatment. A grave prognosis is warranted and, if a definitive diagnosis of mercury poisoning has been made, clinically affected ferrets should be euthanized.

SALT POISONING

The disease is caused by feeding a diet of 100% salted fish.

Epizootiology and Control. The disease in ferrets is caused by feeding an exclusive diet of tuna that has been stored in brine.[49] Of 30 ferrets ingesting the salted tuna 9 were clinically affected, and 8 died. In the reported outbreak, control was achieved by reducing the amount of salted tuna in the diet to 30%. Adequate water intake must also be ensured.

Clinical Signs. Clinical signs of salt poisoning are typical of those seen in other species, particularly pigs, affected with the disease. Animals are markedly depressed and have periodic choriform spasms, seen 24 to 96 hours after ingestion of excessive salty diets. Death ensues shortly thereafter. Diagnosis is based on clinical and pathologic findings, coupled with analysis of dietary management.

Pathologic Findings. Pathology is restricted to the brain, which is edematous and shows coning of the cerebellum. A nonsuppurative eosinophilic meningitis is also present.

ARGININE-FREE DIET

Although this is unlikely to be found as a result of dietary deficiency in commercially prepared diets, an arginine-free diet in ferrets can result in profound clinical and pathologic abnormalities. Most young mammals require dietary arginine for optimum growth. Young ferrets, however, fasted for 16 hours and fed an arginine-free diet, will develop hyperammonemia and encephalopathy within 2 to 3 hours after ingesting such a diet.[55] It is speculated that young ferrets cannot synthesize sufficient amounts of ornithine from precursors other than arginine and become depleted of precursors needed to detoxify ammonia.[56] There is also an increase in serum liver enzyme levels as well as in serum-free fatty acids and liver lipids. Histologically, the liver has accumulations of lipid droplets and swollen mitochondria. These results are accentuated in young ferrets challenged experimentally with influenza virus and treated with aspirin.[56, 57] Clinically, the development of encephalopathy involves lethargy, or uncharacteristic combativeness early in the course of the disease, followed by prostration, coma, and death. Unlike Reye's syndrome in children, repetitive vomiting is not seen.

Adult ferrets (18 months) do not develop hyperammonemia and encephalopathy when fed an arginine-free diet. The disease is easily preventable by feeding adequate arginine in the diet. The course of the disease, once clinically apparent, can be abbreviated by ornithine injections. Sodium benzoate administered intraperitoneally to young ferrets fed an arginine-free diet fails to decrease serum ammonia levels.[55]

ADDITIONAL CONSIDERATIONS

The nutrient requirements of the ferret may be modified by age, growth, caloric intake, physical activity, and special physiologic states, such as pregnancy and lactation. For the ferret to be useful in biomedical research, specific nutrient requirements for each phase of the life cycle must be clearly established, including identification of specific requirements for macronutrients, micronutrients, and trace nutrients, and understanding the various combinations of their interactions. In addition, it is necessary to recognize the signs of nutrient deficiencies and toxicities. Further studies will enlighten the research community, assist veterinary clinicians caring for this species, and encourage future investigations of optimum nutrition in the ferret. Hopefully such work will lead to the widespread use of the ferret as an animal model, and provide an effective means of studying a number of physiologic and toxicologic reponses to elucidate similar mechanisms in humans.

REFERENCES

1. Marino, T.A., and Severdia, J.: The early development of the AV node and bundle in the ferret heart. Am. J. Anat., *167*:299, 1983.
2. Breisch, E.: A quantitative ultrastructural study of cardiac hypertrophy and regression. Anat. Rec., *190*:347, 1980.
3. Marino, T.A., Biberstein, D., and Severdia, J.B.: The ultrastructure of the atrio-ventricular junctional tissues in the newborn ferret heart. Am. J. Anat., *161*:383, 1981.
4. Wen, G.Y., Sturman, J.A., and Shek, J.W.: A comparative study of the tapetum, retina and skull of the ferret, dog and cat. Lab. Anim. Sci., *35*:200, 1985.
5. Thorpe, P.A., and Herbert, J.: The accessory optic system of the ferret. J. Comp. Neurol., *170*: 295, 1976.
6. Braekevelt, C.R.: Fine structure of the retinal epithelium, Bruch's membrane (complexus basalis) and choriocapillaris in the domestic ferret. Acta. Anat., *113*:117, 1982.
7. Vinegar, A., Sinnett, E.E., Kosch, P.C., and Miller, M.L.: Pulmonary physiology of the ferret and its potential as a model for inhalation toxicology. Lab. Anim. Sci., *35*:246, 1985.
8. Vinegar, A., Sinnett, E.E., and Kosch, P.C.: Respiratory mechanics of a small carnivore: The ferret. J. Appl. Physiol., *52*:832, 1982.
9. Sweet, C. et al.: Differential distribution of virus and histological damage in the lower respiratory tract of ferrets infected with influenza viruses of differing virulence. J. Gen. Virol., *54*:103, 1981.
10. Bird, R.A., Sweet, C., Husseini, R.H., and Smith, H.: The similar interaction of ferret alveolar macrophages with influenza virus strains of differing virulence at normal and pyrexial temperatures. J. Gen. Virol., *64*:1807, 1983.
11. Chevance, L.G.: Scanning and transmission electron microscopy study of ferret respiratory mucosa infected with influenza A virus. Ann. Microbiol. (Paris), *129*:177, 1978.
12. Kauffman, C.A., Bergman, A.G., and O'Connor, R.P.: Distemper virus infection in ferrets: An animal model of measles-induced immunosuppression. Clin. Exp. Immunol., *47*:617, 1982.
13. Fox, J.G. et al.: Proliferative colitis in ferrets (*Mustela putorius*). Am. J. Vet. Res., *43*:858, 1982.
14. Fox, J.G., Ackerman, J.I., and Newcomer, C.E.: Ferret as a potential reservoir for human campylobacteriosis. Am. J. Vet. Res., *44*:1049, 1983.
15. Koshimizu, K., Kotani, H., and Syukuda, Y.: Isolation of mycoplasmas from experimental ferrets (*Mustela putorius*). Jikken Dobutsu, *31*:299, 1982.
16. Hoar, R.M.: Use of ferrets in toxicity testing. J. Am. Coll. Toxicol., *3*:325, 1984.
17. Brantom, P. G., Gaunt, I.F., and Hardy, J.: One-year toxicity study of Orange G in the ferret. Fed. Cosmet. Toxicol., *15*:379, 1977.
18. Beach, J.E.: The ferret for non-rodent toxicity studies—a pathologist's view. Arch. Toxicol. [Suppl.], *5*:279, 1982.
19. McLain, D.E. et al.: Congenital malformations and variations in reproductive performance in the ferret: Effects of maternal age, color and parity. Lab. Anim. Sci., *35*:251, 1985.

20. McLain, D.E., Roe, D.A.: Fetal alcohol syndrome in the ferret (*Mustela putorius*). Teratology, *30*:203, 1984.

21. McLain, D.E., and Roe, D.A.: Nutrient composition of a natural ferret diet and the reproductive response to several purified diet formulations. Fed. Proc., *43A*:1318, 1983.

22. Haddad, R., Rabe, A., and Dumas, R.: Neuroteratogenicity of methylazoxymethanol acetate: Behavioral deficits of ferrets with transplacentally induced lissencephaly. Neurotoxicology, *1*:171, 1979.

23. Frederick, K., and Babish, J.G. Compendium of recent literature on ferrets. Lab. Anim. Sci., *35*:299, 1985.

24. Rammell, C.G., Brooks, H.V., Bentley, G.R., and Savage, G.P.: Fitch diets in New Zealand: An analytical survey. N. Zeal. Vet. J., *33*:207, 1985.

25. Horwitz, W. (ed.): Official Methods of Analysis of the Association of Official Analytical Chemists. 13th Ed. Washington, DC, Association of Official Analytical Chemists, pp. 1018.

26. Reeves, J.B., and Weihrauch, J.L. (eds.): Composition of Foods: Fats and Oils: Raw, Processed, Prepared. Washington, DC, United States Department of Agriculture, Handbook No. 8-4, 1979.

27. National Research Council, Committee on Animal Nutrition, Board on Agriculture and Renewable Resources: Nutrient Requirements of Dogs. Washington, DC, National Academy of Sciences, Handbook No. 8, 1974.

28. National Research Council, Committee on Animal Nutrition, Board on Agriculture and Renewable Resources: Nutrient Requirements of Cats. Washington, DC, National Academy of Sciences, Handbook No. 13, 1978.

29. National Research Council, Committee on Animal Nutrition, Board on Agriculture and Renewable Resources: Nutrient Requirements of Mink and Foxes. Washington, DC, National Academy of Sciences, Handbook No. 7, 1968.

30. Warner, R.G. et al.: Niacin requirements of growing mink. J. Nutr., *95*:563, 1968.

31. Allen, R.P., Evans, E.V., and Sibbald, I.R.: Energy: Protein relationships in the diets of growing mink. Can. J. Physiol. Pharmacol., *47*:733, 1964.

32. Sinclair, D.G., Evans, E.V., and Sibbald, I.R.: The influence of apparent digestible energy and apparent digestible nitrogen in the diet on weight gain, feed consumption, and nitrogen retention of growing mink. Can. J. Biochem. Physiol., *40*:1376, 1962.

33. Ontko, J.A., Wuthier, R.E., and Phillips, P.H.: The effect of increased dietary fat upon the protein requirement of the growing dog. J. Nutr., *62*:163, 1957.

34. Holman, R.T.: Essential fatty acid deficiency. Prog. Chem. Fats and Other Lipids, *9*:275, 1968.

35. Harris, P.L., and Embree, N.D.: Quantitative consideration of the effect of polyunsaturated fatty acid content of the diet upon the requirements for vitamin E. Am. J. Clin. Nutr., *13*:385, 1963.

36. Weisse, H.F., Hansen, A.E., and Coon, E.: Influence of high and low caloric intakes on fat-deficiency of dogs. J. Nutr., *76*:73, 1962.

37. Naismith, D.J., and Cursiter, M.C.: Is there a specific requirement for carbohydrate in the diet? Nutr. Soc. Proc., *31*:94A, 1972.

38. Leoschke, W.L.: Mink Nutrition Research at the University of Wisconsin. Madison, University of Wisconsin, Research Bulletin 222, 1960.

39. Helgebostad, A., Svenkerud, R.R., and Ender, F.: Sterility in mink induced experimentally by deficiency of B6. Acta Vet. Scand., *4*:228, 1963.

40. Warner, R.G., Bassett, C.F., and McCarthy, B.: The determination of the Minimum Nutrient Requirements of Mink Using Purified Diets. Milwaukee, WI, Mink Farmers' Research Foundation Progress Report, 1962.

41. Stout, F.M., Adair, J., and Oldfield, J.E.: Aberrant iron metabolism and the cotton fur abnormality in mink. J. Nutr., *72*:46, 1960.

42. Bunce, G.E., Jenkins, K.J., and Phillips, P.H.: The mineral requirements of the dog. III. The magnesium requirement. J Nutr., *76*:17, 1962.

43. Vitale, J.J., Hellerstein, E.E., Nakamura, M., and Lown, B.: Effects of magnesium-deficient diets upon puppies. Circ. Res., *9*:387, 1961.

44. Abbrecht, P.H.: Cardiovascular effects of chronic potassium deficiency in the dog. Am. J. Physiol., *223*:555, 1972.

45. Brooks, H.V., Rammell, C.G., Hoogenboom, J.J.L., and Taylor, D.E.S.: Observations on an outbreak of nutritional steatitis (yellow fat disease) in fitch (*Mustela putorius furo*). N. Z. Vet. J., *33*:141, 1985.

46. Lalor, R.J., Leoschke, W.L., and Elvehjem, C.A.: Yellow fat in the mink. J. Nutr., *45*:183, 1951.

47. Mason, K.E., and Hartsough, G.R.: Steatitis or yellow fat in mink and its relation to dietary fats and inadequacy of vitamin E. J. Am. Vet. Med. Assoc., *119*:72, 1951.

48. Stowe, H.D., and Whitehair, C.K.: Gross and microscopic pathology of tochopherol-deficient mink. J. Nutr., *81*:287, 1963.

49. Diseases of the fitch. Surveillance, *11*:2, 1984.

50. Straube, E.F., and Walden, N.B.: Zinc poisoning in ferrets (Mustela putorius furo). Lab. Anim., *15*:45, 1981.

51. Straube, E.F., Schuster, N.H., and Sinclair, A.J.: Zinc toxicity in the ferret. J. Comp. Pathol., *90*:355, 1980.

52. Hanko, E., Erne, K., Wanntorp, H., and Borg, K.: Poisoning in ferrets by tissues of alkyl mercury-fed chickens. Acta Vet. Scand., 11:268, 1970.

53. Borg, K., Wanntorp, H., and Ernek Hanko, E.: Mercury poisoning in Swedish wildlife. J. Appl. Ecol. (Suppl.), 3:171, 1966.

54. Smart, N.A., and Lloyd, M.K.: Mercury residues in eggs, flesh and livers of hens fed on wheat treated with methyl mercury dicyanodiamide. J. Sci. Food Agric., 14:734, 1963.

55. Thomas, P.E., and Desmukh, D.R.: Effect of arginine-free diet on ammonia metabolism in young and adult ferrets. J. Nutr., 116:545, 1986.

56. Desmukh, D.R., and Thomas, P.E.: Arginine deficiency, hyperammonemia and Reye's syndrome in ferrets. Lab. Anim. Sci., 35:242, 1985.

57. Desmukh, D.R., Thomas, P.E., McArthur, B., and Sarnaik, A.P.: Serum glutamate-dehydrogenase and ornithine carbamyl transferase in Reye's syndrome. Enzyme, 33:171, 1985.

chapter 6

HOUSING AND MANAGEMENT

J. G. Fox

Housing, management, and breeding practices for ferrets are in many ways analogous to those of other carnivores, and many of the principles discussed in this chapter can also be applied to the dog and cat.

HOUSING

A number of factors need to be considered in regard to safe and adequate housing for the ferret.

PHYSICAL FACILITIES AND ENVIRONMENT

Under proper environmental conditions, the ferret can be housed indoors as well as outdoors.

Temperature and Humidity

Although ferrets can be maintained outdoors at temperatures as low as 7 to 10°C, and for experimental purposes in a refrigerated room, low temperature and high humidity should be avoided.[1] Similarly, elevated temperatures, above 30°C (90°F), cannot be tolerated; because of poorly developed sweat glands the ferret is susceptible to heat prostration. Clinical signs of hyperthermia include open-mouthed breathing, panting, eventual flaccidity, and occasional vomiting. Particular care must be exercised when transporting ferrets in poorly ventilated vehicles. Optimum temperatures for the ferret appear to be 4 to 18°C (40–65°F), with a humidity range of 40 to 65%; unweaned ferrets should be maintained at a minimum temperature of 15°C (59°F). The optimum temperature range recommended by the Council of Europe Convention for ferrets is 15 to 21°C.[2]

Lighting

Lighting is set at 12:12 light:dark cycle in conventional housing to maintain stock animals. Light can be manipulated to control breeding cycles. Ferrets are seasonal breeders and, by increasing daylight or by exposure to longer periods of artificial light when housed indoors, estrus can be induced in females and sexual activity can be stimulated in immature males (see Chap. 8, Reproduction, Breeding, and Growth).

Air Handling

Like most laboratory animals, ferrets utilized for biomedical research should be housed under laboratory conditions, in rooms with 10 to 15 air exchanges of nonrecirculated air per hour.[3] This is particularly important in ferrets for husbandry reasons because of their musky odor, and for disease prevention because of their susceptibility to respiratory viral infections. In addition, because of the ferret's strong odor, efforts should be made to minimize transmission of their scent to rodents maintained in the same vivarium. Because of the rodent's fear of ferrets (stimulated by olfactory senses), any trace of ferret scent may interrupt breeding cycles or disturb other physiologic processes. Pets should be maintained in nondrafty areas, and should not be housed in extremely warm or cold areas.

CAGING

Various primary enclosures have been described to house ferrets. Most of them, however, consist of metal rod framework, similar to the design used to house rabbits and cats. The flooring may be solid or may consist of metal cross braces, allowing urine and some feces to collect in a drop pan (Fig. 6–1). If small numbers of ferrets are maintained in a vivarium, rabbit cages can be modified to house ferrets. Basically, a specially made wire grid can be secured to the front of the cage to prevent escape (Fig. 6–2). Caging standards for the ferret were not specified in the NIH Guide,[3] but the size described by Wilson,[4] 49 × 46 × 46 cm, meets the space requirements cited by the Royal Society of England.[2]

Ferrets prefer a small enclosure as a nesting area; if paper or cardboard sheets are used as contact bedding, they are often found nestled beneath them. A solid-bottomed plastic rodent cage can be modified to serve as a nesting area.[5]

Solid plastic caging can also be used to house ferrets. One cage described measures 37 × 24 × 25 cm, with the bottom covered with sawdust to facilitate cleaning.[2] I suggest, however, that this type of cage be used only for short-term housing. I have successfully used solid-bottomed rodent caging for weanling ferrets, and find them useful for helping the ferret to maintain its body temperature.

Because of ferrets' tendency to lick and bite their enclosures, careful attention should be given to monitoring ferrets for trauma to the teeth and gums. Zinc toxic-

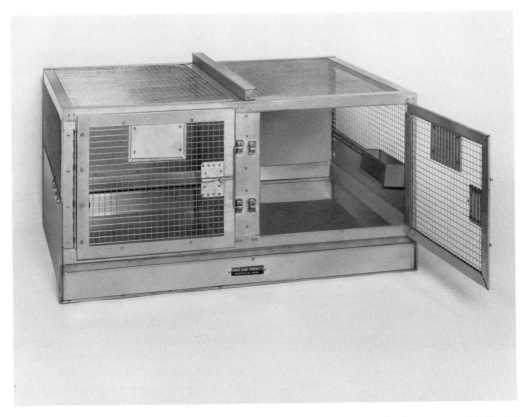

Fig. 6–1. Ferret cages with removable drop pan. The suspended wire grid floor has been removed to illustrate the drop pan. The cage is 32″ wide × 23″ deep × 16″ high. (Courtesy of Fenco Cage Products, Boston.)

ity has been noted, caused by ferrets licking zinc compounds from the galvanized bars of the caging, a result of steam sterilization (82°C for 20 min; see Chap. 5, Nutrition).[6]

Ferrets may be housed singly or in groups by sex. Estrous females should not be housed together, however, nor should females that have been mated, because of sexual play eliciting ovulation or pseudopregnancy (see Chap. 18, Use of the Ferret in Behavioral Research).[7] Also, in group housing, sexually active males should be removed because of their tendency to fight.

FOOD AND WATER

Nutritional needs and dietary habits of the ferret are addressed separately (see Chap. 5, Nutrition). For husbandry aspects, however, a selected number of issues in dietary requirements will be mentioned here.

Food

Ferrets are carnivores, and have historically been fed a diet of meat or meat-by-products. Because of the large body of literature available on the nutritional requirements of another commercially reared mustelid, the mink, many recommendations about the ferret's dietary needs are extrapolated from those cited for the mink. Feral ferrets are known to exist on various small mammals, particularly mice. One laboratory in England, which has used ferrets extensively for physiology and anatomy studies, has successfully maintained their ferrets on dead mice

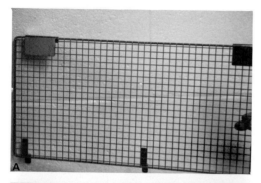

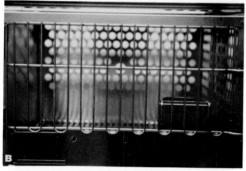

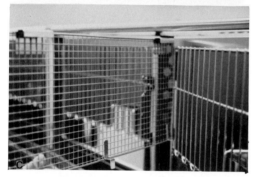

Fig. 6–2. Rabbit cage modified for ferrets. *A,* Removable stainless steel wire grid. *B,* Door of rabbit cage. *C,* Grid being placed on door to prevent escape. (Courtesy of Lab Products, Inc., Maywood, New Jersey.)

and rats.[2] In many research settings, however, and certainly with household pet ferrets, this diet is not practical nor considered aesthetically pleasing. Most ferrets are therefore fed a combination of commercially available cat and dog food, both in the canned moist form and the prepared pelleted form. We have successfully maintained a nonbreeding research colony (average daily census, 50–150 animals) for 8 years on pelleted cat food sup-

plemented with various canned cat food products. Similar results have been obtained by others who have used dog food and, in some cases, pelleted mink chow. The use of raw chicken, beef, horsemeat, or their by-products is discouraged because of the likelihood of *Campylobacter, Salmonella, Listeria, Mycobacterium, Clostridium,* and *Streptococcus* group C contamination (see Chap. 10, Bacterial and Mycoplasmal Diseases). More recently, specially formulated ferret pelleted diets have become commercially available (see Chap. 5, Nutrition).

The ferret usually consumes 140 to 190 g of semimoist food daily. On a dry weight basis, daily food consumption for male and female ferrets is 43 g/kg body weight.[8] Mean food passage time as measured by a dye marker in the feed is 182 minutes, indicating a relatively short digestive tract. Ferrets with free access to food will eat nine or ten meals a day.[9] Care should be exercised to ensure that ferrets, especially males, do not become obese; therefore, restricted food intake is recommended.

Water

Potable fresh water should be available ad libitum. This is supplied either in stainless steel water bowls or in water bottles equipped with stainless steel sipper tubes. When using a pelleted diet, mixing the diet with water not only provides another source of water but in our experience makes this form of diet more palatable for the ferret. In the study by Andrews and Illman, water intake was noted for adult male ferrets at 39 ± 6 ml/day, and for adult females at 17 ± 2 ml/day; according to the authors, however, the ferret readily consumes milk, and the low water intake was a result of supplementing these animals with milk, 418 ± 40 ml/day for males and 312 ± 46 ml/day for females.[2] Average daily water intake in adult ferrets is estimated at 75 to 100 ml.[11] Bread and milk is sometimes fed regularly, but it predisposes the ferret to periodontal disease and loose feces.[10]

SANITATION

Food and water bowls should be changed daily. If water bottles with stainless steel sipper tubes are used, they should be replaced with clean sanitized bottles two or three times weekly.

Because of the musky odor produced by the sebaceous and anal glands, and the constant need to minimize microbial cross contamination, caging should be routinely sanitized with appropriate disinfectants or with 180°F water that can destroy vegetative microorganisms. In a research setting this is accomplished by sanitizing the caging at least weekly; if using suspended grid flooring the drop pans, preferably constructed of stainless steel, should be cleaned and sanitized daily. Ferrets usually prefer to defecate in one corner of the cage because of behavioral traits; like the cat, they can be trained to use a litter tray, which allows easy removal of excreta between weekly sanitation of cages.[4, 12]

MANAGEMENT

There are several factors to be considered in the proper management of ferrets.

HANDLING AND RESTRAINT

The ferret, unlike another closely related mustelid, the mink, is considered to be inquisitive and to have a gentle disposition. The animal is often handled without protective gloves, and in pet settings is commonly allowed free access to the household; caging can be used at night, though, or for periods when the owner wants the animal to be confined. Ferrets that are hungry or ill, particularly males and females with litters, can exhibit aggressive behavior and bite unsuspecting handlers. Frequent handling, as well as neutering animals at 8 to 10 weeks or 6 to 8 months, minimizes aggressive behavior. It should be cautioned, however, that some pet ferrets allowed free access to the household have been known to traumatize infants severely.

If injecting ferrets with medication, or performing a physical examination that may alarm the animal, it is wise for the person holding the animal to wear protective gloves and to grasp the animal firmly at the nape of the neck with one hand and to extend and support the body with the other hand (Fig. 6–3). Alternatively, the ferret can be handled safely by one person for subcutaneous injection (Fig. 6–4).

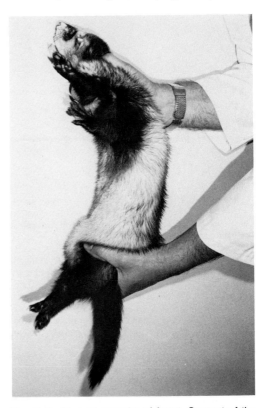

Fig. 6–3. Manual restraint of ferret. Support of the hindquarters and restraint of the head are important components.

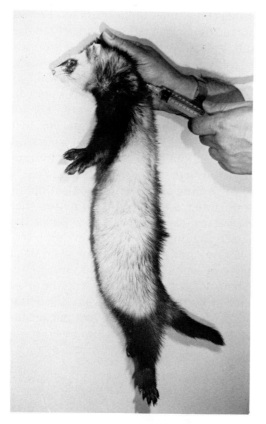

Fig. 6–4. Restraint of ferret by technician administering vaccine via subcutaneous injection.

Appropriate tranquilizers or anesthetics can be used effectively when handling fractious animals (see Chap. 16, Anesthesia and Surgery).

IDENTIFICATION

Subtle coat color difference, body size, or behavioral traits are often sufficient to distinguish a particular ferret from a small group of cohorts. If, however, large numbers of animals are utilized, individual markings or tags on the animals are required. In our experience, ear tags have been used successfully for a number of years. The ear tags can be placed in young ferrets; the procedure is atraumatic, and the pinna of the ear reacts minimally. If an occasional tag is lost another can be inserted easily. Ear notching or tattooing the ear can be attempted, but the size of the pinna poses limitations to these procedures.[1] The albino ferret can be marked with indelible dyes. Alternatively, the inner thigh can be tattooed; ferrets must of course be anesthetized during this manipulation. In pet ferrets, collars are sometimes used.

REFERENCES

1. Hammond, J., Jr., and Chesterman, F.C.: The ferret. *In* UFAW Handbook on the Care and Management of Laboratory Animals. 4th ed. London, Churchill Livingstone, 1972.
2. Andrews, P.L.R., and Illman, O.: The ferret. *In* UFAW Handbook on the Care and Management of Laboratory Animals. 6th ed. Edited by T. Poole. London, Longman's Scientific and Technical, 1987.
3. U.S. Department of Health and Human Services: Guide for the Care and Use of Laboratory Animals. Washington, D.C., Public Health Service, NIH No. 8523, 1985.
4. Wilson, M.S., and Donnoghue, P.N.D.: A mobile rack of cages for ferrets (*Mustela putorius furo*). Lab. Anim., 16:278, 1982.
5. Ryland, L.M., and Gorham, J.R.: The ferret and its diseases. J. Am. Vet. Med. Assoc., 173:1154, 1978.
6. Straube, E.F., and Wilson, N.B.: Zinc poisoning in ferrets (*Mustela putorius furo*). Lab. Anim., 15:45, 1981.
7. Beck, F., et al.: Comparison of the teratogenic effects of mustine hydrochloride in rats and ferrets. The value of the ferret as an experimental animal in teratology. Teratology, 13:151, 1976.
8. Bleavins, M.R., and Auberich, R.J.: Feed consumption and food passage time in mink (*Mustela vison*) and European ferrets (*Mustela putorius furo*). Lab. Anim. Sci., 31:268, 1981.
9. Kaufman, L.W.: Foraging cost and meal patterns in ferrets. Physiol. Behav., 25:139, 1980.
10. Cooper, J.E.: Ferrets. *In* Manual of Exotic Pets. Edited by J.E. Cooper, M.F. Hutchison, O.F. Jackson, and R.J. Maurice. Cheltenham, England, British Small Animal Veterinary Association, 1985.
11. Moody, K.D., Bowman, T.A., Lang, C.M.: Laboratory management of the ferret for biomedical research. Lab. Anim. Sci., 35:272, 1985.
12. Bissonnette, T.H.: Ferrets. *In* The Care and Breeding of Laboratory Animals, pp. 234–255. 3rd ed. Edited by E.J. Farris. New York, John Wiley & Sons, 1965.

chapter 7

NORMAL CLINICAL AND BIOLOGIC PARAMETERS

J. G. Fox

BIOLOGIC DATA USED IN CLINICAL EVALUATION

Certain biological data are routinely used for assessment of the animals' health or for husbandry needs. These data are provided in tabular form for easy reference (Table 7–1). (Also see Chapters 2, 4, 5, and 8 for further details.)

IMMUNE RESPONSE

Infant ferrets have nearly undetectable immunoglobulin levels but, by day 9, their serum has 77, 29, and 13%, respectively, of the adult mean serum levels of IgG, IgA, and IgM.[1]

ONTOGENY OF HUMORAL IMMUNE RESPONSE

The postpartum transfer of immunoglobulin occurs across the intestinal mucosa via the products of lactation (Fig. 7–1). All three classes of immunoglobulin are present in the ferret's milk, but at lower concen-

TABLE 7–1. SELECTED NORMATIVE DATA

Parameter	Value
Adult weight	
Male	1–2 kg
Female	600–900 g
Life span (average)	5–11 years
Body temperature	38.8°C (37.8°–40°C)
Chromosome number (diploid)	40
Dental formula	2 (I 3/3, C 1/1, P 4/3, M 1/2)
Vertebral formula	$C_7 T_{15} L_5 S_3 Cd_{14}$
Age of sexual maturity	6–12 months
Length of breeding life	2–5 years
Gestation	42 ± 2 days
Litter size	8, average (range, 1–18)
Birth weight	6–12 g
Eyes open	34 days
Onset of hearing	32 days
Weaning	6–8 weeks
Food consumption, semimoist	140–190 g/24 hr
Water intake	75–100 ml/24 hr
Urine volume	26–28 ml/24 hr
Urine pH	6.5–7.5
Cardiovascular/Respiratory:	
Arterial blood pressure	
Mean systolic	Female, 133, male, 161 mm Hg (conscious)
Mean diastolic	110–125 mm Hg (anesthetized)
Heart rate	200–400 beats/min
Cardiac output	139 ml/min
Circulation time	4.5–6.8 sec
Blood volume	Male, 60, female, 40 ml (approx.)
Respirations	33–36/min

trations than in the adult ferret's serum. Although IgG levels in the milk may vary from animal to animal, they do not vary with time in any one ferret and do not correlate with adult serum IgG levels. IgG transmucosal uptake occurs for the first 30 days of the ferret's life. Like IgG levels, IgM milk levels do not vary in animals infected with respiratory syncytial virus (RSV) when compared to uninfected ones.[2] IgM levels do not appear to rise or fall with IgG milk levels of IgG serum content in the infant ferret. Interestingly, there is strong evidence to suggest a dichotomous population consisting of ferrets whose milk has unstable levels of IgA and an-

other group with relatively stable levels.[2] When these two groups are divided on the basis of their IgA stability in milk, the stable ferrets (i.e., those with stable IgA milk levels), have a geometric mean value of 21 ± 4% of the pooled serum standard, and the unstable group has a geometric mean value of 41 ± 14% of the pooled serum standard. These two populations of ferrets are significantly different (sine test, p = 0.015).

The infant ferret gastrointestinal tract can uptake IgG from its mother's or maternal milk selectively across a five-fold concentration gradient to reach serum concentrations in 7-day-old ferrets that are 100-fold or greater than those in near-term fetal sera.[2] The other two classes, IgM and IgA, are not concentrated in milk, and hence do not approach adult serum levels during the first 2 weeks of life.

MATERNALLY ACQUIRED IMMUNITY TO VIRAL DISEASES

The in vivo protective effect of trans-mucosal antibody to RSV has been demonstrated experimentally in the ferret.[2] Acquired immunity to RSV may be seen in 3-day-old ferrets challenged intranasally with RSV. The level of protection correlates with the maternal serum-neutralizing titer. The protection is specific for RSV, and is effective only in infants who nursed on dams previously infected with RSV. The protective effect of IgG-specific RSV antibody in milk disappears after weaning, and most transmucosal transport of the RSV-specific antibody occurs during the first 8 days of life.

CELL-MEDIATED IMMUNITY

A number of factors pertaining to cell-mediated immunity in the ferret have been studied in several laboratories.

Delayed Dermal Hypersensitivity

In a study to measure delayed hypersensitivity, 3- to 12-month-old ferrets were immunized twice, 12 days apart, with 500 U of streptokinase (SK) in complete Freund's adjuvant.[4] Skin tests were performed using purified protein derivative (10,000 tuberculin units in 0.1 ml 0.9% saline solution or 400 U SK. Skin test responses to both SK and PPD are characterized by induration, with little erythema (the maximal response is observed at 32 hours, Fig. 7–2). Skin biopsy at 30 hours shows mononuclear cell infiltration and dermal edema. Six weeks after immuni-

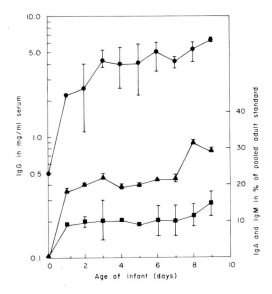

Fig. 7–1. The time course of postpartum transfer of immunoglobulins of each class via products of lactation to infant ferrets. The bars indicate ranges. (Modified from Suffin, S.C., et al.: Ontogeny of the ferret humoral immune response. J. Immunol., *123*:6, 1979.)

zation the skin tests remained positive, and the experiment was terminated.

Although delayed hypersensitivity is elicited in ferrets, it is not as easily demonstrated as in the guinea pig, human, or nonhuman primate. Footpad swelling after antigen injection is not an effective correlate to cellular immunity in the ferret, as in the other species.[3]

Lymphocyte Transformation

Three different sera were tested to study their in vitro effect on mononuclear cell proliferation. Peripheral blood lymphocytes from 12 different ferrets were used. Proliferation of lymphocytes was supported by human, ferret, and fetal calf sera.[4] Because of its commercial availability and consistent results, fetal calf sera were utilized for further in vitro studies. In this study, peripheral blood mononuclear cells from 10 ferrets were incubated for 2 to 5 days for mitogen response and for 4 to 8 days for specific

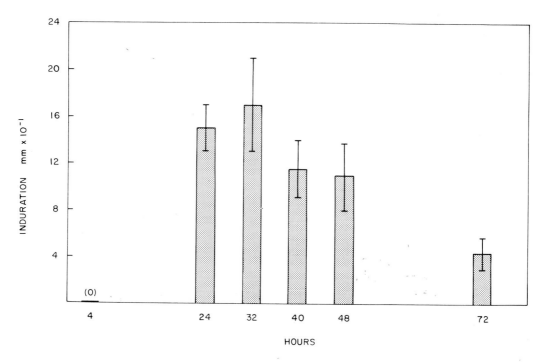

Fig. 7–2. Delayed hypersensitivity to PPD (200 μg = 10,000 tuberculin units) in 22 ferrets immunized with complete Freund's adjuvant. The top of each bar represents the mean difference in induration between the skin test site and normal skin; the brackets show the standard error of the mean. Responses were similar up to 6 weeks following immunization. (Modified from Kauffman, C.A.: Cell-mediated immunity in ferrets: Delayed dermal hypersensitivity, lymphocyte transformation, and macrophage inhibitory factor production. Dev. Comp. Immunol., 5:125, 1981.)

antigens. Mitogen responses were maximal at day 2 for concanavalin A (ConA), day 3 for pokeweed mitogen (PWM), and at day 2 or 3 for phytohemagglutinin-M (PHA). Proliferative responses to SK were the highest at day 5.[3] These results are similar to previously reported maximal proliferation responses in unseparated peripheral blood leukocytes in ferrets.[4] Splenic lymphocytes responded, as did peripheral lymphocytes. Kauffman has suggested that results obtained using a technique that separates out complement receptor-bearing cells indicate that spleen cells responding to PHA and ConA are non-B cells and may be T lymphocytes. Another report stated that ferret splenic lymphocytes respond poorly to mitogenic stimulation.[5]

Lymphocyte Subpopulations

When researchers used a technique that attaches complement to zymogen particles, 16.7% of peripheral blood lymphocytes and 15% of splenic lymphocytes exhibited receptors for complement.[6] Receptors for the Fc portion of IgG, measured by an assay using antibody-coated sheep erythrocytes, were found in 11.7% of peripheral blood lymphocytes and 34.8% of splenic lymphocytes.[6] It is probable that these cells, identified by Fc complement, are B lymphocytes; monocytes are excluded because they have phagocytized latex particles. Using an indirect fluorescent antibody technique, researchers visualized surface immunoglobulin in 13.4% of peripheral lymphocytes and 10.3% of splenic lymphocytes. They could not demonstrate rosetting of T lymphocytes, even though erythrocytes of 16 animal species were used.

Macrophage Migration Inhibitory Factor (MIF)

Kauffman and associates used mononuclear cells from ferret blood or spleen to demonstrate the production of splenic lymphocyte MIF for up to 8 weeks following immunization with SK.[3] They did not produce MIF with peripheral blood leukocytes, however, possibly because of the small cell yield. Using an indirect method, others have also demonstrated MIF activity in stimulated ferret lymphocytes.[7]

VIRAL-INDUCED IMMUNOSUPPRESSION

Distemper infection in ferrets, similar to distemper in dogs and measles in humans, can result in a significant suppression of cell-mediated immunity. To induce immunosuppression, Kauffman and colleagues produced a mild systemic illness in a group of ferrets by inocula-

TABLE 7–2. HEMATOLOGIC VALUES OF NORMAL FERRETS

Parameter		Albino Ferrets*		Fitch Ferrets†		Fitch Ferrets, Male‡	
		Male	Female	Male	Female	Orbital	Cardiac
PVC (%)	Mean	55.4	49.2	43.4	48.4	52.1	53.1
	Range	44–61	42–55	36–50	47–51	47–57.5	48–59
Hemoglobin (g/dl)	Mean	17.8	16.2	14.3	15.9	16.8	16.9
	Range	16.3–18.2	14.8–17.4	12–16.3	15.2–17.4	14.5–18.5	15.4–18.5
RBC ($\times 10^6/mm^3$)	Mean	10.23	8.11			11.3	11.3
	Range	7.3–12.18	6.77–9.76			9.7–12.4	10.1–13.2
Platelets ($10^3/mm^3$)	Mean	453	545				
	Range	297–730	310–910				
Reticulocytes (%)	Mean	4.0	5.3				
	Range	1–12	2–14				
WBC ($\times 10^3/mm^3$)	Mean	9.7	10.5	11.3	5.9	6.3	6.2
	Range	4.4–19.1	4.0–18.2	7.7–15.4	2.5–8.6	2.8–13.4	1.7–11.9
Differential (%)	Mean			0.9	1.7		
Bands	Range			0–2.2	0–4.2	0–2	0–1
Neutrophils	Mean	57.0	59.5	40.1	31.1		
	Range	11–82	43–84	24–78	12–41	22–75	24–72
Lymphocytes	Mean	35.6	33.4	49.7	58.0		
	Range	12–54	12–50	28–69	25–95	20–72	26–73
Monocytes	Mean	4.4	4.4	6.6	4.5		
	Range	0–9	2–8	3.4–8.2	1.7–6.3	0–4	1–4
Eosinophils	Mean	2.4	2.6	2.3	3.6		
	Range	0–7	0–5	0–7	1–9	0–3	0–3
Basophils	Mean	0.1	0.2	0.7	0.8		
	Range	0–2	0–1	0–2.7	0–2.9		
MCV	Mean					46.3	47.1
	Range					42–55.9	42.6–51
MCH	Mean					14.9	15.0
	Range					14–16.4	13.7–16
MCHC	Mean					32.3	32.0
	Range					26.9–35	30.3–34.9

* Data from Thornton, et al.[11]
† Data from Lee, et al.[12]
‡ Data from Fox, et al.[13]

TABLE 7–3. SERUM CHEMISTRY VALUES OF NORMAL FERRETS

Parameter		Albino Ferrets*	Fitch Ferrets†	Fitch Ferrets, Male‡	
				Orbital	Cardiac
Sodium (mmol/L)	Mean	148	152	152	154
	Range	137–162	146–160	153–164	152–156
Potassium (mmol/L)	Mean	5.9	4.9	4.5	4.4
	Range	4.5–7.7	4.3–5.3	4.1–5.2	4.1–4.9
Chloride (mmol/L)	Mean	116	115	121	121
	Range	106–125	102–121	118–125	118–126
Calcium (mg/dl)	Mean	9.2	9.3	9.2	8.5
	Range	8.0–11.8	8.6–10.5	7.5–9.9	8.7–9.4
Inorganic phosphorus (mg/dl)	Mean	5.9	6.5	5.8	5.6
	Range	4.0–9.1	5.6–8.7	4.8–7.2	52–7.6
Glucose (mg/dl)	Mean	136	101	115	115
	Range	94–207	62.5–134	99–125	107–138
BUN (mg/dl)	Mean	22	28	16	15
	Range	10–45	12–43	11–25	11–25
Creatinine (mg/dl)	Mean	0.6	0.4	0.6	0.5
	Range	0.4–0.9	0.2–0.6	0.4–0.8	0.4–0.7
Total protein (g/dl)	Mean	6.0	5.9	6.9	6.6
	Range	5.1–7.4	5.3–7.2	6.3–7.7	6.2–7.1
Albumin (g/dl)	Mean	3.2	3.7	4.0	3.9
	Range	2.6–3.8	3.3–4.1	3.3–4.4	3.5–4.2
Total bilirubin (mg/dl)	Mean	<1.0		<1.0	<1.0
				0–0.1	0–0.1
Cholesterol (mg/dl)	Mean	165		165	148
	Range	64–296		129–209	119–201
SAP (IU/L)	Mean	23	53		
	Range	9–84	30–120		
ALT (IU/L)	Mean		170	108	109
	Range		82–289	86–145	78–149
SGOT (IU/L)	Mean	65		85	117
	Range	28–120		57–165	74–248
CO_2	Mean			23.9	24.9
	Range			16–28	20–28
Globulin (g/dl)	Mean			2.3	2.2
	Range			1.8–3.1	2–2.9
AG (g/dl)	Mean			1.7	1.8
	Range			1.2–2.1	1.3–2.1
LDH	Mean			408	460
	Range			221–618	241–752
Alkaline phosphatase	Mean			44	42
	Range			34–66	31–64
Triglycerides	Mean			19	18
	Range			11–30	10–32

* Combined values for male and female ferrets from Thornton, et al.[11]
† Combined values for male, female, and castrated ferrets from Lee, et al.[12]
‡ Data from Fox, et al.[13]

tion. The lymphocyte transformation to mitogens ConA, PWM, and PHA is suppressed on day 5 postinfection, reaches a nadir by days 8 to 11, and returns to normal by 23 to 30 days postvirus challenge. MIF production is also suppressed, whereas a delayed hypersensitivity skin test response is only slightly diminished in distemper-infected ferrets.[8] These in vitro tests of lymphocyte function were accompanied by a marked lymphopenia.

The immunosuppression induced by distemper virus has obvious clinical implications, as noted by Kauffman's experiments with an attenuated strain. Three ferrets died of gram-negative bacillary pneumonia.[8] It is not known whether neutrophil function is affected in distemper infection in ferrets, nor if other viral infections in ferrets can cause similar cell-mediated immunosuppression. Nevertheless, other viral infections in humans can cause cell-mediated immunity depression.[9,10] The exact mechanisms that cause distemper-induced immunosuppression are unknown.

HEMATOLOGY AND SERUM CHEMISTRY

To date there have been limited analyses of normal hematology and serum chemistry in ferrets. In one study from England,

TABLE 7–4. SEX AND STRAIN DIFFERENCES OF SOME HEPATIC DRUG-METABOLIZING ENZYMES IN THE FERRET

Parameter	Albino Ferret		Fitch Ferret		Rat	
	Male	Female	Male	Female	Male	Female
Liver wt/body wt × 100	3.4 ± 0.4	3.4 ± 0.3	4.4 ± 0.2	4.1 ± 0.1	4.2 ± 0.1	4.3 ± 0.1*
Benzpyrene-hydroxylase (nmol/g liver/hr)	3.1 ± 0.4	3.4 ± 0.5	4.0 ± 0.1	3.2 ± 0.5		
Biphenyl-4-hydroxylase (μmol/g liver/hr)	1.1 ± 0.1	1.6 ± 0.1	0.8 ± 0.1	1.2 ± 0.1	1.4	1.5†
Biphenyl-2-hydroxylase (μmol/g liver/hr)	0.11 ± 0.02	0.14 ± 0.01	0.05 ± 0.01	0.08 ± 0.01	<0.1	<0.1†
Ethylmorphine N-demethylase (μmol/g liver/hr)	40 ± 15	26 ± 2	14 ± 2	11 ± 3	14.4 ± 1.5	3.0 ± 0.6*
Aniline hydroxylase (μmol/g liver/hr)	1.0 ± 0.3	1.3 ± 0.1	2.2 ± 0.1	1.2 ± 0.4	0.48 ± 0.06	0.42 ± 0.06*
p-Nitrobenzoate reductase (μmol/g liver/hr)	6.2 ± 1.0	7.5 ± 0.6	4.8 ± 0.2	4.4 ± 0.8	6.5 ± 0.2[3]	
Glucuronyl transferase (μmol/g liver/hr)	0.27 ± 0.01	0.26 ± 0.01	0.30 ± 0.002	0.29 ± 0.02		
NADPH-cytochrome c reductase (nmol/g liver/min)	310 ± 80	280 ± 20	220 ± 10	210 ± 80	1275 ± 50	975 ± 40*
Cytochrome P450 (nmol/g liver)	8.8 ± 0.6	3.3 ± 0.3	3.7 ± 0.2	3.9 ± 0.1	17.5 ± 1.0	10 ± 1.5*
Cytochrome b_5 (nmol/g liver)	3.6 ± 0.3	3.0 ± 0.2	2.8 ± 0.3	2.1 ± 0.5	7.6 ± 0.4‡	
Microsomal protein (mg/g liver)	12 ± 2	8 ± 1	10 ± 1	9.5 ± 1	25 ± 1	20 ± 1*

Results are presented as means ± SEM of three animals.
* Data from El-Defrawny, et al.[15]
† Data from Creaven, et al.[16]
‡ Data from Ioannides and Parke.[17]

28 adult male and 11 albino females were used,[11] and similar analyses on 8 male and 5 female fitch ferrets were undertaken in another study on commercially reared adult ferrets in the United States.[12] More recently, our laboratory compared normal hematology and serum chemistry values on blood collected from the retroorbital plexus and obtained via cardiac puncture.[13] Hematologic values from these three studies are presented in Table 7–2, and are similar to those of the cat, except for the higher erythrocyte count, hemoglobin values, and greater percentages of reticulocytes in the ferret blood. Because the ferret has a slower erythrocyte sedimentation rate, microhematocrit tubes may have to be spun for a longer time than for the dog or cat. A prothrombin time of 14.4 to 16.5 seconds (range) is within the range of those documented in the dog. The mean reticulocyte level for ferrets is 4.0% in males and 5.3% in females, with ranges up to 12 and 14%, respectively.[11]

Table 7–3 presents serum chemistry values on the ferrets used in the previously cited studies.[11–13] These values are in general agreement with normal values seen in dogs and cats. Like other species, ferrets have an age-related decrease in their alkaline phosphatase levels; this bone isoenzyme decreases after the end of rapid bone growth.[12] When ferrets have elevated liver enzyme levels, Aleutian disease must be ruled out.

DRUG METABOLISM

The hepatic microsomal mixed function oxidases and other drug metabolism enzymes have been determined in the developing ferret.[14–17] Biphenyl 4-hydroxylation parallels the activity of NADPH-cytochrome c reductase; both of these enzymes reach a maximum level at 7 to 14 days after birth. Ethylmorphine N-demethylase, aniline hydroxylase, and biphenyl-2-hydroxylase activities are highest at 56 days and are paralleled by cytochrome P_{450}. p-Nitrobenzoate reductase is detectable after 56 days, and is also paralleled by cytochrome P_{450} reductase.

Although no other enzyme parameters differ between the sexes, the hepatic cytochrome P_{450} and ethylmorphine N-demethylase levels are much greater in the male than in the female albino ferret. Levels of cytochrome P_{450}, ethylmorphine N-demethylase, and other enzymes do not differ in the male or female phenotypic fitch ferret.

Cytochrome P_{450} is twice as great and NADPH-cytochrome c reductase is four times greater in the rat than in the ferret. Nevertheless, ethylmorphine N-demethylase and aniline hydroxylase are only a third as active in the rat as in the ferret.

TABLE 7–5. SELECTED URINALYSIS RESULTS IN FERRETS*

Parameter	Male		Female	
	Mean	Range	Mean	Range
Volume (ml/24 hr)	26	8–48	28	8–140
Sodium (mmol/24 hr)	1.9	0.4–6.7	1.5	0.2–5.6
Potassium (mmol/24 hr)	2.9	1.0–9.6	2.1	0.9–5.4
Chloride (mmol/24 hr)	2.4	0.7–8.5	1.9	0.3–7.8
pH		6.5–7.5		6.5–7.5
Protein (mg/dl)		7–33		0–32

Thornton, P.C., et al.: The ferret, *Mustela putorius furo*, as a new species in toxicology. Lab. Anim., *13*:119, 1979.)

* Based on 24-hr urine samples.

Other enzymes measured have approximately equal activity in both species (Table 7–4).

THYROID AND ADRENAL GLAND PARAMETERS

Levels of serum thyroxine, tri-iodothyronine, and cortisol have been measured in ferrets, as have responses to ACTH stimulation and dexamethasone suppression.

SERUM THYROXINE AND TRI-IODOTHYRONINE

In a recent study, serum thyroxine (T_4) and tri-iodothyronine (T_3) values were obtained for normal ferrets by use of a commercial ^{125}I-radioimmunoassay.[18]

Sera from 44 animals, 31 male (27 intact, 4 castrated) and 13 females (10 intact, 3 spayed), were tested. Serum T_4 values ranged from 1.01 to 8.29 $\mu g/dl$ for males (average, 4.5 $\mu g/dl$), and 0.71 to 2.54 $\mu g/dl$ for females (average, 1.38 $\mu g/dl$). Serum T_4 values in adult female ferrets and juvenile ferrets (3 months old) of either sex were similar to the normal T_4 values in the cat, 1.20 to 3.80 $\mu g/dl$. Adult male ferrets, however, both intact and castrated, had higher serum T_4 values that were more comparable to those of the normal dog, 1.52 to 3.60 $\mu g/dl$. Serum T_3 values ranged from 0.45 to 0.78 ng/ml for males (average, 0.61 ng/ml) and 0.29 to 0.73 ng/ml for females (average, 0.53 ng/ml), comparable to those of dogs and cats (0.50–1.50 ng/ml).[18] In another study, adult females had T_3 levels measuring 0.7 ng/ml, whereas their T_4 levels were 45 ng/ml.[28]

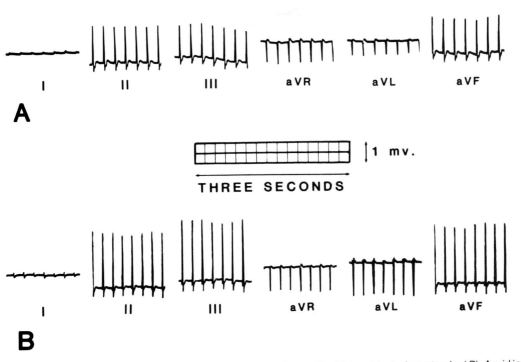

Fig. 7–3. Electrocardiograms in a normal ferret (*A*) and in a ferret with right ventricular hypertrophy (*B*). A grid in the center of the figure is calibrated for measurement of 1 mV and a 3-sec strip in these photographically enhanced images of original recordings. (Smith, S.H., and Bishop, S.P.: The electrocardiogram of normal ferrets and ferrets with right ventricular hypertrophy. Lab. Anim. Sci., *35*:268, 1985.)

SERUM CORTISOL

Cortisol values were obtained from 30 ferrets using a commercial ^{125}I-radioimmunoassay.[19] Sera from 24 males (19 intact, 5 neutered) and 6 females (4 intact, 2 spayed) were tested. Resting serum cortisol values ranged from 0.22 to 2.70 μg/dl for males (average, 0.97 μg/dl), and 0.55 to 1.84 μg/dl for females (average, 0.93 μg/dl). The resting serum cortisol values in both males and females were comparable to those in the cat (1.0–3.0 μg/dl).

RESPONSES TO ACTH STIMULATION AND DEXAMETHASONE SUPPRESSION TESTS

To evaluate or compare applicability of the adrenal function tests used in dogs and cats, an ACTH stimulation test (1 U/kg IM) and a low-dose dexamethasone suppression test (0.1 mg/kg) were performed on three ferrets. Post-ACTH serum cortisol levels increased by an average of 42%. Postdexamethasone se-

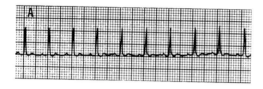

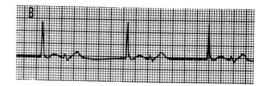

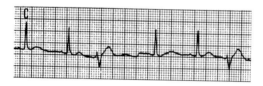

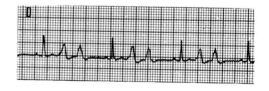

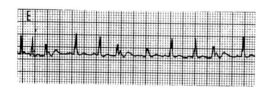

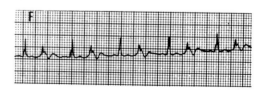

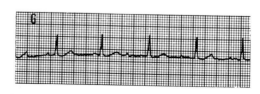

Fig. 7–4. Selected electrocardiograms of ferrets during anesthesia with ketamine (k), ketamine-xylazine (k-x), and ketamine-diazepam (k-d). *A,* Sinus rhythm (k-x). *B,* Bigeminy (k-d). *C,* Trigeminy (k-x). *D,* Ventricular premature contractions (VPCs) in couplet (k). *E,* VPC 3-1 (k). *F,* VPC 1-1 (k). *G,* QRS notching (k-x). (Lead II, paper speed = 50 mm/sec, sensitivity of 1 cm = 1 mV (Moreland, A.F., and Glaser, C.: Evaluation of ketamine, ketamine-xylazine and ketamine-diazepam anesthesia in the ferret. Lab. Anim. Sci., 35:287, 1985.)

TABLE 7–6. ECG VOLTAGE SUMS FOR LEADS I, II, AND III VENTRICULAR WEIGHT RATIO FOR NORMAL ADULT AND RIGHT VENTRICULAR-HYPERTROPHIED FERRETS

Parameter	S Waves (mV)	Total Voltage (mV)	LV:RV Ratio (g:g)
Adult control			
1	1.0	2.0	4.0
2	0.7	4.0	3.96
3	0.5	4.1	4.26
4	0.7	4.1	3.63
5	0.6	4.5	—*
6	0.2	2.2	—
7	1.2	5.3	—
8	1.3	5.9	—
9	0.7	3.6	—
10	0.8	5.1	—
11	0.6	4.0	—
12	0.8	4.4	3.81
13	0.9	5.6	4.19
14	0.9	4.6	3.88
15	0.6	3.3	3.52
16	1.5	7.1	4.16
17	1.1	4.0	3.44
18	0.9	3.7	3.89
19	1.3	7.0	4.05
Mean ± SD	0.86 ± 0.32	4.45 ± 1.35	3.90 ± 0.26
Adult RV hypertrophy			
1	0.5	2.7	—
2	0.9	4.3	3.12
3	1.4	7.0	2.34
4	1.1	6.4	3.33
5	1.5	6.9	2.57
6	0.7	4.3	—
7	1.9	8.5	—
8	0.6	4.5	—
9	1.5	8.1	—
10	0.9	4.6	—
11	1.5	6.2	—
12	0.9	4.8	—
13	0.8	3.5	—
14	0.8	5.1	—
15	1.5	7.5	3.10
16	1.1	6.4	2.22
17	0.9	4.4	2.97
18	0.0	3.5	2.22
19	1.3	3.6	2.80
20	1.2	5.4	2.03
Mean ± SD	1.05 ± 0.44	5.39 ± 1.65†	2.67 ± 0.43

(Smith, S.H., and Bishop, S.P.: The electrocardiogram of normal ferrets and ferrets with right ventricular hypertrophy. Lab. Anim. Sci., *35*:268, 1985.)

* A dash indicates that the individual animal was used for cell isolation studies, precluding any possibility for separate ventricular weight to be measured.

† $p \leq 0.030$.

rum cortisol values decreased by an average of 27% 6 hours postinjection. These responses, like those of the thyroid function tests, were similar to the published results for the normal dog and cat and confirmed the efficacy of these tests when used on ferrets.[19]

URINALYSIS

To evaluate the results of ferret urinalysis, Thornton and associates collected 24-hour selected samples from 40 males and 24 females (Table 7–5).[12] Trace amounts of blood were detected in the urine of three males; the hematuria found in females was invariably associated with estrus. Hematuria in the male, although not commented on by the authors, may have been due to the urethritis or cystitis seen occasionally in male ferrets. Most ferrets had protein in their urine; quanti-

TABLE 7–7. ECG DATA FOR 27 CLINICALLY NORMAL FERRETS*

Parameter	Value
Average age	5.2 months
Male:female ratio	1.25
Heart rate	233 ± 22 bpm
Rhythm	
Normal sinus rhythm	67%
Sinus arrhythmia	33%
Mean electrical axis	
(frontal plane)	+77.22 ± 12°
P (II) duration	0.024 ± 0.004 sec
P (II) amplitude	0.122 ± 0.007 mV
P–R interval	0.047 ± 0.003 sec
Q (II) (6 of 27 had Q waves)	0.10 ± 0.001 mV
QRS (II) duration	0.043 ± 0.003 sec
R (II) amplitude	1.46 ± 0.84 sec
R (I)/RAVF	0.236 ± 0.08
S (II) amplitude	0.125 ± 0.025 mV
S-T segment duration	0.036 ± 0.016 sec
Q-T duration	0.12 ± 0.04 sec
T (II) duration	0.05 ± 0.02 sec
T (II) amplitude	0.22 ± 0.12 mV

(Edwards, J.: Unpublished data, 1987.)
* All patients sedated with ketamine-xylazine combination.

fication of protein by the ponceau B dye method[20] in 12 males and 12 females yielded values in the range of 7 to 33 and 0 to 32 mg/dl, respectively. It was speculated that high systolic pressure (particularly in males), coupled with thicker intrarenal arterial walls, may have been partly responsible for this proteinuria.[12] Again, urinary tract and genital disease must be ruled out.

ELECTROCARDIOGRAPHIC FINDINGS

Electrocardiography is a common technique used in the clinical evaluation of dogs and cats. Texts describing this specialty have been published; refer to these for further details and methodology.[21,22] The electrocardiogram is used in the ferret for various research projects as well as in clinical practice to diagnosis arrhythmias and conduction disturbances, and to ascertain myocardial health. Because the ferret is predisposed to cardiomyopathy and dirofilariasis, it is particularly important to monitor its myocardial status (see Chaps. 12 and 13).[23,24]

Electrocardiograms of normal adult and weanling ferrets have been recorded (Figs. 7–3 and 7–4; Tables 7–6, 7–7, and 7–8). In one study weanlings were induced with ketamine and maintained with 1% halothane.[24] In the same study, adult ferrets were anesthetized with sodium pentobarbitol (25 mg/kg, IP). Electrocardiograms were recorded using leads I, II, III, aVR, aVL, and aVF, with the ferret in right lateral recumbency. In this study the anesthetized ferrets' heart rate was about 300 bpm,[24] whereas in the ketamine-xylazine anesthetized ferret the heart rate was 233 ± 22 bpm.[25] The animals exhibited normal sinus rhythm composed of the expected P wave, QRS complex, and T wave.[24] Heart rates in unanesthetized ferrets and ferrets on various anesthesia protocols are compared in Table 7–9.[26]

TABLE 7–8. RESULTS OF ELECTROCARDIOGRAPH EXAMINATIONS OF FERRETS BEFORE AND DURING ANESTHESIA

Parameter	Unanesthetized	Treatment Group A (Ketamine)	Treatment Group B (Ketamine-Xylazine)	Treatment Group C (Ketamine-Diazepam)
Normal sinus rhythm	14/15*	11/14	9/14	11/14
Ventricular premature contractions	1/15	3/14	5/14	3/14
Other conduction abnormalities (QRS notching)	0/15	2/14	1/14	2/14

(Moreland, A.F., and Glaser, C.: Evaluation of ketamine, ketamine-xylazine, and ketamine-diazepam anesthesia in the ferret. Lab. Anim. Sci., *35*:287, 1985.)
* Numerator, number showing indicated condition; denominator, population in group.

TABLE 7–9. HEART RATE OF FERRETS BEFORE AND DURING ANESTHESIA (bpm)

Parameter	Treatment Group A (Ketamine)	Treatment Group B (Ketamine-Xylazine)	Treatment Group C (Ketamine-Diazepam)
Unanesthetized	250 (160–320)*	250 (160–320)	250 (160–320)
5 minutes postinjection	280 (240–340)	195 (120–240)	300 (280–360)
15 minutes postinjection	320 (260–320)	160 (160–200)	320 (300–360)
30 minutes postinjection	330 (280–360)	150 (120–180)	340 (280–400)
45 minutes postinjection	320 (280–400)	150 (100–200)	350 (320–400)
60 minutes postinjection	340 (280–400)	170 (110–200)	325 (320–330)

(Moreland, A.F., and Glaser, C.: Evaluation of ketamine, ketamine-xylazine, and ketamine-diazepam anesthesia in the ferret. Lab. Anim. Sci., *35*:287, 1985.)
* Mean value; range in parentheses.

The ferret has a consistent mean electrical axis, $+69°$ to $+97°$. In one study, the animals had an axis that was perpendicular to lead I and most positive in lead aVF. The average axis was 86°, with a standard deviation of 6.6°.[24] In another study, the electrical axis was $77 \pm 12°$ (Table 7–7).[25] These findings are, in part, the result of the long narrow shape of these animals, and an axis deviation appears to be the most significant parameter in detecting gross abnormal morphology of the heart in a normal ferret.

Investigators have also induced right heart hypertrophy using pulmonary artery banding. Despite right ventricular hypertrophy the axis of the ECG was not affected, but the overall ECG voltage was increased (Table 7–6; Fig. 7–3).[24]

SEMEN STUDIES

Various properties of ferret semen have been characterized.

COLLECTION OF SEMEN BY ELECTROEJACULATION

Semen can be successfully collected in ferrets by the electroejaculation method.[27] Animals are anesthetized with 50 to 75 μl of a 1:1 combination of zolasepam

TABLE 7–10. SEMEN CHARACTERISTICS OF MALE FERRETS (Based on Three Ejaculates per Male)

Ferret No.	Age (years)	Mean Spermatozoa Concentration (10^6/mm^3)	Mean Semen Volume (ml)	Mean Spermatozoa per Ejaculate (10^6)	Mean Spermatozoa Motility (%)
1	4	0.370 ± .232*	0.022 ± .002*	8.251	76.7
2	3	1.272 ± .314	0.026 ± .001	33.072	88.3
3	3	0.964 ± .207	0.024 ± .006	23.425	91.7
4	3	0.349 ± .111	0.030 ± .007	10.540	62.3
5	2	0.627 ± .140	0.032 ± .008	19.813	44.4
6	1	0.991 ± .494	0.028 ± .008	28.045	55.0
7	1	0.272 ± .148	0.027 ± .003	7.290	88.3
8	1	0.610 ± .219	0.023 ± .006	14.152	71.7
Mean		0.680	0.027	18.074	72.3

Modified from Shump et al.[27]
* Mean ± SE.

(Tilazol), and maintained on their backs with their rear legs extended. A bipolar rectal electrode is inserted at a depth of 3.75 cm and an electrical stimulus of about 4 V and 0.35 mA is applied for 4 seconds, repeated at 10-second intervals using an AC (60 cps) rheostat-controlled stimulator. If unsuccessful after several attempts, the procedure should be discontinued. An average of approximately 12.3 stimuli are required to obtain semen.

SEMEN CHARACTERISTICS

Shump and colleagues studied semen characteristics by collecting samples in prewarmed glass vials (1.25 × 3.75 cm)

from ferrets during their breeding cycle.[27] A few abnormalities in the sperm were noted, including coiled tails and clumping of the spermatozoa. The full results are summarized in Table 7–10.

TESTOSTERONE

In young male adults, the peak testosterone levels occur at day 60-80 (maximum 2.6 ng/ml). As mature adults, testosterone level is correlated with the reproductive activity and inactivity of the ferret. The maximum level (17.7 ng/ml) occurs in spring and early summer, whereas in fall and winter the level declines to about 0.1 ng/ml.[28]

REFERENCES

1. Suffin, S.C., et al.: Ontogeny of the ferret humoral immune response. J. Immunol., 123:6, 1979.
2. Suffin, S.C., et al.: Immunoprophylaxis of respiratory syncytial virus infection in the infant ferret. J. Immunol., 123:10, 1979.
3. Kauffman, C.A.: Cell-mediated immunity in ferrets: Delayed dermal hypersensitivity, lymphocyte transformation, and macrophage migration inhibitory factor production. Dev. Comp. Immunol., 5:125, 1981.
4. Kauffman, C.A., Schiff, G.M., and Phair, J.P.: Influenza in ferrets and guinea pigs. Effect on cell-mediated immunity. Infect. Immunol., 19: 547, 1978.
5. McLaren, C., and Butchko, G.: Regional T- and B-cell response in influenza-infected ferrets. Infect. Immunol., 22:189, 1978.
6. Kauffman, C.A., and Bergman, A.G.: Lymphocyte subpopulations in ferret. Devel. Comp. Immunol., 5:671, 1981.

7. Potter, C.W., et al.: Immunity to influenza in ferrets. IX. Delayed hypersensitivity following infection or immunization with A2/Hong Kong virus. Microbios, *10A*:7, 1974.
8. Kauffman, C.A., Bergman, A.G., and O'Connor, R.P.: Distemper virus infection in ferrets: An animal model of measles-induced immunosuppression. Clin. Exp. Immunol., *47*:617, 1982.
9. Oldstone, M.B.A.: Virus can alter cell function without causing cell pathology: Disordered function leads to imbalance of homeostasis and disease. *In* Concepts in Viral Pathogenesis. Edited by A.L. Hotkins. New York, Springer-Verlag, 1984.
10. Notkins, A. (ed): Viral Immunology and Immunopathology. New York, Academic Press, 1970.
11. Thornton, P.C., Wright, P.A., Sacra, P.J., and Goodier, T.E.W.: The ferret, *Mustela putorius furo*, as a new species in toxicology. Lab. Anim., *13*:119, 1979.
12. Lee, E.J., et al.: Haematological and serum chemistry profiles of ferrets (*Mustela putorius furo*). Lab. Anim., *16*:133, 1982.
13. Fox, J.G. et al.: Serum chemistry and hematology reference values in the ferret (*Mustela putorius furo*). Lab. Anim. Sci., *36*:583, 1986.
14. Ioannides, C., Sweatman, R., Richards, R., and Parke, D.V.: Drug metabolism in the ferret: Effects of age, sex, and strain, Gen. Pharmacol., *8*:243, 1977.
15. El Defrawny-El Masry S., Cohen, G.M., and Mannering, G.J.: Sex-dependent differences in drug metabolism in the rat—I. Temporal changes in the microsomal drug-metabolizing system of the liver during sexual maturation. Drug. Metab. Dispos., *3*:267, 1974.
16. Creaven, P.J., Parke, D.V., and Williams R.T.: A fluorimetric study of the hydroxylation of biphenyl in vitro by liver preparations of various species. Biochem. J., *96*:879, 1965.
17. Ioannides, C., and Parke, D.V.: Development of the hepatic drug-metabolizing enzymes in the ferret. *In* Basic and Therapeutic Aspects of Perinatal Pharmacology. Edited by P.L. Morselli, S. Garattini, and F. Sereni. New York, Raven Press, 1975.
18. Garibaldi, B.A., Pecquet-Goad, M.E., and Fox, J.G.: Serum thyroxine (T_4) and tri-iodothyronine (T_3) radioimmunoassay values in the normal ferret. Lab. Anim. Sci., *37*:544, 1987.
19. Garibaldi, B.A., Pecquet-Goad, M.E., and Fox, J.G.: Serum cortisol radioimmunoassay values in the normal ferret and response to ACTH and dexamethasone-suppression tests. Lab. Anim. Sci., *37*:545, 1987.
20. Pesce, M.A., and Strande, C.S.: A new micromethod for determination of protein in cerebrospinal fluid and urine. Clin. Chem., *19*:1265, 1973.
21. Bolton, G.R.: Handbook of Canine Electrocardiography. Philadelphia, W.B. Saunders, 1975.
22. Tilley, L.P.: Essentials of Canine and Feline Electrocardiography. 2nd Ed. Philadelphia, Lea & Febiger, 1984.
23. Cohen, R.B.: Electrocardiographic techniques in clinical practice. *In* Symposium on Cardiopulmonary Diagnostic Techniques. Vet. Clin. North Am., *13*:217, 1983.
24. Smith, S.H., and Bishop, S.P.: The electrocardiogram of normal ferrets and ferrets with right ventricular hypertrophy. Lab. Anim. Sci., *35*:268, 1985.
25. Edwards, J.: Unpublished data, 1987.
26. Moreland, A.F., and Glaser, C.: Evaluation of ketamine, ketamine-xylazine and ketamine-diazepam anesthesia in the ferret. Lab. Anim. Sci., *35*:287, 1985.
27. Shump, A.U., Aulerich, R.J., and Ringer, R.K.: Semen volume and sperm concentration in the ferret (*Mustela putorius*). Lab. Anim. Sci., *26*:913, 1976.
28. Kastner, R., Kastner, D., and Apfelbach, R.: Developmental patterns of thyroid hormones and testosterone in ferrets. Horm. Metabol. Res., *19*:194, 1987.

chapter 8

REPRODUCTION, BREEDING, AND GROWTH

J. G. Fox

MORPHOLOGY

The ferret has a long body, with short muscular legs and a long tail. The adult ferret's average body length is 44 to 46 cm from the nose to the tip of the tail. Some of its anatomic features resemble those of the cat and dog—the anterior and lateral portion of its skull resembles the cat's, not the dog's. On the other hand, the zygomatic bones of the eye orbits of the ferret and dog are open, while those of a cat are almost closed.[1]

As a result of its behavioral traits and burrowing instincts, the ferret has developed certain anatomic adaptations. It is postulated that, because of its burrowing nature, the ferret's long neck and placement of the carotid arteries may help the ferret maintain sufficient cerebral blood flow when it turns its head in tight confined spaces (see Chap. 2, Anatomy of the Ferret).[2] Also, the compliant chest wall, total lung capacity, and respiratory reserve, which is very large in comparison to body size, are anatomic adaptations. The

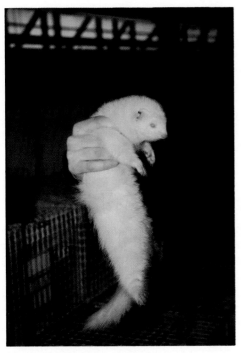

Fig. 8–1. Albino (English) ferret.

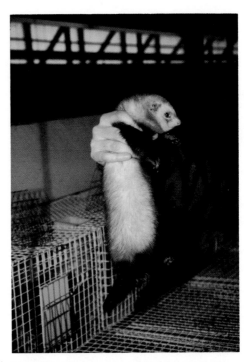

Fig. 8–3. Siamese ferret (brown guard hair).

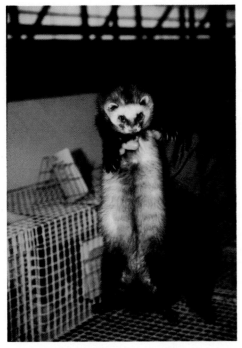

Fig. 8–2. Sable or fitch ferret (black guard hair).

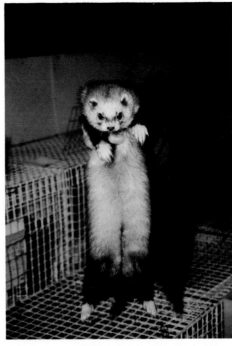

Fig. 8–4. Silver mitt ferret (sable with white chest and feet).

relatively large-diameter airway and long trachea result in a lower central airway and lower pulmonary resistance in comparison to those of other animals of similar size (see Chap. 4, Physiology of the Ferret).[3]

The ferret's short digestive tract is characteristic of other carnivores, but a cecum and appendix are absent in this species. Also, the large intestine is unique, because there is no external anatomic division between the ileum and the colon, and the lower intestine thus appears grossly as one long, undifferentiated organ.[4] Anatomy was discussed in greater detail elsewhere (see Chap. 2).

COAT CYCLES

Using the method described by Hammond and Chesterman,[5] it is sometimes possible to determine parturition dates in the female ferret by removing a pluck of hair from the dorsum of the loin in the proestrous animal. This area will remain hairless until after ovulation or until the end of estrus. The hair regrowth reaches the skin 21 to 24 days after mating, coinciding with or occurring within a week after the first uterine swellings can be ascertained by abdominal palpation.

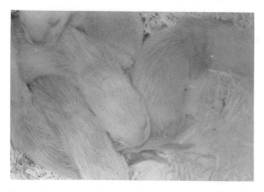

Fig. 8–5. Young fitch ferrets with gray hair coats. The eyes are closed until the fifth week.

Under natural lighting conditions the animals lose hair in October or November, when partial alopecia is noted.[6] In males the hair coat is not fully regrown until the end of the breeding cycle. Hair loss in the female follows the first ovulation of the breeding season and usually follows subsequent ovulations, but the loss is delayed during lactation.

COAT COLORS

Readily available commercial stocks, based on coat color, are albino (English; Fig. 8–1), sable or fitch (black guard hair; Fig. 8–2), Siamese (brown guard hair; Fig. 8–3), silver mitt (sable with white chest and feet; Fig. 8–4), and Siamese-silver mitt (Siamese with white chest and feet).[7] The fitch has the most common coat color, recognized by yellow-buff fur with patches of black or dark brown, particularly on the tail and limbs.[8] The facial fur is somewhat lighter, with a dark mask over the eyes that is less marked in neutered animals. The eyes themselves are usually dark brown.

The albino (with a nonpigmented iris) is also seen frequently, but this coat color is recessive to the pigmented wild phenotype. The pet industry is currently promoting additional coat colors, such as white-footed sable, butterscotch, white-footed butterscotch, spotted, and cinnamon.[9]

GROWTH AND DEVELOPMENT

The ferret has a marked sexual dimorphism in body weight, with the male often weighing twice as much as the female. The male is referred to as a "hob" and the female as a "jill." At birth the ferret "kit" weighs approximately 6 to 12 g. Its eyes are closed, and its body is covered with fine hair. After about 3 days the albino ferret still retains its white hair coat, while the fitch ferret acquires a gray coat (Fig. 8–5). Each animal has a subcutaneous fat pad on the dorsal surface of its neck.[10]

Even before their eyes actually open (at about 34 days), the young animals are moving actively about the cage and appear to have little trouble in identifying their mother. The lactating female is particularly aware of and responsive to the complex variety of her young's vocalizations during their first few weeks of life.[11]

The young ferrets begin to hear sound at about 32 days after birth, whereas cats can hear at 6 days.[12] The deciduous teeth erupt at about 14 days, and emerge completely through the gums at 18 days. The permanent canine teeth appear at 47 to 52 days, prior to the shedding of the deciduous canines at 56 to 70 days.[13] Although ferrets are usually weaned between 6 and 8 weeks of age, they begin to take in solid food as early as 2 to 3 weeks postnatally.

Young ferrets have a voracious appetite, and the female must provide adequate milk for the growing kits; solid food must be provided as early as 3 weeks postpartum. By the time they are eating solid food exclusively the young ferrets

can defecate without stimulation. Prior to this time, the female licks the urogenital area to stimulate both urination and defecation.[10]

Body weight gradually increases in both sexes between 4 and 5 weeks of age. There is then a sharp increase in growth until adult weight is reached, at about 16 weeks of age (Fig. 8–6).[10,14,15] Ferrets, when weaned at 6 to 8 weeks, average about 300 to 450 g in weight. There is no significant body weight difference between males and females until the seventh week of life, and none in body length until the ninth week. Table 8–1 compares organ weights of adult male and female ferrets.

The development of social behavior in the ferret over the first few months of life has been described elsewhere.[16]

SEASONAL WEIGHT FLUCTUATION

Both female and male ferrets experience marked seasonal weight fluctuations, up to 30 to 40% of their body weight, from the loss of subcutaneous fat in the spring

TABLE 8–1. ORGAN WEIGHTS OF FERRETS*

Organ	Weight (per kg body weight)	
	Male	Female
Body weight (g)	1527 (1235–2105)	964 (740–1210)
Brain (g)	4.23 (2.60–6.23)	5.03 (4.05–6.15)
Pituitary (g)	4.09 (0.90–6.20)	5.07 (2.25–8.05)
Heart (g)	3.87 (2.99–5.90)	3.72 (2.43–5.27)
Spleen (g)	4.44 (2.15–8.00)	4.15 (3.04–6.22)
Liver (g)	33.2 (24.5–45.0)	29.4 (19.7–38.0)
Kidneys (g)	4.29 (3.25–5.80)	3.69 (2.87–4.86)
Adrenals (mg)	101 (71–150)	101 (79–139)
Testes (g)	2.02 (0.8–3.8)	
Ovaries (mg)		151 (94–183)
Uterus (mg)		766 (135–2439)

(Thornton, P.C., Wright, P.A., Sacra, P.J., and Goodier, T.E.W.: The ferret, *Mustela putorius furo,* as a new species in toxicology. Lab. Anim., *13*:119, 1979.)
* Mean body weight and organ weight (with ranges) in 28 male and 11 female ferrets.

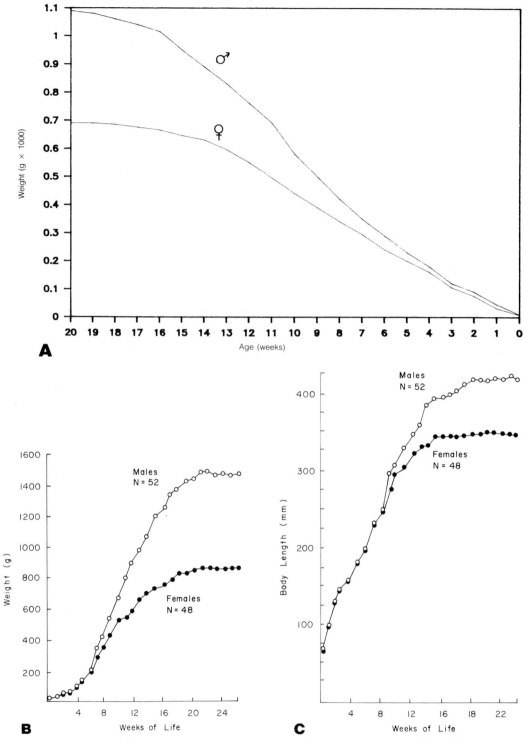

Fig. 8–6. *A,* Growth chart of female and male ferret. Because of fat accumulation in winter, male adults may weigh as much as 1600 g, and female adults may weigh as much as 750 g. *B,* Body weight of male and female European ferrets from birth to 26 weeks of age. *C,* Body length of male and female European ferrets from birth to 26 weeks of age. (Shump, A.U., and Shump, K.A.: Growth and development of the European ferret (*Mustela putorius*. Lab. Anim. Sci., *28*:89, 1978.)

(previously deposited in the fall). Ferrets' coats also undergo seasonal cycling, with molting occurring in the early summer.

LIFE SPAN

The ferret lives approximately 5 to 6 years, but pet ferrets may live longer (8- to 11-year life spans have been recorded).

BIOTIC FACTORS

There are a number of considerations involved in a discussion of the reproduction of ferrets.

SEXING AND SEXUAL MATURITY

One can easily ascertain the sex of a neonate ferret by measuring the anogenital distance. In the male the urogenital opening is on the ventral abdomen; in the female the anogenital distance is short (Fig. 8–7). The male also has an os penis, which can be palpated.

Generally, ferrets reach sexual maturity at 8 to 12 months of age. The adult male usually weighs 1½ to 2 times more than the female. In a population of 1-year-old ferrets, the male body weight was 1000 ± 45 g, whereas that of the female was 580 ± 38 g.[8] These values are similar to those reported for a wild population of ferrets, in which the male weighed 1026 g and the female 505 g.[17] Animals weighing up to 3500 g have been reported,[5] but any weight greater than 1500 g is most likely a result of fat deposition, particularly in the viscera. This obviously makes the animals less desirable for abdominal surgery and may modify their responses to intraperitoneal injections of some drugs, particularly anesthetics. Studies done in wild populations showed that no ferrets weighed more than 1500 g.[8]

In the United States, according to one commercial breeder, ferrets have increased in size by about 20% over the years. Mature males will range from 3 to 5 lb

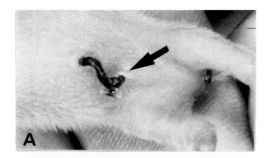

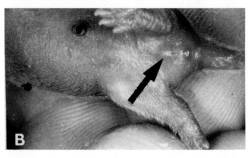

Fig. 8–7. *A*, Male neonate ferret, with urogenital opening on ventral abdomen (*arrow*). The dark structure is a remnant of umbilicus. *B*, Female ferret with narrow anogenital distance. The arrow indicates the genital opening. Note the distance from the umbilical stump.

(1.5–2.5 kg), and mature females from 1.5 to 3 lb (0.75–1.5 kg).[9]

In male ferrets born in June, testicular development commences in December and reaches maturity by February.[18] Functional activity lasts from March until July. The period of quiescence extends from August until December, with redevelopment beginning again in January and reaching a second functional period in March. Immature testes are characterized by a lack of germinal centers, the undifferentiated precursors of Sertoli cells, a lack of tubular lumens, and small interstitial cells. The prepubertal (as well as the redeveloping) testes enlarge because of developing germinal epithelium and tubular lumen, and growth of Sertoli and interstitial cells.[18] The male's sexual activity from December until July (when spermatogenesis is active) is apparent by the descent of the testicles into the scrotum.

Sexual activity continues until 3 years of age. The male's breeding season, from December to July, precedes the female's from March to August (under normal lighting conditions).[5] This time lapse is presumed to be a functional adaptation, allowing for adequate maturation of sperm.[19] The female usually reaches sexual maturity at the same age as the male and is seasonally polyestrous, with the onset of estrus coinciding with an increase in day length.

Mating should occur 14 days after the onset of vulvar swelling. Three to four days after mating, the vulva becomes dry and regresses in size during the following 4 weeks. Within 10 to 14 days after the end of pseudopregnancy, a pregnancy termination due to abortion, or weaning, the vulva will again enlarge, reaching full size in about 10 days. If mating is not delayed a female may have two litters a year, under normal lighting conditions.

PHOTOPERIODS AND REPRODUCTIVE PERFORMANCE

Light cycles play an important part in the reproduction of the ferret.[6] If breeding is required at all times of the year for commercial or biomedical research purposes, half the colony can be maintained on reverse light cycles. Nevertheless, it is also possible to maintain the entire colony on constant short photoperiods (6–8 hours of light daily) and also to have a long-day room available (14–15 hours of light daily). Males on short days are continuously in breeding condition for periods of a year or more. Females on short photoperiods commence estrus at 7 to 8 months but, if on continuous lighting (24 hours), estrus commences at about 1 year. On a 14-hour photoperiod (14:10 light:dark), many females will remain anestrous.[5] Thus, on short photoperiods, males will be available for breeding almost constantly, and females will be breeding according to their dates of birth.

Females who have completed a breeding season of short photodays can be brought into estrus by placing them in a room on a 14-hour light cycle. Young ferrets reared on 6- 8-hour light cycles will breed at $4\frac{1}{2}$ to 5 months if transferred to long-day photoperiods. This transfer must not occur before the ferret is 90 days old, or the ferret will become anestrous before attaining full breeding condition.[5]

In one breeding colony, because of management practices, females began their reproductive life between 7 and 10 months of age and were bred continuously until productivity declined. Females averaged 3.7 litters per year, and were rarely maintained beyond 6 litters or 30 months of age.[7] Rebreeding occurred immediately on onset of postweaning estrus. Under these conditions maternal age and parity, but not coat color, were important predictors of reproductive performance.

ESTROUS CYCLE

The estrous cycle is closely related to seasonal changes. An enlarged pink vulva, which signals the onset of estrus, reaches maximal size in about 1 month after estrus ensues and then regresses in the 2 to 3 weeks following mating.[20] Estrogen levels control this vulvar swelling, as well as changes in vaginal cytology.[21] Behavioral changes during estrus include decreased food intake, reduced sleep, and irritability.

Because the female ferret is an induced ovulator, she will maintain estrus for up to 6 months if not bred. The onset of estrus can be altered and the breeding period prolonged by manipulating the photoperiod, as previously described.[22]

BREEDING

As with many animal species, an estrous female should be taken to the male's cage for breeding purposes. It is helpful to observe the animals during the initial mating process to ensure that fighting and trauma do not ensue. Ferrets copulate vigorously, noisily, and for prolonged periods (10 minutes to 3 hours), with a mean of approximately 1 hour. The male typically grabs the female at the back of the neck and they proceed pressed together, side by side, on the floor. If necessary, they may be separated (see Chap. 19 for further details).

FERTILIZATION AND PREGNANCY

Although ovulation (with 5–13 ova being shed) is induced approximately 30 to 40 hours after coitus,[23] and the trophoblast is implanted 12 to 13 days after coitus (Table 8–2),[19] the deciduous cell reaction to implantation is absent in the ferret and the uterus responds minimally to the presence of an embryo. Although the sperm require only 3 to 11 hours to achieve their fertilization capacity in the reproductive tract, they can survive in the female reproductive tract for 36 to 48 hours.[23] After mating, the vulva regresses in 3 or 4 days and regains normal size in 2 to 3 weeks, although it will take longer initially if estrus was prolonged. Placentation of the ferret is zonal (or discoid), and of the endotheliochorial type.[24]

If fertilization fails, pseudopregnancy ensues after breeding, lasting approximately 40 to 42 days. If the vulva does not recede the female should be rebred. Pregnancy can be detected by abdominal palpation as early as 14 days postfertilization. The fetuses should be about the size of small walnuts.[25]

Females will return to estrus about 2 weeks after the litter is weaned or in the next breeding season, depending on the time of year. On occasion, the female will return to estrus 2 to 3 weeks after the first litter is born. Apparently five is the critical number of corpea lutea or suckling young required to prevent lactational estrus. If lactational estrus does occur it is recommended that the ferret be bred at this estrus, thus diminishing estrogen's inhibitory effect on lactation.[26]

TABLE 8–2. FERRET REPRODUCTIVE DATA

Parameter	Value
Age at puberty	
Female (adult, average 800 g)	7–10 months
Male (adult, average 1500 g)	8–12 months
Minimum breeding age	8–12 months
Estrous cycle	Monestrus, March through August
Duration of estrous cycle	Continuous until intromission
Type of ovulation	Induced by copulation
Ovulation time	30–40 hours after mating
Number of ova	12 (range, 5–13)
Copulation time	Up to 3 hours
Sperm deposition site	Posterior os cervix
Ovum transit time	5–6 days
Viability of sperm in female tract	36–48 hours
Cleavage to formation of blastocoele	Uniform rate
Implantation	12–13 days
Gestation period	42 ± 1 days
Implantation—parturition	30 ± 1 days
Litter size	8 average (range, 1–18)
Size at birth	6–12 g
Return to estrus	Next March,* occasionally postpartum estrus
Weaning age	6 weeks
Solid food eaten	3 weeks, before eyes are open
Breeding life of female	2–5 years
Breeding life of male	2–5 years
Breeding habits	One male to several females; in colony production

* Dependent on lighting cycle.

PARTURITION

Although pregnant females can be maintained together in communal housing it is prudent to house them singly, beginning 2 or 3 weeks prior to parturition. This will help minimize disturbance of

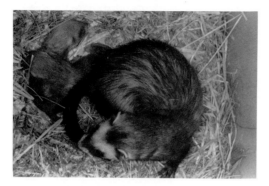

Fig. 8–8. Fitch jill ferret with kits.

the jill, who may be more irritable late in gestation, and thus reduce cannibalism after the birth of her kits.[27] Rowlands observed nest building activity during late pregnancy,[26] but others have not.[8] Either way, nesting boxes can be provided along with nesting material, such as cotton batting, shredded paper, clean hay, or cloth (Fig. 8–8). Females may also use fur pulled from their own bodies for bedding material.[28] Some authors maintain, however, that nesting boxes are unnecessary if

sufficient bedding material (such as sawdust chips) is present in the ferret's cage.

After the kits are born (average weight, 6–12 g; average litter size 8, ranging up to 18), it is important not to disturb the mother and kits for at least several days to prevent cannibalism.[7] It is also important to maintain a narrow variation in environmental temperature because wide diurnal temperature fluctuations (0–22°C) may induce abnormal behavior in lactating jills and cause them to reject their young.[29]

Provided she has sufficient milk, the jill can nurse more kits than she has nipples for (total of eight mammary nipples). If the kits must be fostered, one should remove the jill and allow her kits to mix with the kits of the foster mother. This will help to prevent the foster mother from rejecting her new "adopted" litter (because of olfactory stimuli).

Ferret's milk consists of 23.5% solids; of that 34% is fat, 25.5% protein, and 16.2% is carbohydrate.[30] With proper dilutions, powdered or liquid milk replacers (canine or feline) can be used if foster rearing by bottle feeding is necessary.

REFERENCES

1. Wen, G.Y., Sturman, J.A., and Shek, J.W.: A comparative study of the tapetum, retina, and skull of the ferret, dog, and cat. Lab. Anim. Sci., *35*:200, 1985.
2. Andrews, P.L.R., Bower, A.J., and Illman, O.: Some aspects of the physiology and anatomy of the cardiovascular system of the ferret, *Mustela putorius furo.* Lab. Anim., *13*:215, 1979.
3. Boyd, R.L., and Mangos, J.A.: Pulmonary mechanics of the normal ferret. J. Appl. Physiol., *50*:799, 1981.
4. Bueno, L., and Fioramonti, J.: Is there a large intestine in the ferret? Experientia, *37*:257, 1981.
5. Hammond, J., Jr., and Chesterman, F.C.: The ferret. *In* UFAW Handbook on the Care and Management of Laboratory Animals. 4th ed. London, Churchill Livingstone, 1972.
6. Harvey, N.E., and MacFarlane, W.V.: The effects of day length on coat-shedding cycle, body weight, and reproduction of the ferret. Aust. J. Biol. Sci., *11*:187, 1958.
7. McLain, D.F., et al.: Congenital malformations and variations in reproductive performance in the ferret: Effects of maternal age, color, and parity. Lab. Anim. Sci., *35*:251, 1985.
8. Andrews, P.L.R., and Illman, O.: The ferret. *In* UFAW Handbook on Laboratory Animals. 6th ed. Edited by T. Poole. London, Longman's Scientific and Technical, 1987.
9. Morton, C., and Morton, F.: Ferrets: A Complete Pet Owner's Manual, p. 72. New York, Barrons, 1985.
10. Shump, A.U., and Shump, K.A.: Growth and development of the European ferret (*Mustela putorius*). Lab. Anim. Sci., *28*:89, 1978.
11. Von Solmsen, E., and Abfelbach, R.: Brutpflegewirksame Kimponenten im Weinen neonater Frettchen. Z. Tierpsychol., *50*:337, 1979.
12. Moore, D.R.: Late onset hearing in the ferret. Brain Res., *253*:309, 1982.
13. Berkovitz, B.K.B., and Silverstone, L.M.: The dentition of the albino ferret. Caries Res., *3*:369, 1969.

14. Willis, L.H., and Barrow, M.V.: The ferret (*Mustela putorius furo L.*) as a laboratory animal. Lab. Anim. Sci., *21*:712, 1971.

15. Hahn, E.W., and Wester, R.C.: The Biomedical Use of Ferrets in Research. North Rose, NY, Marshall Research Animals, 1969.

16. Lazar, J.W., and Beckhorn, G.D.: The concept of play or development of social behavior in ferrets. Am. Zool., *14*:405, 1974.

17. Lavers, R.B.: Aspects of the biology of the ferret (*Mustela putorius furo L.*) at Pukepuke Lagoon. Proc. N.Z. Ecol. Soc., *20*:7, 1973.

18. Ishida, K.: Age and seasonal changes in the testis of the ferret. Arch. Histol. Jap., *19*:193, 1968.

19. Ryland, L.M., and Gorham, J.R.: The ferret and its diseases. J. Am. Vet. Med. Assoc., *173*:1154, 1978.

20. Marshall, F.H.A., and Hammond, J., Jr.: Experimental control of hormone action on the estrous cycle in the ferret. J. Endocrinol., *4*:159, 1945.

21. Hamilton, W.J., and Gould, J.H.: The normal estrous cycle of the ferret: The correlation of the vaginal smear and the histology of the genital tract, with notes on the distribution of glycogen, the incidence of growth, and the reaction to intravital staining with trypan blue. Proc. R. Soc. Edinb., *60*:88, 1940.

22. Donovan, B.T.: Light and the control of the estrous cycle in the ferret. J. Endocrinol., *39*:105, 1967.

23. Chang, M.C., and Yanagimachi, R.: Fertilization of ferret ova by deposition of epididymal sperm into the ovarian capsule with special reference to the fertilizable life of ova and the capacitation of sperm. J. Exp. Zool., *154*:175, 1963.

24. Morrow, D.A.: Current Therapy in Theriogenology. W.B. Saunders, Philadelphia, 1980.

25. Conalty, M.L.: Husbandry of Laboratory Animals. London, Academic Press, 1967.

26. Rowlands, I.W.: The ferret. *In* UFAW Handbook on the Care and Management of Laboratory Animals. 3rd ed. Edinburgh, E & S Livingstone, 1967.

27. Bissonnette, T.H.: Ferrets. *In* The Care and Breeding of Laboratory Animals, pp. 234–255. 3rd ed. Edited by E.J. Farris. New York, John Wiley & Sons, 1965.

28. Moody, K.D., Bowman, T.A., and Lang, C.M.: Laboratory management of the ferret for biomedical research. Lab. Anim. Sci., *35*:272, 1985.

29. Anonymous: Diseases of the fitch. Surveillance, *11*:27, 1984.

30. Anonymous: Mother's milk is nature's most perfect food. Eglin, Illinois, Pet-Ag, Inc., 1986.

DISEASES AND CLINICAL APPLICATIONS

chapter 9

DISEASES ASSOCIATED WITH REPRODUCTION

J. G. Fox
R. C. Pearson
J. R. Gorham

DISEASES OF THE JILL

Female ferrets are subject to a number of disorders related to the reproductive process.

ESTROGEN-INDUCED ANEMIA

Etiology. Aplastic anemia is a frequent clinical pathologic finding associated with prolonged estrus in female ferrets. If the jill is not bred she will usually remain in estrus for the duration of the breeding season, and may succumb. The bone marrow depression is attributed to prolonged exposure of hematopoietic tissue to estrogens.[1-3] Hart[3] and Sherrill and Gorham[4] have speculated on the mechanisms by which estrogens may suppress the myeloid, erythroid, and megakaryocytic cell lines. Bernard and colleagues[1] experimentally produced severe bone marrow suppression of all blood cell populations in ferrets, regardless of gender or ovariohysterectomy, by administering high levels of exogenous estrogen.

Epizootiology and Prevention. The incidence of aplastic anemia is highest during the breeding season, occurring in 50% of females experiencing prolonged estrus.[5] The loss of 30% of estrous females in a colony was reported during one breeding season.[1] Aplastic anemia may be avoided by spaying nonbreeding females at 6 to 8 months of age. If females become estrous they may be induced to ovulate by the injection of gonadotropin-releasing hormone (Gn-RH) or human chorionic gonadotropin (HCG), as described earlier.[1,4] The injection may be repeated when a female returns to estrus 40 to 60 days later. Jills should not be allowed to remain in estrus for longer than 1 month. The use of vasectomized hobs is another option in preventing prolonged estrus in ferrets.[6] Breeding of estrous ferrets will also prevent aplastic anemia.

Pathogenesis. Initially there is a leukocytosis followed by leukopenia, anemia, and thrombocytopenia. There is also a coagulopathy associated with prolonged estrus involving a liver-related dysfunction, in addition to the thrombocytopenia.[3] Although ferrets are considered to be highly susceptible to the effects of estrogens,[3] surviving experimental females were found to be less sensitive.[1] The neutropenia may predispose females to bacterial infections such as pyometra, vaginitis,[1] and bronchopneumonia.[2]

Clinical Signs. The clinical signs of bone marrow suppression in ferrets are combined with those seen during estrus. Ferrets have a bilateral symmetric alopecia of the ventral abdomen and tail area, weight loss, vulvar enlargement with a serous to mucopurulent discharge, and possibly a superficial perivulvar dermatitis. Jills experience anorexia, depression, and lethargy, and may also have pneumonia, pyometra, systemic bacterial infection, posterior paralysis, or melena (Fig. 9–1). Examination reveals

pale mucous membranes and possibly a systolic murmur, consistent with anemia.[2] Hemorrhage is the most common cause of death, and coagulopathy is manifested as petechiae or ecchymoses of the skin, buccal mucosa, and conjunctiva, or as melena from gastrointestinal hemorrhage (Fig. 9–2). Subdural hematoma of the spinal cord or brain may result in posterior paralysis or ataxia and depression.[1,4] Ferrets are typically in estrus for 2 months before the first deaths occur.[4]

Clinical Pathology. Sherrill and Gorham[4] studied alterations in the hematologic parameters of ferrets in prolonged estrus. They recorded initial thrombocytosis and neutrophilia followed by thrombocytopenia, neutropenia, lymphopenia, anemia, and hypocellular bone marrow. Females maintained platelet counts of 50,000/μl, with some counts decreasing to 20,000 platelets/μl and less. Hemorrhage occurred when platelet counts fell below 20,000/μl. Bernard and associates[1] noted platelet counts less than 50,000/μl in ferrets given exogenous estrogens. Kociba and Caputo[2] reported decreased platelet numbers in all six pet ferrets they examined. One had a thrombocyte count of less than 7,000/μl. Another was euthanized but the remaining died, despite treatment.

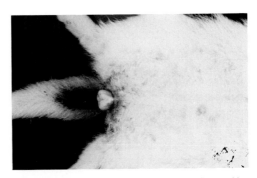

Fig. 9–1. Hyperestrogenism in female ferret. Note the swollen vulva and melena on the tail. (Courtesy of C. Leathers.)

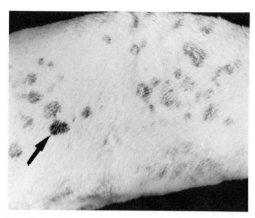

Fig. 9–2. Diffuse subcutaneous petechial to ecchymotic hemorrhages (*arrow*) in female ferret with estrogen-induced bone marrow depression. (Courtesy of J.R. Gorham.)

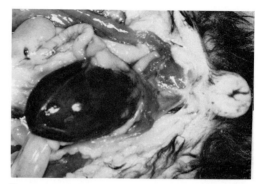

Fig. 9–3. Hemorrhage in the urinary bladder of female ferret with hyperestrogenism. Also note the enlarged vulva.

At some point in estrus all female ferrets will have at least a mild anemia. Initially it is normocytic normochromic, and may progress to a macrocytic hypochromic anemia. Reticulocyte counts provide evidence of inadequate regeneration for the degree of anemia present, and nucleated RBCs have been reported.[2] Clinical signs are not apparent until the PCV falls below 20% and/or the platelets below 50,000/μl; PCVs of less than 10% have been recorded in fatal cases. The low hematocrit, with concurrent low platelets, is accompanied by a decrease in the total serum protein level, even in cases with significant dehydration.[2] Mild anemia is attributed to erythroid hypoplasia, but severe anemia results from a combination of hypoplasia plus hemorrhage caused by the thrombocytopenia.

In severely affected animals, bone marrow cytology reveals decreased erythroid, granulocytic, and megakaryocytic precursors. The hypocellular bone marrow of ferrets in prolonged estrus is comprised of 10 to 20% hematopoietic cells, with the remainder being adipocytes, lymphocytes, RBCs, and hemosiderin-containing macrophages.[4]

Gross Pathology. The most consistent necropsy findings of ferrets with aplastic anemia are pale tissues and generated hemorrhages. The bone marrow is light tan to pale pink or light red. The liver and mucous membranes are markedly pale. Body weight is generally below normal. The blood is thin and watery, and there is evidence of hemorrhage in various areas. Frank blood may be found in the lumen of the stomach and in the small and large intestines. Subcutaneous and subendocardial ecchymoses and petechiae are common findings. Hemorrhage has also been observed in the omentum, urinary bladder, uterus, and periovarian adipose tissue, (Fig. 9–3). Subdural hematoma or hematomyelia is observed at the thoracic, lumbar, and sacral levels of the spinal cords of animals with neurologic signs. Uterine changes from hydrometra (Fig. 9–4) to pyometra (e.g., *Escherichia coli*) or mucoid to mucopurulent vaginitis (e.g., *Corynebacterium* sp.) have been reported.[1] A suppurative bronchopneumonia caused by *Klebsiella* sp. has also been diagnosed.[2]

Histopathology. The most striking histopathologic change is the hypocellularity of the bone marrow (Figs. 9–5 and 9–6).[1] There is no significant hematopoiesis of either the erythroid or granulocytic cell series, and megakaryocytes may be absent in the sections. The changes in the bone marrow reflect those in the peripheral

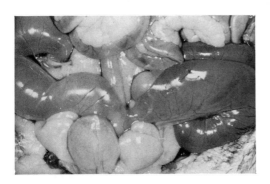

Fig. 9–4. Hydrometra in female ferret with hyperestrogenism.

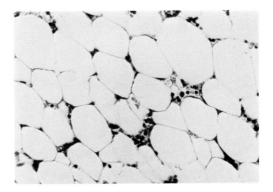

Fig. 9–5. Photomicrograph of bone marrow from an intact estrogen-treated female ferret (H & E stain; × 40). (Courtesy of C. Leathers.)

blood. There are numerous adipocytes and variable numbers of lymphocytes, plasma cells, and hemosiderin-laden macrophages.

Hemosiderosis, indicative of hemorrhage, is seen in the spleen, lymph nodes, liver, and lung. Suppurative bronchopneumonia may be diagnosed.[2] There is mild hepatic lipidosis to significant centrilobular fatty degeneration, and possibly diffuse small areas of extramedullary hematopoiesis.[2,4] Splenic section reveals either diminished or no evident extramedullary hematopoiesis.

As mentioned above, hydrometra, mucometra, or pyometra is present. Cystic endometrial hyperplasia may frequently be diagnosed.[4] Multiple follicles may be found in the ovaries.

Diagnosis. The diagnosis of bone marrow depression is based on the history and clinical presentation of an estrous female (an enlarged, edematous vulva), with a PCV less than 20%. Secondary bacterial infections, such as pyometra and pneumonia, as well as CNS signs, may confuse the diagnosis of the primary disease.

Treatment. By the time of clinical presentation jills are often too severely affected to survive, even with therapy. The prognosis must remain guarded, because the ferret's response to any procedure correlates with the length of estrus before beginning treatment. The first objective is to remove the source of endogenous estrogens, with the condition of the animal dictating whether this is done by medical or surgical means, or by both. Unless the animal is intended for use in breeding, an ovariohysterectomy is the fastest way of removing the estrogenic activity. If the jill's PCV and platelet count are low, blood replacement may be necessary to stabilize the animal for surgery. Care must also be taken to ensure minimal blood loss or hemorrhage during the surgical procedure.

One female with a PCV of 7% was spayed and then transfused with 10 ml fresh whole ferret blood containing 1 ml sodium citrate via a 23-gauge jugular catheter.[7] This female had been in estrus for more than 4.5 months prior to presentation. The ferret eventually recovered after extensive therapy involving anabolic steroids, corticosteroids, amoxicillin, a high-calorie diet, B vitamins, an attempted femoral, intramedullary bone marrow transplant, and a total of 13 blood transfusions over a 5-month period. Signs of nonregenerative anemia persisted for over 3.75 months in this jill.[7]

Ferrets with less severe anemia may be cycled out of heat by administering an IM injection of either 20 µg Gn-RH or 50 to 100 IU HCG. These agents may be used

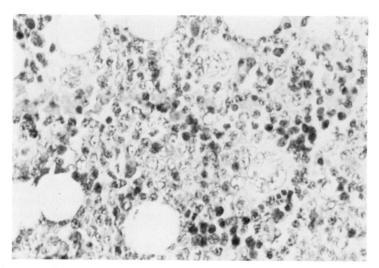

Fig. 9–6. Photomicrograph of bone marrow from an intact ferret without estrogen treatment (H & E stain; × 40). (Courtesy of C. Leathers).

10 or more days after the onset of estrus, with ovulation occurring 35 hours later. Vulvar swelling and turgidity should diminish within 1 week of the injection, and signs of estrus should disappear by 20 to 30 days postinjection.[1,4] A jill will remain anestrous for a pseudopregnancy of 40 to 45 days. If the jill remains in estrus, the injection of either HCG or Gn-RH may be repeated. Megestrol acetate has been used to delay estrus,[8] but its use is discouraged because of the risk of pyometra. The use of tamoxifen citrate, an antiestrogenic drug for women, is contraindicated, because it has estrogenic activity in ferrets.[1] Supportive care in the form of corticosteroids, anabolic steroids, B vitamins, antibiotics for secondary bacterial infections, and blood transfusions is an important adjunct to the removal of endogenous estrogens. Ovariohysterectomy is indicated after the jill is out of estrus and no longer severely anemic.

MASTITIS

Mastitis occurs frequently in laboratory jills and can be caused by various bacteria, including hemolytic *Escherichia*

coli, other coliforms, or gram-positive cocci.

Epizootiology and Control. Mastitis in cattle (and probably ferrets) is generally acquired from the area around the teat canal.[9] In an outbreak of hemolytic *Escherichia coli* mastitis in ferrets, isolation of the organism from rectal swab specimens from clinically normal ferrets suggests that the *E. coli* is part of the normal bacterial flora of the ferret colon.[10] The high level of coliform contamination in the perineal area may have contributed to the early involvement of the inguinal glands reported in this study. Hemolytic *E. coli* (of the same serotype, O4:K23:H5, from the mammary gland, rectal area, and blood) isolated from the oral cavity of suckling kits may also serve as another mode of transmission to unaffected glands and to other jills via cross fostering.[10] Coliform mastitis is not highly contagious in cattle, and infection usually results from environmental contamination such as organisms in sawdust bedding.[11,12] In a large epizootic of mastitis associated with food poisoning in mink resulting from *Staphylococcus aureus* and *E. coli*, the suspected cause was meat from a septicemic bovine carcass fed prior to the epizootic.[13] Humans can also carry *E. coli* and *S. aureus*, and may be considered as a possible source of infectious microorganisms.[14]

Cows are most susceptible to coliform mastitis at or shortly after parturition.[15] Similarly, in ferrets, affected jills are usually in the early stage of lactation. Bovine milk contains an iron-binding protein, lactoferrin, which inhibits multiplication of bacteria with high iron requirements. Lactoferrin activity is highest in the nonlactating cow and is lost just before parturition.[16] The udder is resistant to coliform infection during the nonlactating period, which coincides with the period of highest lactoferrin activity. This same activity may be present in ferret milk, and may be a factor in determining the time of onset of infection.

Clinical Signs. Swelling, discoloration, firmness, and tenderness of affected mammary glands are initially observed (Fig. 9–7). The swelling of affected tissue progresses rapidly, and adjacent glands frequently become involved. Affected jills become anorectic and lethargic, and no longer nurse their young; if the pups are left unattended many will die. Systemic signs in jills are often seen and include pyrexia, diarrhea, nasal discharge, pulmonary rales, fulminant septicemia, and death. The rapid progression of the disease may be attributable to the rapid multiplication of *Escherichia coli* in tissues, with the release and dissemination of endotoxin. At least two toxins are involved in the pathogenesis of *E. coli* infection in the cow.[17]

Diagnosis and Pathology. In mastitis caused by *Escherichia coli* the histopathologic findings vary in severity from case to case, but the basic pathology is similar.[10] The primary lesion is characterized by large areas of coagulative and liquefactive necrosis that involve the

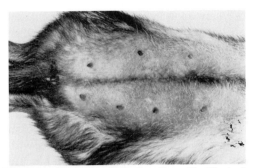

Fig. 9–7. Jill with hemolytic *E. coli* mastitis. The teats are black and necrotic, and the mammary glands are swollen, discolored, and firm.

glandular tissue, as well as the adjacent adipose tissue and muscle. Extensive congestion and edema, with focal areas of hemorrhage, are in the intralobular and perilobular tissue, as well as the adjacent subcutaneous tissues. A moderate leukocytic infiltrate, composed primarily of polymorphonuclear leukocytes, concentrates at the perimeter of the necrotic areas, and permeates lobules with minimal evidence of necrosis. Large numbers of bacteria are in the affected tissues. Thrombosis and necrosis of vessels within and immediately adjacent to areas of inflammation are common findings.

With *Staphylococcus aureus* mastitis described in mink, the mammary glands are suppurative, with lactiferous ducts distended with purulent exudate, marked inflammatory edema of connective tissue, cellular debris, inflammatory cells, and desquamation of alveolar cells.[13] Cocci are readily observed in affected tissues.

Diagnosis is based on clinical signs and on isolation of the causative agent. Serotyping or phage typing of the organism may be helpful in establishing the source and spread of the organism in an affected colony of animals.

Treatment. Immediate and aggressive therapy is warranted if *Escherichia coli* mastitis is to be successfully treated. Antibiotics, ampicillin, 10 mg/kg twice daily, and gentamicin, 5 mg/kg once daily, can be used if the disease is recognized early. In our experience, antibiotic therapy combined with wide surgical resection of the involved glands is the most effective treatment of the disease. The affected glands and adjacent tissues are widely excised; the skin is closed over ¼-inch Penrose drains with a simple interrupted pattern of nonabsorbable suture material. Protective bandages are applied to the surgical site. Broad-spectrum antibiotics injected subcutaneously or intramuscularly are used to treat mastitis caused by gram-positive cocci.

PYOMETRA

Pyometra in the ferret has many clinical and pathologic features similar to those documented in the dog and cat.

Epizootiology and Control. The disease is often documented in breeding colonies of ferrets or colonies in which ferrets are used for biomedical research,[18–20] and is also recognized in pet ferrets.[21] Pyometra was undoubtedly more prevalent prior to the recognition that prolonged estrus in the ferret produces aplastic anemia[2] (see discussion on aplastic anemia).

Clinical Signs and Pathology. It is important to ascertain whether the animal with pyometra is suffering from estrogen-induced bone marrow depression. Signs of hyperestrogenism include pancytopenia, enlarged vulva, purpuric hemorrhages, and melena. Animals with pyometra are depressed, lethargic, and sometimes febrile. Purulent discharge from the vagina may be present, and enlarged uterine horns may be diagnosed by abdominal palpation and radiography. Various microorganisms may be cultured from infected uteri, including *Escherichia coli*, *Staphylococcus*, *Streptococcus*, (including S. group C), and *Corynebacterium*.

Affected enlarged uteri have the lumen filled with purulent exudate. Endometrial glands are dilated and cystic. Cells lining glands are desquamated, and lumens of glands are engorged with polymorphonuclear cells. The endometrial stroma also contains a mixed cell inflammatory infiltrate, often with focal abscess formation.

Treatment. If hyperestrogenism is diagnosed conservative treatment for that disease should be initiated, along with antibiotic therapy to treat the pyometra. Once the animal has cycled out of estrus after HCG treatment, or by breeding the female ferret, ovariohysterectomy is indicated. Blood transfusions and intensive supportive care may be required if the animal is pancytopenic.[1,7]

Diagnosis. Pyometra is diagnosed by clinical signs, determination of prolonged estrus, and demonstration of enlarged uteri. Purulent exudate caused by various microorganisms is often present within the vaginal canal. A neutrophilia may be present in cases of pyometra, uncomplicated by estrogen-induced aplastic anemia. In cases of pyometra with concurrent hyperestrogenism, however, pancytopenia may be observed.

ECLAMPSIA

Eclampsia (pregnancy toxemia) occurs in some pregnant jills before whelping, and can kill unborn pups as well as the pregnant jill.[22] The disease may be similar to the condition in guinea pigs, in which diet and stress may precipitate the toxemia. The only characteristic postmortem tissue lesion is an excessively fatty yellow liver (Fig. 9–8). More definitive studies are needed to determine the etiology and importance of this disease in pregnant ferrets.

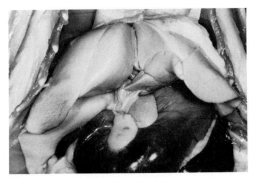

Fig. 9–8. Fatty liver of near-term pregnant ferret. Also note the hemorrhagic gravid uterus.

VAGINITIS

Vaginitis, a result of irritation from foreign bodies, can occur, particularly in estrous females, because of mucous secretion and adherence of bedding material to the vulva.

Epizootiology and Control. The disease is sporadic but may occur frequently if estrous females are maintained on hay or straw, particularly if the bedding contains grass awns or seeds. It may also be seen in ferrets maintained on wood bedding. *Streptococci* and enteric organisms (e.g., hemolytic *Escherichia coli* or *Klebsiella pneumoniae*) can establish a secondary bacterial infection. Control of the disease depends on removal of offending contact bedding from the ferret's enclosure, commencing 3 weeks pre-estrus and continuing until after mating. Alternate bedding could include shredded newspaper, or cloth or cotton matting.

Clinical Signs. Females have a yellow mucopurulent vulvar discharge. Physical examination often reveals the presence of foreign material (usually bedding) within the vagina. *Streptococci* or enteric bacteria are sometimes isolated on bacterial culture. Occasionally, ferrets also have a metritis and are febrile.

Treatment. Removal of the foreign body, coupled with the use of broad-spectrum antibiotics, is usually accompanied by clinical recovery.

NURSING SICKNESS (Agalactia)

A condition known as nursing sickness occurs in dams before the fifth or sixth week of lactation. Affected females show signs at about the time of weaning, and sometimes after the kits are removed. Clinical signs include inappetence, weight loss, weakness, and incoordination.[22, 23] Death follows an interval of coma. In some cases the liver of affected jills is yellow, with a greasy texture. A hemolytic anemia may also be seen. Females should be watched closely for signs of emaciation and dehydration during lactation. The cause is unknown, but evidence on some ferret farms in New Zealand suggests that peroxidative stress associated with diets rich in polyunsaturated fatty acids predispose jills to this disease.[24] Another report noted that it is more common in jills during the first part of the breeding season, particularly when estrus was induced outside the normal breeding season.[25] Providing the kits with food and water at 2 weeks of age may preclude the onset of nursing sickness. Care must be exercised, however, to monitor supplemental food intake in the kits; overeating and an inability to digest food properly can result in diarrhea and rectal prolapse.

MILK FEVER (Hypocalcemia)

This condition was reported in one commercial ferret farm in New Zealand.[24] It occurred in primiparous jills 3 to 4 weeks postparturition. Signs included posterior paresis, hyperesthesia, and convulsions. A rapid clinical response was achieved with an intraperitoneal injection of calcium borogluconate. The condition can be controlled by use of a calcium supplement in the diet.

PSEUDOPREGNANCY

If implantation is not successful after mating, pseudopregnancy can develop. Pseudopregnancy can occur if there is an improper hormonal balance in the ferret caused by reduced light intensity 1 month before the initiation of breeding. It is important, therefore, to verify the light intensity of artificial lighting in breeding units or the light intensity during the spring on commercial farms. If breeding ferrets is continued in late summer, artificial light can extend hours of light.

Pseudopregnancy can also result from using immature males younger than 6 months of age. It is advisable to ensure sperm viability in breeding males and to ensure that males have fully descended testes.[26] After mating the vulval swelling recedes, the abdomen enlarges, and the jill will remain pseudopregnant for 41 to 43 days. The corpus luteum in the pseudopregnant ferret usually functions as long as those in pregnant animals. Nesting behavior and mammary enlargement will be variable. A lack of palpable fetuses, establishes the diagnosis.

MORTALITY AND DISEASES OF THE NEONATE KIT

Strict attention to proper nutrition and environment are important in maintaining the health of neonates. Various causes have been linked to neonatal deaths in ferret breeding colonies. Although mortality in ferrets was as high as 70% in one particular colony,[18] modern husbandry has reduced this percentage dramatically. It can still occur, however, with alarm-ing frequency in commercially reared ferrets.[24]

NEONATAL MORTALITY

Kits are prone to dehydration, hypothermia, and hypoglycemia. Losses occurring within a 3-day period often result from pups eaten with the placenta, failure of the jill to nurse the pups, and entanglement of the pup in the uneaten placenta.[27] Disturbance of the female at parturition or shortly thereafter may contribute to maternal neglect of the pups.

In a recent study on neonatal mortality in a commercial breeding operation, there was a 7% mortality between days 4 to 14 of lactation, coinciding with the onset of a neonatal infection of unconfirmed etiology.[28] Although the mortality rate did not differ between parturition and day 4, primiparous (11.4%) and one (9.0%) or two (5.8%) previous parity females, the mortality rate between days 4 and 14 of lactation was significantly greater in primiparous females (14.8%) versus that in one and two previous parity females combined (2.0%).[28] These data strongly suggest an infectious etiology. Rotavirus-induced diarrhea should be placed in the differential diagnosis (see Chap. 11).

In the same study, neonatal death within 24 hours was attributed to malformations, premature births, stillborns, breech presentations, cannibalism, and accidental death.[28]

UMBILICAL CORD PROLAPSE

In one study, prolapsed umbilicus occurred at a rate of 11.6 and 29.1/100 litters in kits in two separate cohorts. Potential causes were umbilicus and attached placenta becoming entangled in bedding material, possible trauma induced by jills attempting to free tangled kits, or congenital conditions.[28]

UMBILICAL CORD INFECTION AND SEPTICEMIA

It is important to disinfect the kits' umbilical stumps properly, soon after parturition. Ascending umbilical cord infections caused by *Escherichia coli* or other pathogens can produce septicemia and death in neonates. Signs of kit septicemia include dehydration, distressful crying, anorexia, bloating, and hypothermia. Treatment follows the principles of treatment of the condition in puppies and kittens. It consists of providing external heat to the jill and her kits or removal of the kits to an incubator, administering subcutaneous Ringer's solution, and oral dosing with broad-spectrum antibiotics. Ensuring ingestion of colostrum may prove to be beneficial in combatting this infection.[29, 30]

Environmental conditions, such as type of bedding, humidity, and ventilation, and bacterial contamination resulting from inadequate sanitation may predispose kits to umbilical cord infection or septicemia. Septicemia may also be associated with metritis and mastitis in the jill. Jills with repeated episodes of mastitis and/or metritis should be culled from the colony.

INTERCURRENT DISEASE

Bacterial (e.g., *Campylobacter jejuni*, *Escherichia coli*) or viral (e.g., rotavirus) illness can also contribute to morbidity and mortality in pups (see Chaps. 10 and 11). It is also important to recognize incipient mastitis in lactating jills, and to remove them promptly from the colony, if possible, with affected animals being treated appropriately. Fostering of kits may be necessary.

REFERENCES

1. Bernard, S.L., Leathers, C.W., Brobst, D.F., and Gorham, J.R.: Estrogen-induced bone marrow depression in ferrets. Am. J. Vet. Res., 44:657, 1983.
2. Kociba, G., and Caputo, C.A.: Aplastic anemia associated with estrus in pet ferrets. J. Am. Vet. Med. Assoc., 178:1293, 1981.
3. Hart, J.E.: Endocrine factors in hematological changes seen in dogs and ferrets given estrogens. Med. Hypotheses, 16:159, 1985.
4. Sherrill, A., and Gorham, J.R.: Bone marrow hypoplasia associated with estrus in ferrets. Lab. Anim. Sci., 35:280, 1985.
5. Ryland, L.M., Bernard, S.L., and Gorham, J.R.: A clinical guide to the pet ferret. Compend. Cont. Ed., 5:25, 1983.
6. Ireland, E.R.: Controlling ferret fertility. Vet. Rec., 117:320, 1985.
7. Ryland, L.M.: Remission of estrus-associated anemia following ovariohysterectomy and multiple blood transfusions in a ferret. J. Am. Vet. Med. Assoc., 181:820, 1982.
8. Howard, J.W.: Control of estrus in ferrets. Vet. Rec., 104:291, 1979.
9. Jain, N.C.: Common mammary pathogens and factors in infection and mastitis. J. Dairy Sci., 62:128, 1979.
10. Liberson, A.J. et al.: Mastitis caused by hemolytic *Escherichia coli* in the ferret. J. Am. Vet. Med. Assoc., 183:1179, 1983.
11. Schultze, W.D., and Thompson, P.D.: Intramammary coliform infection after heavy external contamination of teats. Am. J. Vet. Res., 41:1396, 1980.
12. Bramley, A.J., and Neave, F.K.: Studies on the control of coliform mastitis. Br. Vet. J., 131:160, 1975.
13. Trautwein, G.W., and Helmboldt, C.F.: Mastitis in mink due to *Staphylococcus aureus* and *Escherichia coli*. J. Am. Vet. Med. Assoc., 149:924, 1966.
14. Fox, J.G. et al.: Selected zoonotic diseases. In Laboratory Animal Medicine. Edited by J.G. Fox, B.J. Cohen, and F.M. Loew. New York, Academic Press, 1984.
15. Bauer, A.W. et al.: Antibiotic susceptibility testing by a standardized single disk method. Am. J. Clin. Pathol., 45:493, 1966.

16. Welty, F.K., Smith, K.L., and Schanbacher, F.L.: Lactoferrin concentration during involution of the bovine mammary gland. J. Dairy Sci., *59*:224, 1976.

17. Brooker, B.E., Frost, A.J., and Hill, A.W.: At least two toxins are involved in *Escherichia coli* mastitis. Experimentia, *37*:290, 1981.

18. Seamer, J., and Chesterman, F.C.: A survey of diseases in laboratory animals. Lab. Anim., *1*:117, 1967.

19. Hammond, J.: Ferret mortality on a pellet diet. J. Anim. Tech. Assoc., *12*:35, 1961.

20. Hammond, J.: The ferret as a research animal. Carnivore Genet. Newsletter, *6*:126, 1969.

21. Boever, W.J., and Warmbrodt, J.: Pyometra in a domestic ferret. Modern Vet. Pract. *55*:717, 1974.

22. Ryland, L.M., and Gorham, J.F.: The ferret and its diseases. J. Am. Vet. Med. Assoc., *173*:1154, 1978.

23. Bernard, S.L., Gorham, J.R., and Ryland, L.M.: Biology and diseases of ferrets. *In* Laboratory Animal Medicine. Edited by J.G. Fox, B.J. Cohen, and F.M. Loew. New York, Academic Press, 1984.

24. Diseases of the fitch. Surveillance, *11*:28, 1984.

25. Rowland, I.W.: The ferret. *In* UFAW Handbook on the Care and Management of Laboratory Animals. 3rd Ed. London, Baillière, Tindall and Cox, 1967.

26. Shump, A.U., and Shump, K.A.: Semen volume and sperm concentration in the ferret. Lab. Anim. Sci., *26*:913, 1976.

27. Hammond, J., and Chesterman, F.C.: The ferret. *In* UFAW Handbook on the Care and Management of Laboratory Animals. 4th Ed. London, Churchill Livingstone, 1972.

28. McLain, D.E. et al.: Congenital malformations and variations in reproductive performance in the ferret: Effect of maternal age, color, and parity. Lab. Anim. Sci. *35*:251, 1985.

29. Ringler, D.H., and Peter, G.K.: Dogs and cats as laboratory animals. *In* Laboratory Animal Medicine. Edited by J.G. Fox, B.J. Cohen, and F.M. Loew. New York, Academic Press, 1984.

30. Glickman, L.T.: Preventative medicine in kennel management. *In* Current Veterinary Therapy VII. Edited by R.W. Kirk. W.B. Saunders, Philadelphia, 1980.

chapter 10

BACTERIAL AND MYCOPLASMAL DISEASES

J. G. Fox

ACTINOMYCOSIS

This disease has rarely been reported in ferrets, and has been referred to as lumpy jaw. The disease in ferrets has similarities to lumpy jaw in cattle and faciocervical actinomycosis in humans.[1,2] The organism was once thought to be a transitional form between fungus and bacteria, but is now recognized as a bacteria that causes a funguslike infection. The disease in humans (and other animals) is caused by *Actinomyces israelii,* and in cattle by *A. bovis.*[3,4] Other *Actinomyces* species have been associated with disease, but may reflect only normal oral flora invading compromised tissue. All species of this bacteria are gram-positive and nonacid-fast, anaerobic to microaerophilic organisms.

Epizootiology and Control. The occurrence of this disease is probably rare; its predilection for the cervical area reflects entry of the organism through damaged oral mucosa. Feeding ferrets on carcasses with bones may increase the likelihood that actinomycosis, if present in oral flora, could infect animals through cuts and abrasions created by the sharp, jagged ends of the bones. The fungus may also be swallowed or inhaled. The source of clinical disease is considered to be endogenous, although animal bites may transmit the organism. Given the few cases reported in the ferret, susceptibility to *Actinomyces* is probably low.

Clinical Signs and Pathology. Cervical masses with sinus tracts containing thick, greenish-yellow, purulent material were recorded in one case of actinomycosis. The masses enlarged and the animal had difficulty breathing. On histology the cervical masses had abscesses with colonies and sinuses with the characteristic morphology of *Actinomyces* located throughout the tissue. In a second case the animal died without apparent clinical signs. On autopsy firm nodules were found beneath the visceral pleura of the lung. The posterior mediastinal lymph nodes were twice as large as normal, with abscesses containing greenish granules present on the cut surface. Histologically, the abscesses contained typical colonies of *Actinomyces*.[5] Three other cases of swelling of the neck suggestive of lumpy jaw have been diagnosed in ferrets used for research purposes.[1]

The cervical masses in the ferret caused by *Actinomyces* must be distinguished from neoplasia and two other conditions previously reported in the ferret. Ferrets housed outdoors can develop granulomatous masses and sinuses in the cervical region caused by myiasis, produced by the larval stage of *Hypoderma bovis*. Similarly, staphylococcal or streptococcal cervical cellulitis secondary to mandibular osteomyelitis and associated dental disease can be encountered in ferrets.[5]

Diagnosis. Isolation of *Actinomyces* from aspirated exudate is required for definitive diagnosis. Alternatively, histologic demonstration of actinomycetic organisms in specially stained tissue sections establishes the morphologic diagnosis.

Treatment. Sustained treatment with penicillin in high doses is effective in treating the disease in humans. Tetracyclines are also effective. Antibiotic treatment should be supplemented with surgical drainage of the abscess, local débridement, and topical application of antibiotics and antiseptics.

BOTULISM

Botulism is a neuroparalytic disease usually caused by consumption of foods containing toxin(s) produced by one or more of a group of anaerobic spore-forming bacteria.[6]

Epizootiology and Control. Botulism in animals raised for fur production has been documented for decades. Outbreaks in mink have shown mortality rates of 90% caused by ingestion of type C toxin.[7] Similar high mortality rates were documented in mink infected with *Clostridium botulinum* type A.[8] Deaths in ferrets attributed to ingestion of wild carcasses of birds containing *C. botulinum* toxin type C were also recorded in England.[9, 10]

The disease in ferrets in part depends on the occurrence of the clostridial spores in the soil. For example, spores of *Clostridium botulinum* type B are far more prevalent in the soil of the midwestern United States than are the spores of other *Clostridium* species. Feeding of uncooked food and of food contaminated with soil contaminated with clostridial spores greatly increases the occurrence of the disease. Experimentally, ferrets are susceptible to infection by *C. botulinum* types A and B, highly susceptible to type C, but refractory to type E.[11, 12] Toxoids are available, and annual vaccinations are recommended for ferrets produced commercially. The disease is prevented by exclusion of diets containing clostridial toxin.

Clinical Signs and Pathology. Ferrets orally inoculated experimentally with types A and B toxins develop signs within 12 to 72 hours, and death ensues in 1 to 7 days.[11] Clinical signs initiate with blepharospasm, photophobia, lethargy, and urinary incontinence. Rapid weight loss, ataxia, paralysis, and prostration are also noted as the disease progresses. Interestingly, the course of the disease is variable and, to a considerable degree, independent of the amount of toxin administered to the animal. Clinical recovery can occur without treatment. The female ferret appears to be more susceptible to the effects of the toxin than males, which may be due to the female's smaller size.

Congestion of the liver, spleen, and kidney, with subcapsular hemorrhage of the spleen is common. Focal hemorrhage in the cerebellum is also noted with consistency. Histologically, there is marked lymphoid depletion in the spleen with necrosis of the center of the follicles, follicular hyperplasia of mononuclear cells, disruption of the normal reticular pattern, and a marked increase in multinuclear giant cells. This also occurs to a lesser extent in the lymph nodes. Congestion with distension of capillaries and veins, with occasional hemorrhage, is seen in the liver. Hemorrhage in the cerebellum is also noted.

Diagnosis. This is based on the clinical history of ingestion of spoiled or improperly handled food, followed by development of central nervous system symptoms and rapid weight loss. Gross lesions and histologic changes in affected ferrets are similar with ingestion of toxins A and B, and severity depends on the length of illness.[11] Definitive diagnosis is based on demonstrating the presence of botulinum toxin. Numerous methods have been published for the detection of *Clostridium botulinum* and its toxins from foods, clinical specimens, and materials such as soil.[13, 14] When diagnosing botulism it may be possible to demonstrate the toxin directly in the blood, serum, or gastrointestinal tract of ferrets, and in the remains of the contaminated food. An understanding of the properties of this organism and the factors affecting its growth and toxin production is essential for successful isolation and identification.[6]

Treatment. Once botulinum poisoning is suspected, supportive therapy is essential. Antitoxins are not routinely available.

CAMPYLOBACTERIOSIS

Campylobacteriosis is a diarrheal disease caused by a gram-negative microaerophilic bacterium, *Campylobacter jejuni* or, less frequently, *C. coli*. The organism is cited as an important cause of diarrhea in humans and has been linked to diarrhea in the ferret, dog, cat, mink, and nonhuman primates.[15]

Epizootiology and Control. *Campylobacter jejuni* is now included with *Salmonella* and *Shigella* as a leading cause of diarrhea in humans. Previously, *Campylobacter* was relegated to the role of a pathogen or commensal in domestic animals. With the heightened interest in *C. jejuni* as a human pathogen, there have been several reports linking the disease in humans to pets.[16] Many of these outbreaks of diarrhea were associated with dogs, puppies, and kittens recently obtained from animal shelters or pounds. Clinical signs in pets preceded the onset of diarrhea in humans who lived in the same household, and who also had *C. jejuni* isolated from their feces.

In a study on proliferative colitis in ferrets, only 9% (4 of 47) of clinically healthy ferrets were positive for *Campylobacter jejuni*, whereas 50% (9 of 18) of clinically ill animals were positive for the organism.[17] In a subsequent study on the prevalence of *C. jejuni* in ferrets, however, most ferrets positive for *C. jejuni* were asymptomatic carriers. Ferrets from two commercial sources were screened; 8 of 10 cultures from vendor 1 were positive and 43 of 73 from vendor 2 had *C. jejuni* isolated from nondiarrheic feces.[18] It is not known how long ferrets naturally infected with *C. jejuni* shed the organism in their feces, but experimentally infected ferrets have shed the organism for as long as 16 weeks after inoculation.[19] This long-term shedding of *C. jejuni* may present an occupational hazard to laboratory animal personnel or to those in households with pet ferrets.

As with most enteric pathogens, fecal-oral spread and foodborne and waterborne transmission appear to be the principal avenues for infection; these include ingestion of contaminated meat products, particularly poultry, and of unpasteurized milk. Outbreaks of diarrhea in mink kits caused by *Campylobacter jejuni* and *C. coli* were recently described.[20] The likely source of infection was the feeding of uncooked chicken offal. Nosocomial infections are also a possible mode of transmission, as is exposure to other pets (dogs, cats, hamsters, birds, and rabbits) and to rural farm animals that may shed the organism.[17,21]

Two widely adopted serotyping schemes used today to identify *Campylobacter jejuni* and *C. coli* are the passive hemagglutination assay and the slide agglutination assay. Similar serotypes are recognized in both animals and humans.[22,23] Serotypes commonly isolated from humans were also isolated from ferrets. Although *C. jejuni* appears to be prevalent among ferrets, it is not known whether all serotypes found in ferrets cause diarrhea in humans. Increased awareness of the potential of infection from ferrets as well as from dogs and cats (and other domestic and laboratory animals) to humans, and the utilization of reliable serotyping systems, will allow a more complete understanding of the role played by animal hosts in the epidemiology of *Campylobacter* infection in humans.

Clinical Signs and Pathology. Clinical diarrhea has been experimentally induced in ferrets inoculated orally with *Campylobacter jejuni*.[24] As in cases of *Campylobacter* infection in dogs and cats, ferrets can be asymptomatic carriers. Clinical diarrhea appears to occur more frequently in animals less than 6 months of age. In addition, animals may be more susceptible to clinical infection if stressed by experimental regimes, hospitalization, concurrent disease, pregnancy, shipment, or surgery. The pathogenic mechanisms responsible for the clinical alterations and laboratory changes found in infected animals are poorly understood. The typical presenting clinical signs, in our experience, include mucus-laden watery or bile-streaked diarrhea (with or without blood and leukocytes) of several days duration, and partial anorexia.[24,25] In natural outbreaks of colitis and experimental production of colitis in mink kits with *C. jejuni*, there was yellow-white mucoid diarrhea, often blood-tinged, and the animals were febrile.[20] Rectal prolapses in mink kits were also seen. Adults were not affected. Elevated temperature and leukocytosis may also be present. In certain cases, diarrhea in ferrets can persist for more than 4 weeks, or may be intermittent.[24,25]

Abortion caused by *Campylobacter jejuni* was reported in the mink. It is probable, under similar conditions, that *C. jejuni* could induce abortions in ferrets.[26] *C. jejuni* has also been linked to proliferative colitis in ferrets, but Koch's postulate has not been fulfilled (see later discussion on proliferative colitis).

Diagnosis. Because of slow growth requirements and the need for microaerophilic conditions, standard methods used for culture require selective media that incorporate various antibiotics to suppress competing fecal microflora, or filtration techniques are employed. *Campylobacter jejuni* grows well at 42°C in an atmosphere of 5 to 10% carbon dioxide and an equal amount of oxygen. Cultures are incubated for 48 to 72 hours; colonies of *C. jejuni* are round, raised, translucent, and sometimes mucoid. The organism can be identified by a series of biochemical tests readily available in diagnostic laboratories. Hippurate hydrolysis distinguishes *C. jejuni* from *C. coli*.

Treatment. In humans, erythromycin has been shown to clear *Campylobacter jejuni* from the feces of patients with acute enteritis[27] and from the feces of convalescent carriers[28] within 48 hours. In vitro studies of sensitivities to numerous antimicrobials indicate that *C. jejuni* is routinely sensitive to erythromycin, the aminoglycosides, tetracycline, chloramphenicol, furazolidone, and clindamycin. Erythromycin is considered the drug of choice in human *C. jejuni* infection on the basis of the frequency with which the organism is susceptible, the ease of drug administration, and the lack of serious drug toxicity.[29] Ampicillin and metronidazole, and sulfa combinations, are less effective therapeutically. Several antibiotics are ineffective: penicillin, polymyxin B, cephalosporins, trimethoprim, and vancomycin.[30–32] Many *Campylobacter* strains produce a ß-lactamase,[33] which accounts for their resistance to penicillin.

A therapeutic trial was undertaken in an attempt to eliminate *Campylobacter jejuni* from 16 carrier ferrets. Despite the uniform sensitivity of in vitro *C. jejuni* isolates from ferrets to erythromycin, erythromycin given orally did not eliminate the carrier state in this study.[25] There are several possibilities why erythromycin therapy failed to eliminate the *C. jejuni* carrier state in the ferret. The dosage used in the study was based on the recommendations for erythromycin therapy in children with severe infections.[27] Consequently, interspecies differences in pharmacokinetics may account for the therapeutic failure. The lack of significant differences in the pre- and posttherapy mean inhibitory concentrations (MIC) of antibiotic values of *C. jejuni* strains indicate that the emergence of resistant strains did not contribute to therapeutic failure in this study.[25] Reinfection of the ferrets with *C. jejuni* could also have occurred. One day after erythromycin treatment 6 of the 16 ferrets were negative, which may indicate elimination of the organism from the enteric bacterial flora of the caudal part of the intestine. Subsequent intestinal recolonization of 5 of these 6 ferrets was via exposure to and ingestion of *C. jejuni* from a contaminated environment. Unfortunately, with available microbiologic techniques and housing of ferrets under standard laboratory conditions, it is impossible to make a clear-cut distinction between a chronic carrier (with lack of therapeutic response) and reinfection.[25]

Erythromycin, 220 g/ton of feed, however, appeared to control colitis associated diarrhea in two outbreaks caused by *Campylobacter* in weaning mink kits. Supportive treatment included warming and hydrating the animals, and frequent changing of bedding to keep the kits dry.[20] It is therefore recommended to treat symptomatic ferrets with *Campylobacter jejuni* present in diarrheic feces. Reculture of ferrets after treatment is recommended; precautions should also be taken to minimize zoonotic potential as well as spread of the organisms to other ferrets, household pets, or other laboratory animals maintained in the same vivarium.

CAMPYLOBACTER-LIKE ORGANISMS

Usually, for practical purposes, the normal stomach is considered to be bacteriologically inert because of the bactericidal effect of low gastric pH. Therefore, until recently, bacteria and their role as a cause of gastric disease received little attention. Several recent reports in humans are of the opinion that a newly recognized bacteria, *Campylobacter pylori*, causes gastritis, rather than gastritis permitting secondary infection by the bacteria.[34, 35] *Campylobacter*-like organisms (CLO) have been isolated from gastric lesions in ferrets.[36, 37] Using Warthin-Starry stain, these were seen on the glandular epithelium of ferrets with gastric lesions from which CLO were isolated. It must be cautioned, however, that CLO are also isolated from apparently normal gastric tissue. Of 33 ferrets from 1 to 173 days old (with 26 less than 45 days old) cultured for gastric CLO, only 2 of 33 ferrets (one 24 days old and one 31 days old) were positive for gastric CLO. In another series of 27 ferrets, all older than 1 year, 25 were positive for gastric CLO. This indicates that colonization with gastric CLO in ferrets, as in humans, appears to be age-dependent.[19]

The organism is isolated from gastric tissue and not from gastric fluid. Tissue is homogenized and plated on a selective *Campylobacter* medium, or tissue is filtered through a 0.65-μ filter and plated on Mueller-Hinton agar with 10% horse serum. The CLO from ferrets has similar but not identical biochemical features to those of *C. pylori*, particularly in regard to the production of large amounts of urease (Table 10–1). Because ferrets are now recognized as having significant gastric disease, further studies are warranted to evaluate the cause and importance of CLO-associated gastritis and gastric ulcer disease in ferrets (see Chap. 14).

PROLIFERATIVE COLITIS

This disease entity was first reported in research ferrets in 1983,[17] and again in 1986 in a pet ferret.[38]

Epizootiology and Control. During a 4-month period, 31 of 156 ferrets used in a biomedical research program developed protracted diarrhea.[17] Nine of these were examined by necropsy and histology and were found to have proliferative colitis, with six having intermittent clinical signs for 6 weeks or longer. *Campylobacter jejuni* was isolated from six of the nine ferrets, and all nine had CLOs in the apical portion of their epithelial cells. The pet ferret had similar clinical signs and histologic findings.[38] Because it is not known if the organism is responsible for the disease, however, control measures are difficult to implement. *Campylobacter*

TABLE 10–1. BACTERIOLOGIC PROPERTIES OF *CAMPYLOBACTER*-LIKE ORGANISMS (CLO)*

Bacteriologic Property	C. jejuni	C. coli	C. pylori	CLO from Ferret
Growth at 42° C	Yes	Yes	Variable	Yes
Growth at 37° C	Yes	Yes	Yes	Yes
Susceptibility to antimicrobials				
Nalidixic acid (30-μg disk)	S†	S	R	S
Cephalothin (30-μg disk)	R	R	S	R
Hippurate hydrolysis	Yes	No	No	No
Number of flagella	1	1	≤4	≤4
Urease production	No	No	Yes	Yes
NO₂	Yes	Yes	No	Yes

(Fox, J.G. et al.: *Campylobacter*-like organisms isolated from gastric mucosa of ferrets. Am. J. Vet. Res., 47:236, 1986.)

* Isolated from the gastric mucosae of ferrets compared with those of *Campylobacter jejuni, C. coli,* and *C. pyloridis.*

† S, susceptible; R, resistant.

species have been implicated in proliferative diseases in other animals, including hamsters, swine, guinea pigs, and rats. Experimental reproduction of proliferative bowel lesions with *Campylobacter* in these animals, when attempted, has met with equivocal results. It should be cautioned, however, that with *C. jejuni*, fecal-oral spread and food- and waterborne transmission appear to be the principal avenues for infection (see earlier discussion).

Clinical Signs and Pathology. Ten animals ranging in age from 4 to 6 months were seen clinically because of diarrhea, body weight loss, and partial prolapse of the rectum (Table 10–2). Fecal material was usually blood-tinged, often discolored green, and contained mucus. The diarrhea persisted on an intermittent basis for more than 6 weeks. Seven of the ten animals exhibited more than a 100-g

weight loss during the first 2 to 4 weeks of illness. Affected males lost 12 to 54% of their body weight, and affected females lost 30 to 54%. CNS signs of ataxia and muscular tremors were observed in several ferrets.

Pathology. The gross morphologic changes observed are relatively subtle in most cases, and could be easily overlooked (Fig. 10–1), but the histologic changes are distinctive. The ferret does not have a cecum, and thus lacks a readily identifiable division between the small and large intestines (Fig. 10–2). Limited studies indicate that the transition from villous to nonvillous mucosa occurs in the area analogous to the transverse colon in humans and other animals. Proliferative colitis in the ferret consistently shows marked proliferation of mucosal cells and intracytoplasmic *Campylobacter*-like organisms within the apical portion of the epithelium (Figs. 10–3 and 10–4).

The lesions observed in the colon mimic the pathologic changes described by numerous investigators for the proliferative lesion in the ileum of hamsters, and are referred to by various synonyms: "wet tail," proliferative ileitis, atypical ileal hyperplasia, hamster enteritis, and enzootic intestinal adenocarcinoma.[39–42] They also mimic the proliferative lesions described by many in the ileum of swine, also referred to as various syndromes

TABLE 10–2. FERRETS WITH PROLIFERATIVE COLITIS*

Clinical Data	Number of Affected Ferrets
Age at onset of diarrhea	
4–6 months	10
Partial rectal prolapse	10
Diarrhea	
Mucohemorrhagic	7
Greenish, mucoid	3
CNS signs: ataxia, muscular tremors	5
Weight loss, >100 g in 2–4 weeks	8
Rectal cultures	
Campylobacter jejuni	6
Salmonella species	0
Sex incidence	
Males	7
Females	3
Disposition of animals	
Died	4
Euthanized	6
Duration of illness	
6–18 weeks	7
Less than 3 weeks	3

*Ten ferrets seen clinically were used in this study.

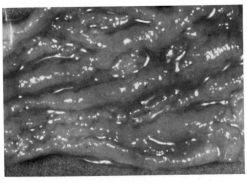

Fig. 10–1. Proliferative colitis in a ferret, showing colonic mucosa with thickened longitudinal folds.

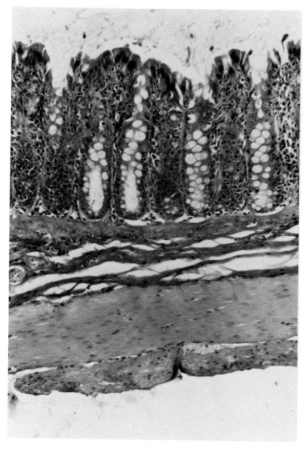

Fig. 10–2. Normal ferret colon with straight tubular arrangement of glands and usual component of goblet cells (H & E stain; × 240).

(e.g., intestinal adenomatosis, adenomatous intestinal hyperplasia, proliferative ileitis, and proliferative hemorrhagic enteropathy).[43,44] The major difference between the lesion in the ferret and that in the hamster and pig is the location in the colon; the lesion in the hamster and pig is primarily in the ileum, with occasional extension to the colon and jejunum.[40,42] The microscopic features in the ferret of epithelial hyperplasia, glandular irregularity, reduced goblet cell production, and variability in type and severity of inflammatory cell infiltrate are all features of the lesion in the hamster and pig.

Recently, by utilizing fluorescent antibody techniques, "omega" (Ω) *Campylobacter* antigen was demonstrated at the site of bacterial colonization within hyperplastic epithelial cells of six colons from ferrets affected with proliferative colitis (Fig. 10–5).[45] The same *Campylobacter* Ω antigen is present within the affected epithelia of tissue from porcine intestinal adenomatosis and hamster proliferative ileitis.[46] Penetration of the intestinal glands through the muscularis mucosa into the submucosa and tunica muscularis is a common feature reported in the hamster,[39,40] and was observed to some degree in all ferrets with proliferative colitis. Gross and microscopic findings indicate an increase in thickness of the tunica muscularis; this may be due to hypertrophy of the muscle fibers, although this has not been confirmed.

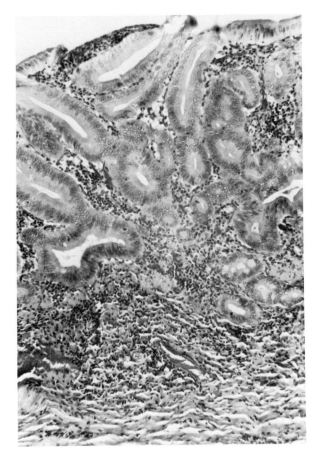

Fig. 10–3. Hyperplastic colonic mucosa in a ferret, with irregular glands and a moderate mononuclear cell infiltrate in the lamina propria (H & E stain; × 240).

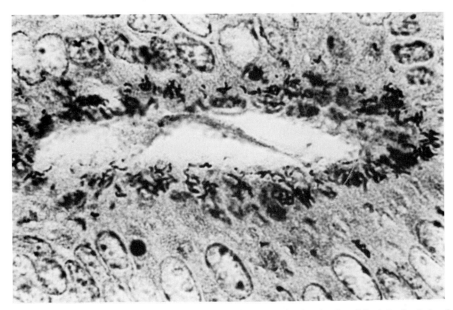

Fig. 10–4. Comma-shaped organisms clustered in the apical cytoplasm of cells of the intestinal glands in the colon of a ferret with proliferative colitis, (Warthin-Starry stain; × 2400).

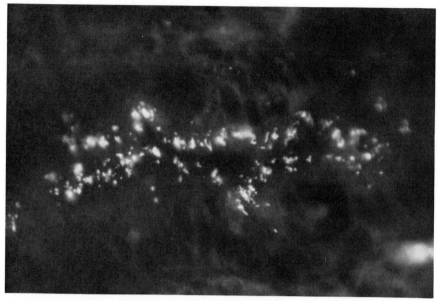

Fig. 10–5. Proliferative colitis in a ferret, showing intracellular *Campylobacter* Ω antigen (paraffin trypsinized section stained with 1080/76 antisera conjugated fluorescein sheep antirabbit serum; × 450).

Diagnosis. Diagnosis is based on a grossly enlarged, palpable colon; biopsy of affected tissue reveals a hyperplastic mucosa. Until the etiology is known, preventive measures are unavailable, and a guarded prognosis is warranted.

Treatment. Death occurred in two affected animals after they were given broad-spectrum antibiotics (chloramphenicol or gentamicin) and fluid therapy, and in two others after marked weight loss and diarrhea of 5 days' duration. Also, six ferrets treated with supportive parenteral fluids and antibiotics during periodic episodes of diarrhea responded temporarily, but subsequently relapsed and required euthanasia. Recently however, therapy with chloramphenicol, 25 mg/lb twice daily for 10 days, has resulted in remission of clinical signs and regression of histologic lesions in ferrets previously affected with the disease.[47]

SALMONELLOSIS

Salmonella, a gram-negative bacteria, can be isolated on selective enteric media from infected tissues and feces. Salmonellosis, although seldom reported in the literature, most likely occurs in ferrets with a frequency that dictates its inclusion in the list of differential diagnoses in ferrets with nonspecific signs of gastroenteritis or suspected infective abortions.

Epizootiology and Control. The fur farming industry has historically referred to the disease in ferrets and minks as food poisoning. The prevalence of salmonellosis in ferrets is unknown; prior to isolation of the organism from the liver and spleen of an asymptomatic animal in 1947, the organism, according to the literature, had not been isolated in ferrets.[48] Its occurrence in ferrets depends largely on exposure to different salmonella serotypes present in various raw meats and meat by-products. It must be cautioned that animal pet foods may also be contaminated with salmonella.[49,50] Morbidity and mortality rates vary, but one report cited a morbidity of 10% in a group of infected ferrets. In this recent outbreak of enteritis in a small group of ferrets, *Salmonella typhimurium* was isolated from a ferret who died of enteritis and from another with clinical signs of bloody diarrhea. The source of this outbreak, however, is unknown. Because of the highly contagious nature of the infection, the spread of the disease to other ferrets should be precluded by strict attention to disinfection of the premises and to the personal hygiene of those handling infected ferrets. Clinically ill ferrets or asymptomatic carriers of *Salmonella* may serve as primary sources of infection to humans.

Clinical Signs and Pathology. Infected ferrets can be asymptomatic carriers of *Salmonella* or, depending on host resistance and infecting strain, may be clinically affected, usually presenting with lethargy and varying degrees of symptomatology commonly associated with gastroenteritis. *S. newport*, when fed experimentally to three ferrets on a marginal nutritional intake, produced lassitude, anorexia, and muscular trembling in one ferret on day 1 after inoculation; on day 2 it had bloody feces, and on day 3 it died.[51]

Salmonella typhimurium, isolated from the spleen and liver of an asymptomatic ferret, was inoculated (presumably orally) into two ferrets.[48] The animals became febrile and emaciated; they exhibited conjunctivitis with a clear watery discharge, and one animal had balanitis. Ten days after inoculation one animal was moribund; both animals were euthanized. Tarry intestinal contents were present in both animals, and petechial hemorrhage was noted in the gastric mucosa in one ferret. Although the authors stipulated that the temperature curve noted in the animals was not characteristic of distemper, they could not exclude the possibility that the

animals were also infected with other organisms.[48] It should be noted, however, that cats and guinea pigs can present clinically with *Salmonella*-associated conjunctivitis.[52,53] Ferrets naturally infected with salmonellosis (uncomplicated by concurrent infection) also demonstrate severe conjunctivitis, tarry stools, and typhoidlike temperature fluctuations.[54]

Accompanying signs often seen with *Salmonella*-associated gastroenteritis may include dehydration, anorexia, moderately elevated temperature, pale mucous membranes, and malaise. Although not documented in ferrets, cats are seen with a lowered white blood cell count, with marked neutropenia and lymphopenia; acute septicemias with thrombocytopenia and nonregenerative anemia are also occasionally noted.[55]

Morbidity and mortality rates vary, but in a recent outbreak of salmonellosis in ferrets maintained for biomedical research, 2 of 20 ferrets with blood-tinged diarrhea had *Salmonella typhimurium* isolated from their feces. Abortion has also been noted in mink infected with *S. choleraesuis*.[51] The source was traced to the feeding of infected raw pork livers to the mink.

Gross and microscopic findings are similar to those seen in other animals infected with clinical salmonellosis. Gross examination of experimentally or naturally infected ferrets reveals hyperemic serosal vessels of the intestine, distended gallbladder, and small intestine filled with dark red, semisolid material. Histologically, the gastrointestinal tract has congestion of the gastric mucosa, with a layer of mucus consisting of inflammatory cells and desquamated epithelium.[51] The small intestine has a similar exudate on the mucous layer, with tips of villi sloughed in the lumen of the intestine. The small intestine may have marked macrophage and lymphocyte infiltration in the submucosa, lamina propria, and mucous epithelium. The liver, spleen, and mesenteric lymph nodes routinely contain areas of necrosis, which can be detected grossly as yellowish-white foci of varying size. Although not pathognomonic, the necrotic foci (the so-called "paratyphoid nodules") are often visible on the surface or in cut sections of the liver. Splenomegaly is also encountered.

Thrombosis of abdominal vessels is sometimes encountered, and may be consistent with the syndrome of disseminated intravascular coagulation. In cases of septicemia, ecchymoses and petechiae can be noted on the visceral and parietal pleura, peritoneum, endocardium, epicardium, and meninges.

Diagnosis. *Salmonella* is a gram-negative rod of the family *Enterobacteriaceae*. The organism grows readily on enrichment media, such as GN broth, selenite broth, and tetrathionate broth. Plating media used are *Salmonella-Shigella* agar, brilliant green agar, eosin-methylene blue agar, and MacConkey agar. The organism can be recovered from liver, heart blood, spleen, and intestinal contents, and occasionally from bone marrow.

Treatment. It is important not only to recognize the clinical syndrome of salmonellosis but also to isolate, identify, and establish antibiotic sensitivities to the *Salmonella* serotype causing the disease. *Salmonella* isolates from ferrets may be resistant to a number of the antibiotics used routinely in veterinary medicine. Serotypes recovered from clinically ill or asymptomatic ferrets may have multiple antibiotic-resistant patterns. *Salmonella* isolates can often transfer part or all of the antibiotic resistance pattern present on plasmids to susceptible *Escherichia coli*.[56] The improper selection and utilization of an antibiotic will limit the success of clinical treatment and may also increase the amount, duration, and antibiotic resistance pattern of shedding *Salmonella* organisms.[57, 58]

Similar to treatment of the disease in cats, careful attention to the management of fluids and to the electrolyte balance assists in the successful recovery of clinically affected ferrets. Of particular importance is the treatment of the hypoglycemia that can result from endotoxemia. To counteract intestinal vasoconstriction, acepromazine (1 mg/kg) is recommended.[59] Glucocorticoids and, in selected cases, blood therapy are also recommended for treatment of endotoxic shock. Elimination of stress, treatment of concurrent diseases, and supportive therapy with nutrients and vitamins are also essential.

Investigators have been successful in treating experimentally infected ferrets. Six of twelve ferrets infected with *Salmonella typhimurium* were treated with sulfathalidine in their food for 4 days (1 g/day/kg body weight). Three days following treatment, *S. typhimurium* was isolated in four of six untreated ferrets, but not from ferrets treated with sulfathalidine.[54] Sulfathalidine administered by the same authors in a controlled experiment to a colony of 77 ferrets for an outbreak of salmonellosis resulted in a decrease of ferrets shedding *S. typhimurium*; the organism was isolated from 40 (52%) prior to treatment and from only 12 (15.5%) posttreatment. Treatment also dramatically increased weight gain and general health of the ferrets. Autogenous vaccine, however, failed to protect against natural infection with the disease.

LEPTOSPIROSIS

Leptospirosis in animals was diagnosed in 1850, 30 years before recognition of the disease in humans. *Leptospira grippotyphosa* and *L. icterohaemorrhagiae* have been isolated from ferrets,[60] and leptospires in ferrets have been postulated as a zoonotic threat.[61]

Epizootiology and Control. The historic use of ferrets to control rats and mice in domestic or farm settings certainly allowed ferrets to be exposed to leptospires shed in rodent urine. Fur-bearing animals maintained in commercial operations, including ferrets, can contract leptospirosis. The incidence in captive fur bearers is relatively low, but it may occur either as individual cases or as epidemics.[60,62] Given the high incidence of the disease in domestic animals and dogs, pet ferrets exposed to these animals are probably at risk for contracting the disease, although reports of the disease in ferrets are fragmentary.

Free-living members of the *Mustelidae*, including nine stoats (*M. erminea*), nine ferrets (*M. putorius*), and four weasels (*M. nivalis*) inhabiting farmland in the north island of New Zealand, were surveyed for evidence of leptospiral infection. None of the animals examined had evidence of infection using serology (using 12 different leptospiral antigens) as well as culture of kidneys.[63] Interestingly, even though there was a high prevalence of endemic infection with *L. ballum* occurring in house mice (*Mus musculus*), ship rats (*Rattus rattus*) as well as other rat populations in New Zealand, and the fact that *Mustelidae* utilize these species of rodents as a major food source, infection with this serotype was not demonstrated. In Denmark, 10% of the stoats examined had serologic titers to serovars *poi pomona* and *sejroe*. However, 11 polecats (*M. putorius*) and 16 weasels examined were negative.[64] In Great Britain, a similar survey indicated weasels have had serologic titers to serovars *sejroe* and *bratislava*.[65,66]

A properly produced vaccine, if warranted, should protect ferrets against clinical disease and development of a carrier state. To date, however, leptospirosis vaccine has not been recommended for ferrets raised commercially, maintained as pets, or used for research purposes.

LISTERIOSIS

Listeriosis is classified as a mildly infectious but highly fatal disease that affects several species of animals, including humans.[67] The etiologic agent, *Listeria monocytogenes*, is a gram-positive, non-spore-forming rod that is motile at room temperature and hemolytic, characteristics that separate it from other similar diphtheroid bacteria. It is usually isolated from the CNS of symptomatic animals or from infected tissues. Occasionally it is isolated from the organs of asymptomatic hosts.

Epizootiology and Control. The prevalence of the organism in ferrets is unknown. It was isolated from a group of ferrets previously inoculated with a suspension of bacteriologically sterile lung tissue from distemper-infected ferrets.[66] The lungs and spleens of the ferrets were subsequently found to harbor *Listeria monocytogenes*, both by culture and by intracerebral inoculation into hamsters.[68] It was also isolated from another mustelid, the sable, *Mustela zibellina*.[69] Recently, the organism was isolated from the pleural fluid of an immunosuppressed ferret suffering from Cushing's disease and cardiomyopathy.[70] Pneumonia and hepatitis in this animal were attributed to listeria infection.

Ingestion of contaminated food or inhalation are suspected as modes of transmission. The organism may be isolated from water, soil, dust, animal feed, and various domestic and wild animals. It is not known whether in utero infection occurs in ferrets, as it does in humans. Asymptomatic ferrets may play a role in the dissemination of the disease, but experimental evidence or other reports in the literature concerning this hypothesis are lacking. It is known, however, that asymptomatic listeria fecal carriers have been reported in both humans and animals.

Clinical Signs and Pathology. Neither clinical signs nor pathology due to the organism have been described for the ferret, but they are presumed to be the same as those encountered in other species—that is, predominantly confined to the CNS, or associated septicemia. The disease is frequently superimposed on other debilitating diseases, especially in patients receiving steroid therapy or immunosuppressive drugs.[3,70]

Diagnosis. If a ferret presents with CNS signs, it is without question prudent to quarantine the animal and to consider rabies in the differential diagnoses. Minimal handling is therefore warranted. If rabies exposure can be definitely excluded, a cerebral spinal fluid culture should be performed. *Listeria* grows aerobically and tests positive for catalase and the Voges-Proskauer reaction. It is important not to confuse this organism and misidentify it as a diphtheroid contaminant. Cold enrichment techniques may be used for increased sensitivity in isolating listeria.

Treatment. Treatment, if initiated, consists of broad-spectrum antimicrobial agents, including penicillin and ampicillin. In vitro listeria isolates are also usually sensitive to chloramphenicol, tetracycline, erythromycin, and cephalothin.

TUBERCULOSIS

The ferret appears to be highly susceptible to certain strains of *Mycobacterium*, including avian, bovine and human strains. Clinical illness may be vague or asymptomatic and may therefore escape detection, thus offering the potential for spread of the disease to other animals and for zoonotic infection in pet owners or laboratory personnel.

Epizootiology and Control. Only scattered reports of tuberculosis in ferrets appear in the literature; these are almost exclusively in ferrets maintained for research in England and Europe during the period 1929 to 1953.[71,72] One investigator reported that, among thousands of necropsies performed on ferrets obtained from dealers, 60% were infected with the tubercle bacillus, most commonly avian strains and less frequently bovine strains.[73,74] The disease continues to be recognized in New Zealand ferret farms.[75]

The ferret can be infected either naturally or experimentally by bovine, avian, and human tubercle bacillus. Tuberculosis was recorded in ferrets during the period when the feeding of unpasteurized milk, raw poultry, and meat (including meat by-products) was routinely performed. Feeding of infected carcasses or milk to ferrets undoubtedly contributed greatly to tuberculosis in ferrets during this era. Chicken offal used in preparing mink ration, which is also fed to ferrets, can be a possible source of infection.[76] Efforts to eliminate tuberculosis in commercially reared livestock and chickens, in the United States and worldwide, have effectively reduced the incidence of tuberculosis in ferrets. In addition, the general use of commercially prepared dog and cat food as the sole food source for ferrets also has appreciably reduced the possibility of introducing this disease into the ferret population. Infected wild birds shedding tubercle bacilli in feces should be prevented from contaminating feed supplies and outdoor areas housing ferrets.

Clinical Signs and Pathology. Documentation of this aspect of the disease in ferrets is sketchy. Systemic infection caused by the bovine strain results in generalized weight loss, loss of appetite, lethargy, and death. In one well-documented case of tuberculosis caused by a bovine strain of tuberculosis, the animal first had difficulty walking, with the hind legs splayed; the extent of paralysis progressed, and the animal was killed and necropsied. Tubercle bacillus isolated from this animal was inoculated intramuscularly into another ferret. The second ferret remained normal until 6 months later, when it developed paralysis of the adductor muscles of the thigh; eventually, all muscles of the limbs were affected.[74] In ferrets, splenomegaly, hepatomegaly, and intestinal nodules can also be detected by palpation in cases with disseminated, multiple organ involvement.

Disseminated disease is more likely with *Mycobacterium bovis*, whereas the human and avian tubercle strains usually produce only local, indolent tubercular lesions. The lesions produced by *M. bovis* are characterized by minimal cellular reaction, with numerous acid-fast bacilli in the lesions. These reactions are associated with an impaired cell-mediated immune response.[77] In vitro phytohemagglutinin (PHA) responses of normal versus *M. bovis*-treated peripheral leukocytes demonstrate that *M. bovis* suppression of PHA correlates with the cytotoxicity of *M. bovis* for ferret peripheral leukocytes. *M. bovis* concentrations of 10^6/ml and below enhance PHA response, but more than 10^6 organisms/ml suppress it.[78] Thorns and Morris speculated that the cytotoxic activity of high concentrations of *M. bovis*, and associated in vitro suppression of PHA-stimulated leukocytes, may play a role in the pathogenesis of the *M. bovis* disease in ferrets, producing a depression of specific and nonspecific cell-mediated immunity, which explains the lack of cellular tissue reactions seen in naturally occurring *M. bovis* disease in ferrets.[78]

Diagnosis. Nodular lesions, if calcified, can be demonstrated radiographically. Laparotomy, with biopsy of involved abdominal lymph nodes or other organs and isolation of mycobacterial organisms, will establish a definitive diagnosis of tuberculosis. Experimentally, ferrets inoculated with Freund's complete adjuvant (FCA, containing killed *M. tuberculosis*) react to an intradermal injection of 10,000 U (200 μg) of tuberculin (see Chap. 7, Fig. 7–2).[79] In other studies in ferrets inoculated with FCA, and with 10^4 and 10^5 U of tuberculin, skin reactions were elicited 14 days postinoculation (PI).[80] Skin tests carried out 4 weeks after immunization and inoculation with FCA were negative. In ferrets experimentally infected with *M. bovis*, however, a minimal tuberculin response to purified protein derivative (10 μg/ml) was observed only 36 hours PI, and no response was observed at 7 and 15 days PI.[81] The tuberculin skin test was used to eliminate natural cases of tuberculosis in controlling tuberculosis in a breeding colony of ferrets.[82] Unfortunately, the type and dosage of tuberculin were not detailed. Depending on the infecting mycobacterium strain, reaction to a tuberculin test using PPD may be minimal. For example, Pulling[83] found that mink from a tuberculous colony tested by intradermal injection of bovine tuberculin did not show a delayed hypersensitivity reaction.

Treatment. Because of the zoonotic risk associated with tuberculosis, infected ferrets should be euthanized. If other ferrets are at risk they should be tuberculintested (which may or may not be helpful), or other diagnostic tests should be performed to ascertain their disease status. Personnel at risk should also be screened with appropriate tuberculin tests.

BACTERIAL PNEUMONIA

Various bacterial organisms have been implicated in either primary or secondary bacterial pneumonias. *Streptococcus zooepidemicus*, group C, and group G streptococcus were cited as causes of primary pneumonia, and were also isolated from pneumonic lungs of ferrets who died during an influenza epidemic.[84, 85] *S. pneumoniae*, diagnosed as a cause of pleuritis and pneumonia in mink, should also be considered in a differential diagnosis of bacterial pneumonia in ferrets.[86] Gram-negative bacteria, such as *Escherichia coli, Klebsiella pneumoniae*, and *Pseudomonas aeruginosa* were isolated from suppurative lung lesions of ferrets.[87, 88] *Bordetella bronchiseptica* was isolated from diseased lungs of dead neonatal ferrets.[89] *Listeria monocytogenes* was also isolated from consolidated inflammatory lung tissue and pleural effusion of a ferret suffering from Cushing's syndrome and cardiomyopathy.[70]

Clinical Signs and Pathology. Signs of pneumonia, including nasal discharge, dyspnea, increased abdominal respiration, fever, lassitude, and anorexia, either singly or in combination, may be observed. In certain cases, fulminant pneumonia with sepsis results in acute death without pre-existing clinical signs. A peracute respiratory disease, presumed to be bacterial (e.g., *Bordetella bronchiseptica*), was observed in 7- to 10-day-old kits. The kits had dyspnea, open-mouthed breathing, and serous to suppurative nasal discharge. Without antibiotic treatment the ferrets died within a 24-hour period.[89]

Bacterial pneumonia is usually characterized by a suppurative inflammatory process, affecting either the bronchial tree and surrounding tissue or major portions of the lobes of the lung. Lungs infected with streptococcus Group C have purulent material in the bronchi, and have raised yellow to white patches of varying size (up to several millimeters in diameter) on the dorsal and marginal surfaces of the lungs.[84]

Diagnosis. Diagnosis is based on clinical signs of pneumonia and on culture of the organism from clinical specimens, such as tracheal exudate or affected lung tissue at necropsy. Animals stressed from concurrent infectious disease such as influenza, debilitated from chronic illness such as cardiomyopathy, or immunosuppressed from therapy, metabolic disease, or surgery, may be more susceptible to bacterial pneumonias. Differential diagnoses include pleural effusion caused by *Dirofilaria immitis* or dilative cardiomyopathy, pulmonary mycosis, primary or secondary neoplasia, or malignant hyperthermia.

Treatment. If bacterial isolation is successful, it is essential to perform the appropriate in vitro antibiotic susceptibility tests. Generally, penicillin or synthetic penicillins are effective against gram-positive bacteria, such as *streptococcal* organisms. For gram-negative organisms, gentamicin (5 mg/kg once daily) is used. Tribrissen, trimethoprim, and sulfadiazine (30 mg/kg) is also effective in treating bacterial pneumonia caused by gram-negative organisms that demonstrate in vitro antibiotic susceptibility to this combination of antimicrobial agents. For neonatal ferrets, nebulization therapy using gentamicin is recommended to treat bacterial pneumonias.

ABSCESSES

Etiology. *Staphylococcus, Streptococcus* (groups C and G), *Pasteurella, Corynebacterium, Actinomyces* and hemolytic *Escherichia coli* cause abscesses and localized infections of the lung, uterus, vulva, skin, and oral cavity.

Epizootiology and Control. Penetrating injuries such as bite wounds inflicted during mating and puncture wounds in the mouth from ingested bones and foreign bodies can result in abscess formation. In most cases the infection is walled off, and few systemic signs are observed. Sound management practices can reduce the incidence of abscess formation by reducing exposure to sharp objects in the cage and feed, and by limiting the contact time between the male and female during breeding.

Clinical Signs. Abscesses are detected as fluctuant swellings that may be accompanied by draining tracts. These must be distinguished from cutaneous myiasis.

Diagnosis. Aspirating, draining, or biopsying the affected swelling will aid in differentiating inflammation from neoplasia or parasitic infestation. Culture and antibiotic sensitivity tests of microorganisms isolated from the abscess will assist both in diagnosis and treatment of localized bacterial infections.

Treatment. Drainage of localized abscesses and application of topical antiseptics are usually effective in treating the abscess.

If this procedure does not eliminate the infection, however, systemic antibiotics should be initiated.

INFECTION BY *MYCOPLASMA MUSTELIDAE*

A new organism, *Mycoplasma mustelidae*, has been isolated from normal lungs of mink kits. The new mycoplasma was different from all previously accepted mycoplasmas, and hence was given a new species name.[90] This mycoplasma, along with ureaplasma strains, was originally isolated from three mink farms in Denmark. *Mycoplasma* has also been isolated from the oral and nasal cavities of clinically normal ferrets in Japan.[91] Its pathogenicity and importance as a clinical entity in ferrets await further studies.

REFERENCES

1. Andrews, P.L.R., Illman, O., and Mellerish, A.: Some observations of anatomical abnormalities and disease states in a population of 350 ferrets (*Mustela furo L.*) Z. Versuchstierkd., *21*:346, 1979.
2. Harding, A.R.: Ferret Facts and Fallacies. Columbus, OH, A.R. Harding, 1943.
3. Benenson, A.S. (ed.): Control of Communicable Diseases in Man. 13th Ed. Washington, D.C., American Public Health Association, 1981.
4. Pine, L.: Actinomyces and microaerophilic actinomycetes. In Infectious Diseases and Medical Microbiology, Chap. 48. 2nd Ed. Edited by A.I. Braude, C.E. Davis, and J. Fierer. Philadelphia, W.B. Saunders, 1986.
5. Skulski, G., and Symmers, W. St. C.: Actinomycosis and torulosis in the ferret. J. Comp. Pathol., *64*:306, 1954.
6. Hobbs, G., et al.: Detection and isolation of *Clostridium botulinum*. In Isolation and Identification Methods for Food Poisoning Organisms. Edited by J.E. Corry, D. Roberts, and F.A. Skinner. New York, Academic Press, 1982.
7. Quartrup, E.R., and Holt, D.L.: Case report of botulism type C in mink. J. Am. Vet. Med. Assoc., *97*:167, 1940.
8. Hall, I.C., and Stiles G.W.: An outbreak of botulism in captive mink on a fur farm in Colorado. J. Bacteriol, *36*:282, 1938.
9. Blandford, T.B., Roberts, T.A., and Ashton, W.L.G.: Losses from botulism in mallard duck and other water fowl. Vet. Rec., *85*:541, 1969.
10. Harrison, S.G., and Borland, E.D.: Deaths in ferrets (*Mustela putorius*) due to *Clostridium botulinum* type C. Vet. Rec., *93*:576, 1973.
11. Moll, T., and Brandly, C.A.: Botulism in mouse, mink and ferret with special reference to susceptibility and pathological alterations. Am. J. Vet. Res., *12*:355. 1951.
12. Quartrup, E.R., and Gorham, J.R.: Susceptibility of fur-bearing animals to toxins of *Clostridium botulinum* types A, B, C, and E. Am. J. Vet. Res., *10*:268, 1949.
13. Hobbs, G., Williams, K., and Willis, A.T.: Basic methods for the isolation of clostridia. In Isolation of Anaerobes. Edited by D.A. Shapton, and R.G. Board. New York, Academic Press, 1971.
14. Notermans, S., Dufrenne, J., and Kozaki, S.: Enzyme-linked immunosorbent assay for detection of *Clostridium botulinum* type E. Appl. Environ. Microbiol., *37*:1173, 1979.

15. Fox, J.G.: Campylobacteriosis: A new disease in laboratory animals. Lab. Anim. Sci., *32*:625, 1982.

16. Blaser, M.G., La Force, F.M., and Wilson, N.A.: Reservoirs for human campylobacteriosis. J. Infect Dis., *141*:665, 1980.

17. Fox, J.G., et al.: Proliferative colitis in ferrets. Am. J. Vet. Res., *43*:858, 1982.

18. Fox, J.G., Ackerman, J.I., and Newcomer, C.E.: Ferret as potential reservoir for human campylobacteriosis. Am. J. Vet. Res., *44*:1049, 1983.

19. Fox, J.G., et al.: Gastric mucosa in the ferret: Bacteriologic and pathologic findings. Presented at the Fourth International Workshop on *Campylobacter* Infections. Goteborg, Sweden, June 1987.

20. Hunter, D.B., et al.: *Campylobacter* colitis in ranch mink in Ontario. Can. J. Vet. Res., *50*:47, 1986.

21. Prescott, J.F., and Bruin-Mosch C.W.: Carriage of Campylobacter jejuni in healthy and diarrheic animals. Am. J. Vet. Res., *42*:164, 1982.

22. Penner, J.L., and Hennessy, J.N.: Passive hemagglutination technique for serotyping *Campylobacter fetus* subsp. *jejuni* on the basis of soluble heat-stable antigens. J. Clin. Microbiol., *12*:732, 1980.

23. Lior, H., et al.: Serotyping of *Campylobacter jejuni* by slide agglutination based on heat-labile antigenic factors. J. Clin. Microbiol., *15*: 751, 1982.

24. Fox, J.G., et al.: *Campylobacter jejuni* infection in the ferret: An animal model of campylobacteriosis. Am. J. Vet. Res., *48*:85, 1987.

25. Fox, J.G., Moore R., Ackerman, I.I.: Canine and feline campylobacteriosis: Epizootiology and clinical and public health features. J. Am. Vet. Med. Assn., *183*:1420, 1983.

26. Hunter, D.B., Prescott, J.F., Pettit, S.R., and Snow, W.E.: *Campylobacter jejuni* as a cause of abortion in mink. Can. Vet. J., *24*:398, 1983.

27. Karmali, M.A., and Fleming, P.C.: *Campylobacter* enteritis in children. J. Pediatr., *94*:527, 1979.

28. Blaser, M.T., Wells, J.G., and Feldman, R.A.: Epidemiology of endemic and epidemic *Campylobacter* infections in the United States. *In* Campylobacter: Epidemiology, Pathogenesis, and Biochemistry. Edited by D.G. Newell. Lancaster, England, MTP Press, 1982.

29. Blaser, M.T., and Reller, L.B.: *Campylobacter* enteritis. N. Engl. J. Med., *305*:1444, 1981.

30. Chow, A.W., Patten, V., and Bednorz, D.: Susceptibility of *Campylobacter fetus* to twenty-two antimicrobial agents. Antimicrob. Agents Chemother., *13*:416, 1978.

31. Vanhoof, R., et al.: Susceptibility of *Campylobacter fetus* subsp. *jejuni* to twenty-nine antimicrobial agents. Antimicrob. Agents Chemother., *14*:533, 1978.

32. Vanhoof, R., et al.: Bacteriostatic and bactericidal activities of 24 antimicrobial agents against *Campylobacter fetus* subsp. *jejuni*. Antimicrob. Agents Chemother., *18*:188, 1980.

33. Wright, E.P., and Knowles, M.A.: ß-Lactamase production by *Campylobacter jejuni*. J. Clin. Pathol., *33*:904, 1980.

34. Marshall, B.J.: *Campylobacter pyloridis* and gastritis. J. Infect. Dis., *153*:650, 1986.

35. Goodwin, C.S., et al.: Unusual cellular fatty acids and distinctive ultrastructure in a new spiral bacterium (*Campylobacter pyloridis*) from the human gastric mucosa. Microbiol., *19*:257, 1985.

36. Fox, J.G., et al.: *Campylobacter*-like organisms isolated from gastric mucosa of ferrets. Am. J. Vet. Res., *47*:236, 1986.

37. Fox, J.G., Goad, M.E.P., and Hotaling, L.I.: Gastric ulcers in ferrets (abstract). Lab. Anim. Sci., *36*:562, 1986.

38. Fox, J.G., and Leathers, C.: Proliferative colitis in a pet ferret. J. Am. Vet. Med. Assoc., *189*: 1475, 1986.

39. Jacoby, R.O., Osbaldiston, G.W., and Jonas, A.M.: Experimental transmission of atypical ileal hyperplasia of hamsters. Lab. Anim. Sci., *25*:464, 1975.

40. Boothe, A.D., and Cheville, N.F.: The pathology of proliferative ileitis of the golden hamster. Pathol. Vet., *4*:31, 1967.

41. Frisk, C.S., and Wagner, J.E.: Hamster enteritis: A review. Lab. Anim., *11*:79, 1977.

42. Jonas, A.M., Tomita, Y., and Wyand, D.S.: Enzootic intestinal adenocarcinoma in hamsters. J. Am. Vet. Med. Assoc., *147*:1102, 1965.

43. Rowland, A.C., and Lawson, G.H.K.: Porcine intestinal adenomatosis, a possible relationship with necrotic enteritis, regional ileitis and proliferative hemorrhagic enteropathy. Vet. Rec., *97*:178, 1975.

44. Dodd, D.C.: Adenomatous intestinal hyperplasia (proliferative ileitis) of swine. Pathol. Vet., *5*:333, 1968.

45. Fox, J.G., and Lawson, G.H.K.: *Campylobacter*-like omega intracellular antigen in proliferative colitis in ferrets. Lab. Anim. Sci., *38*:34, 1988.

46. Lawson, G.H.K., Rowland, A.C., and MacIntyre, N.: Demonstration of a new intracellular antigen in intestinal adenomatosis and hamster proliferative ileitis. Vet. Microbiol., *4*:303, 1985.

47. Krueger, K.L., Murphy, J.C., Fox, J.G.: Treatment of Proliferative Colitis in Ferrets. J. Am. Vet. Med. Assoc. (In press.)

48. Morris, J.A., and Coburn, D.R.: The isolation of *Salmonella typhimurium* from ferrets. J. Bacteriol., *55*:419, 1948.

49. Galton, M.M., Harless, M., and Hardy, A.V.: *Salmonella* isolations from dehydrated dog meals. J. Am. Vet. Med. Assoc., *126*:57, 1955.

50. Thornton, H.: The public health danger of unsanitized foods. Vet. Rec., *91*:430, 1972.

51. Gorham, J.R., Cordy, D.R., and Quartrup, E.R.: *Salmonella* infection in mink and ferrets. Am. J. Vet. Res., 10:183, 1949.

52. Fox, J.G., and Gallus, C.M.: *Salmonella*-associated conjunctivitis in a cat. J. Am. Vet. Med. Assoc., 171:845, 1977.

53. Fox, J.G., Beaucage, C.M., Murphy J.C., and Niemi, S.M.: Experimental salmonella-associated conjunctivitis in cats. Can. J. Comp. Med., 48:87, 1984.

54. Coburn, D.R., and Morris, J.A.: The treatment of *Salmonella typhimurium* infection in ferrets. Cornell Vet., 39:198, 1949.

55. Krum, S.H., Stevens D.R., and Hirsh, D.C.: *Salmonella arizonae* bacteremia in a cat. J. Am. Vet. Med. Assoc., 170:42, 1977.

56. Beaucage, C.M., and Fox, J.G.: Transmissible antibiotic resistance in *Salmonella* isolated from random-source cats purchased for use in research. Am. J. Vet. Res., 40:849, 1979.

57. Wilcock, B., and Olander, H.: Influence of oral antibiotic feeding on the duration and severity of clinical disease, growth performance, and pattern of shedding in swine inoculated with *Salmonella typhimurium*. J. Am. Vet. Med. Assoc., 172:472, 1978.

58. Aserkoff, B., and Bennett, J.V.: Effect of antibiotic therapy in acute salmonellosis on the fecal excretion of salmonellae. N. Engl. J. Med., 281:636, 1969.

59. Timoney, J.F., Niebert, H.C., and Scott, F.W.: Feline salmonellosis. A nosocomial outbreak and experimental studies. Cornell Vet., 68:211, 1975.

60. Tortem, M.: Leptospirosis. *In* CRC Handbook Series in Zoonoses, Sect. A, Vol. I. Edited by J.H. Steele. Cleveland, OH, CRC Press, 1979.

61. Hammond, J., and Chesterman, F.C.: The ferret. *In* UFAW Handbook on the Care and Management of Laboratory Animals. 4th Ed. London, Churchill Livingstone, 1972.

62. Sulzer, C.R. (ed.): Leptospiral Serotype Distribution Lists—Supplement to the 1966 Publication. Edited by M.M. Galton. Atlanta, Centers for Disease Control, 1975.

63. Hathaway, S.C., and Blackmore, D.K.: Failure to demonstrate the maintenance of leptospires by free living carnivores. N.Z. Vet. J., 29:115, 1981.

64. Fennestad, K.L., and Borg-Petersen, C.: Leptospires in Dannish wild mammals. J. Wildlife Dis., 8:343, 1972.

65. Michna, S.W., and Campbell, R.S.F.: Leptospires in wild animals. J. Comp. Pathol., 80:101, 1970.

66. Twigg, G.I., Cuerden, C.M., and Hughes D.M.: Leptospires in British wild mammals. Symp. Zool. Soc. (London), 24:75, 1968.

67. Armstrong, D.: *Listeria monocytogenes*. In Principles and Practices of Infectious Diseases. Edited by G.L. Mandell, R.G. Douglas, Jr., and J.E. Bennett. New York, Wiley Medical Publications, 1985.

68. Morris, J.A., and Norman, M.C.: The isolation of *Listeria monocytogenes* from ferrets. J. Bacteriol., 59:313, 1950.

69. Eremeev, M.N., and Stepanenk, N.D.: Listeriosis in Russian sables. Veterinariya (Moscow), 39:57, 1962.

70. Fox, J.G., et al.: Hyperadrenocorticism syndrome in a ferret. J. Amer. Vet. Med. Assoc., 191:343, 1987.

71. Dunkin, G.W., Laidlaw, P.P., and Griffith, A.S.: Note on tuberculosis in the ferret. J. Comp. Pathol., 42:46, 1929.

72. Hughes, D.L.: The ferret. *In* UFAW Handbook on the Care and Management of Laboratory Animals. Edited by A.N. Worden. London, Bailliere, Tindall and Cox, 1947.

73. MacIntyre, A.B.: Personal communication, 1951.

74. Symmers, W.S.T.C., Thomson, A.P.D., and Iland, C.N.: Observations on tuberculosis in the ferret (*Mustela furo L.*) J. Comp. Pathol., 63:20, 1953.

75. Diseases of the fitch. Surveillance, 11:27, 1984.

76. Canadian Council on Animal Care: Guide to the care and use of experimental animals. 2:83, 1984.

77. Morris, J.A., Stevens, A.E., Little, T.W.A., and Stuart, J.D.: Lymphocyte unresponsiveness to PPD tuberculin in badgers infected with *Mycobacterium bovis*. Res. Vet. Sci., 25:390, 1978.

78. Thorns, C.J., and Morris, J.A.: Suppression and enhancement of transformation of ferret peripheral blood mononuclear cells by mycobacteria. Res. Vet. Sci., 36:34, 1984.

79. Kauffman, C.A.: Cell-mediated immunity in ferrets: Delayed dermal hypersensitivity, lymphocyte transformation, and macrophage migration inhibitory factor production. Devel. Comp. Immunol., 5:124, 1981.

80. Potter, C.W., et al.: Immunity to influenza in ferrets. IX. Delayed hypersensitivity following infection or immunization with AZ/Hong Kong virus. Microbios, 10A:7, 1974.

81. Thorns, C.J., Morris, J.A., and Little, T.W.A.: A spectrum of immune responses and pathological conditions between certain animal species to experimental *Mycobacterium bovis* infection. Br. J. Exp. Pathol., 63:562, 1982.

82. Grinham, W.E.: The management of a breeding colony of ferrets. J. Anim. Tech. Assoc., 2:3, 1952.

83. Pulling, F.B.: An outbreak of bovine tuberculosis in mink and treatment with rimifon. J. Am. Vet. Med. Assoc., 121:389, 1952.

84. Andrews, P.L.R., Illman, O., and Mellers, L.: Some observations of anatomical abnormalities and disease states in a population of 350 ferrets. Z. Versuchstierkd., 21:346, 1979.

85. Bell, F.R., and Dudgeon, J.A.: An epizootic of influenza in a ferret colony. J. Comp. Pathol., 58:167, 1948.

86. Hoff, H., and Woxholtt, C.: Diplokokk-foringsin sjon hos mink. Nord. Vet. Med., 4:1201, 1952.

87. Liberson, A.J., et al: Mastitis caused by hemolytic *Escherichia coli* in the ferret. J. Am. Vet. Med. Assoc., 183:1179, 1983.

88. Kociba, G., and Caputo, C.A.: Aplastic anemia associated with estrus in pet ferrets. J. Am. Vet. Med. Assoc., 178:1293, 1981.

89. Marshall, G.: Unpublished observations, 1985.

90. Salih, M.M., Friis, N.F., Arseculeratne, S.N., and Freundt, E.A.: *Mycoplasma mustelidae,* a new species from mink. Int. J. Systematic Bacteriol., 33:476, 1983.

91. Koshimizu, K., Kotani, H., and Syakudo, Y.: Isolation of mycoplasmas from experimental ferrets (*Mustela putorius*). Exp. Anim., 31:299, 1982.

chapter 11

VIRAL AND CHLAMYDIAL DISEASES

J. G. Fox

R. C. Pearson

J. R. Gorham

ALEUTIAN DISEASE

Aleutian disease is a common persistent infection diagnosed in mink, but also occasionally reported in ferrets. A number of excellent reviews on Aleutian disease are available.[1,2] The persistent viremia, rapid viral replication after inoculation, genetic makeup of the host, immune mediated pathology, and hypergammaglobulinemia influence the clinical course and pathogenesis of Aleutian disease in the mink, and may similarly determine the extent of the disease in the ferret.[3] The disease is caused by a parvovirus, Aleutian disease virus (ADV).

Epizootiology and Control. Aleutian disease is probably present in most, if not all, commercially raised mink, and is also found in feral mink. In addition, ADV antibody is present in feral skunks and occasionally in raccoons and foxes.[4,5] Ferrets have a strain of parvovirus that causes a persistent infection, mild histopathologic lesions, and a hypergammaglobulinemia.[1,6] Ferret ADV will persistently infect mink, but does not produce histopathologic lesions.[5]

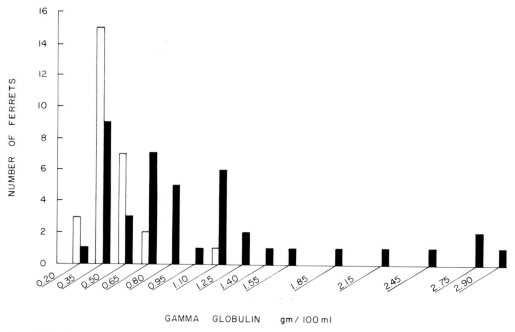

Fig. 11–1. The distribution of serum gamma globulin in normal ferrets (*open bars*) and in those naturally infected with ADV (*solid bars*). The infected ferrets have significantly greater (P < 0.0005) serum gamma globulin levels than normal ferrets. (Porter, H.G., Porter, D.D., and Larsen, A.E.: Aleutian disease in ferrets. Infect. Immunol., *36*:379, 1982.)

In a study involving respiratory syncytial virus in ferrets, 214 adult female ferrets were tested for serum antibody to the Utah-1 mink strain of ADV. When tested by immunofluorescence at a dilution of 1:10, 90 (42%) had ADV antibody.[6] A representative number of 28 antibody-free and 42 antibody-positive ferrets were also tested for serum gamma globulin level. Those with antibody titer to ADV had significantly higher levels of gamma globulin when compared to those without ADV antibody titer (p < 0.0005; Fig. 11–1).

When the highly virulent Utah-1 strain of ADV was injected into ferrets, virus was recovered from the spleen up to 180 days postinfection,[6] and antibody was shown in 19 of 22 ferrets, although the antibody titer was low. Other investigators inoculated a weakly pathogenic Pullman strain of mink ADV into ferrets; 11 developed ADV antibody, whereas only 2 developed hypergammaglobulinemia.[3] In another study, mink ADV inoculated into ferrets produced a low-level persistent infection, but gammaglobulin levels were not elevated.[7] Spontaneous Aleutian disease in ferrets raised commercially has been noted on several occasions.[7,8] Spleen homogenate from a ferret with naturally occurring Aleutian disease, when inoculated into 12 ferrets, induced hypergammaglobulinemia in 4 of the 12 in 6 months; 5 of 15 mink inoculated with the suspension died of the disease.[3]

In a natural outbreak of Aleutian disease in ferrets used for biomedical research, four had a chronic progressive wasting disease, diagnosed as Aleutian disease by histopathologic and serologic findings. The ferrets had been housed in pens that had housed mink infected with Aleutian disease 2 years previously.[9]

Transmission of the virus from ferret to ferret or from ferret to mink (or to other

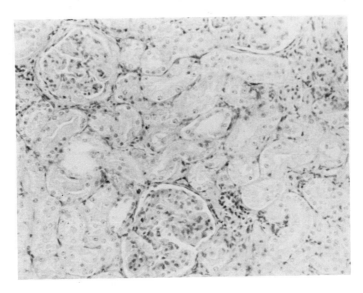

Fig. 11–2. Membranous glomerulonephritis in a ferret attributed to Aleutian disease (H & E stain; × 240).

susceptible hosts) could occur by contact with the handler's gloves or apparatus, because urine as well as other bodily fluids contain the virus.[10] Formalin, a phenolic disinfectant detergent, and sodium hydroxide were active against ADV in the presence of organic material.[11]

The most effective control of Aleutian disease on commercial mink farms is the culling of all mink with ADV antibody, using the counterimmunoelectrophoresis (CIEP) test.[12] Similar programs may be applicable in infected ferret breeding colonies.

Clinical Signs and Pathology. The use of CIEP indicates that ferrets, as well as mink and other species, may have detectable levels of ADV antibody for considerable periods of time without showing clinical signs. Nonspecific signs can include generalized malaise and weight loss; if severely debilitated, stress may precipitate death. In New Zealand clinical signs of progressive posterior paralysis, muscle wasting, urinary incontinence, and tremors were documented.[13] Histologic lesions in the meninges, perivascular cuffing with lymphocytes and plasma

cells, and focal demyelination were observed. The lesions are consistent with those seen in an immune-mediated host response, and Aleutian disease may play a role in the pathogenesis of these lesions.[13] In one laboratory, ferrets infected with ADV of mink origin did not have detectable illness for 136 days of observation.[7] Certain ferrets, however, had massive hepatic periportal lymphocyte infiltrates. Similar hepatic lesions were noted in ferrets raised on a ranch that had ADV-infected mink.[7]

In a subsequent study by the same researchers, ferrets housed with mink and ferrets infected with ADV had hypergammaglobulinemia and typical lesions of Aleutian disease, consisting of bile duct proliferation and plasmacytic and lymphocytic infiltrates in the liver. Also noted were enlargement of the thymus (not observed in Aleutian disease in mink), splenomegaly, lymphadenopathy with interstitial infiltrates of lymphocytes and plasma cells in the kidney, and vasculitis in the meninges, myocardium, and lung.[8, 14] Others have documented similar findings in Aleutian disease in ferrets, but the lesions were not as severe.[3] In a natural

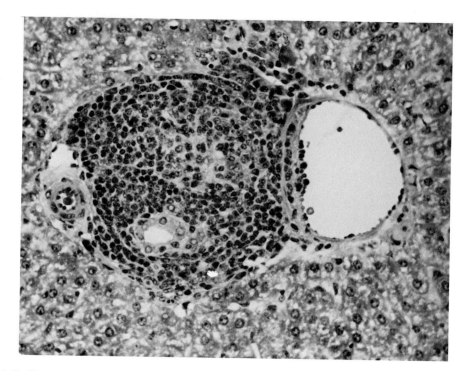

Fig. 11–3. The portal triad of a ferret experimentally infected with ferret ADV for 182 days. A dense lymphoid cell aggregate around the bile duct is present, with characteristics of a lymphoid follicle (H & E stain; × 340). (Porter, H.G., Porter, D.D., and Larsen, A.E.: Aleutian disease in ferrets. Infect. Immunol., *36*:379, 1982.)

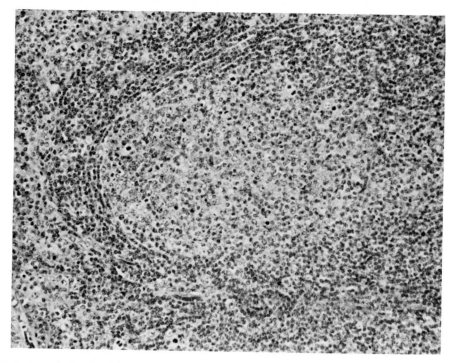

Fig. 11–4. A markedly stimulated lymphoid follicle in an abdominal lymph node from a ferret experimentally infected with ferret ADV (H & E stain; × 228). (Porter, H.G., Porter, D.D., and Larsen, A.E.: Aleutian disease in ferrets. Infect. Immunol., *36*:379, 1982.)

TABLE 11–1. LESIONS OBSERVED IN CONTROL FERRETS AND IN THOSE INOCULATED WITH MINK (UTAH-1) OR FERRET STRAINS OF ADV

Finding*	Control Ferrets (No Inoculation)	Animals Inoculated With Mink ADV	Animals Inoculated With Ferret ADV†
Periportal lymphoid cell infiltration	6/13 (46%)	28/32 (88%)†	12/12 (100%)
Periportal lymphoid cell infiltration ≥ 2+	1/13 (8%)	11/32 (34%)	6/12 (50%)
Stimulation of lymphoid tissue	4/13 (31%)	21/32 (66%)†	9/12 (75%)
Stimulation of lymphoid tissue ≥ 2+	0/13 (0%)	9/32 (28%)†	7/12 (58%)

(Porter, H.G., Porter, D.D., and Larsen, A.E.: Aleutian disease in ferrets. Infect. Immunol., *36*:379, 1982.)
* The presence and severity of tissue lesions were scored on an arbitrary 0 to 3+ scale.
† Significantly different from uninoculated ferrets ($p < 0.05$) using a 2 by 2 X^2 analysis.

outbreak of Aleutian disease in ferrets, presumably transmitted by mink, kidneys of infected ferrets had markedly thickened glomerular basement membranes and proliferation and swelling of mesangial cells. These ferrets also had fibrinoid necrosis and mononuclear cell infiltration of arterioles in the heart, kidneys, liver and lung.[9] The hypergammaglobulinemia (defined as >20% of total serum protein) directed against Aleutian disease antigen(s) in ferrets appears to progress more slowly, producing little clinical manifestation of disease, probably because the disease in ferrets most often affects the glomeruli minimally (Fig. 11–2).[3,15]

The rarity of glomerulonephritis and arteritis in ferrets may represent insufficient antigen for antibody-antigen complex formation and deposition. Serial ferret-to-ferret transmission of a ferret strain of ADV demonstrated experimentally that ADV causes a periportal lymphoid infiltrate (Fig. 11–3) and stimulation of the lymphoid tissues in some experimentally infected ferrets (Fig. 11–4, and Table 11–1).[6] Most ferrets with the highest ADV antibody titers also had the greatest increase in serum gamma globulin levels, and the most severe tissue lesions.[6] Similar tissue lesions are also seen in ferrets inoculated with mink strains of ADV. Unlike previous observations, prolifera-

tion of bile ducts were not seen in ferrets inoculated with either mink or ferret ADV.[6] Kenyon and colleagues[7] enumerated several practical considerations regarding the periportal lymphocytic infiltrates: (1) infiltrates in asymptomatic animals may be misinterpreted when these ferrets are used in various experiments; (2) complications may arise as a result of contamination with ADV if the ferrets are used as sources for vaccines or other biologic products; and (3) commercial ranchers should be warned of the hazard of rearing mink in close proximity to ferrets, or, alternatively, ferrets should not be raised in close proximity to ADV-infected mink.

Diagnosis. Diagnosis is based on histopathologic examination of target organs such as the liver, kidney, spleen, and lymph nodes. Hypergammaglobulinemia (>20% total serum protein) is considered to be diagnostic of Aleutian disease. ADV antibody can be detected by indirect immunofluorescence, CIEP, and complement fixation.[6,15,16] The CIEP test, which uses purified virions as antigens, has a sensitivity of about 5 μg antibody/ml, and is the standard diagnostic test of the disease in mink.[2] This test may not be sensitive enough, however, to diagnose low levels of circulating antibody in infected ferrets.[17] Diagnosis is confirmed by virus isolation.

Treatment and Prevention. There is no treatment for Aleutian disease, nor is there a vaccine for prevention. Affected animals in research or commercial settings should be euthanized to decrease the spread of the virus to other susceptible ferrets and mink. Supportive therapy should be instituted in pets, and a guarded prognosis given to the client.

BOVINE RHINOTRACHEITIS VIRUS

The bovine rhinotracheitis virus belongs to the class Herpesvirus. Its members are widespread in nature, infect various mammalian species, and can be host-specific.

Epizootiology and Control. The virus was first isolated from tissues (liver, spleen, and lung) of a normal ferret and mink. The isolated virus was indistinguishable from the infectious bovine rhinotracheitis (IBR) virus using serologic neutralization tests. The mustelids' diet contained 5% uncooked beef tripe, as well as occasional supplementation with other raw beef byproducts.[18] It was surmised that the source of the infection was ingestion of virus-laden raw beef. The mechanism whereby the virus infected the spleen was unknown.

Clinical Signs and Pathology. Under natural conditions clinical signs and pathology are not associated with this disease. IBR virus, however, causes significant pathology in experimentally infected ferrets (see Chap. 17, Viral Disease Models).

CANINE DISTEMPER

Canine distemper infection in ferrets is caused by a large RNA paramyxovirus that is antigenically related to measles and rinderpest viruses. It is viable at a pH range of 4.5 to 9.0. Canine distemper virus (CDV) in ferret lung suspension retains infectivity when kept for 48 hours at 25°C.[19] When frozen, CDV retains viability for years. It is inactivated by heat, visible light, 0.75% phenol, 0.2% Roccal, 2 to 5% NaOH, and 0.1% formalin. There is only one serotype of CDV, but there are several strains that influence the incubation period and disease duration. The mortality rate approaches 100% with all recognized strains.

Epizootiology and Control. As demonstrated experimentally, distemper infection is commonly transmitted by aerosol exposure. Infectious airborne droplets can traverse a distance of 1.5 m.[20] Direct contact may transmit the virus, because the virulent virus is shed in the conjunctival and nasal exudates, urine, feces, and skin scurf. Artificially aerosolized urine from infected ferrets is infectious for ferrets.[21] Fomites may harbor CDV, as demonstrated by the viability of CDV recovered after 20 minutes from a handler's gloves.[20] Transplacental infection by virulent CDV in the dog has been demonstrated, but attenuated CDV does not cross the placenta in ferrets.[22,23] Virulent CDV may be able to cross the placenta in ferrets as well, because attenuated CDV vaccine strains are not shed from any body secretions.[21] Because viremia occurs, blood-sucking arthropods are potential (but unproven) vectors.

Although effective modified live virus vaccines are available, distemper is still prevalent. Unvaccinated dogs and wild species of the families Canidae (e.g., coyote, wolf, fox), Mustelidae (e.g., mink, ferret, marten, weasel, otter, skunk, badger) and Procyonidae (e.g., raccoon, lesser panda, kinkajou, coati) serve as reservoirs of the disease.[24] A recent outbreak of distemper in Wyoming occurred in a North American black-footed ferret colony, and was probably introduced by a reservoir host (Chap. 1).

Clinical Signs and Pathology. The incubation period for distemper infection is 7 to

10 days postexposure. An early sign is anorexia followed by a rash on the chin 10 to 12 days postinoculation (DPI) that is eventually noted around the anus and the inguinal area (Fig. 11–5). Initially, the animals appear to be photophobic. A serous ocular discharge rapidly becomes mucopurulent. Brown crusts form on the lips, chin, nose, and around the eyes, causing the eyelids to adhere (Fig. 11–6). Affected ferrets may have a generalized orange-tinged dermatitis.

Death may occur as early as 12 to 16 DPI with ferret-adapted CDV, or from 21 to 35 days with wild canine strains. Ferrets that survive the catarrhal phase may die later because of the neurotropic form of distemper. Neurotropic signs include hyperexcitability, excess salivation, muscular tremor, convulsions, and coma.

In addition to the nasal and ocular discharge and the generalized dermatitis, few consistent gross lesions occur with distemper infection. Occasionally, the spleen is enlarged; the lungs may be congested or consolidated in patches, or the entire lobe may be affected.

Inclusion bodies are generally intracytoplasmic but may also be intranuclear, and are usually present in epithelial cells of the tracheal and urinary bladder mucosae (Fig. 11–7). These are eosinophilic with hematoxylin and eosin staining, spherical or ovoid in shape, and may contain refractile particles.[24] Canine distemper viral inclusion bodies may also be observed in the epithelial cells of the skin, gastrointestinal tract, and salivary and adrenal glands, as well as in lymph nodes and spleen.

CDV is a pantropic virus, and viremia occurs 2 DPI, persisting until the virus is neutralized by antibody or until the ferret succumbs. Virus is demonstrated in nasal tissue, lung, spleen, and cervical lymph nodes at 2 DPI, spreading via the blood.[25–27] CDV has been demonstrated in the nasal exudate at 5 to 13 DPI.[20] Virus titers are higher in the lungs and nasal tissue. Moderate titers are seen in the brain and liver; lowest titers are recorded in spleen, kidney, urinary bladder, skeletal muscles, adrenals, and thyroid.[25]

The immunosuppressive action of CDV on lymphocytes has been studied.[28, 29] Ferrets were infected with a moderately

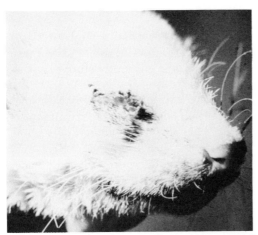

Fig. 11–5. Nasal and ocular discharge associated with canine distemper. (Ryland, L.M., Bernard, S.L., and Gorham, J.R.: A Clinical Guide to the Pet Ferret. The Compendium on Continuing Education, Vol. 5, pp. 25–32. Lawrenceville, NJ, Veterinary Learning Systems, 1983.)

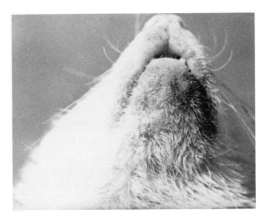

Fig. 11–6. Chin rash in a ferret with canine distemper. (Ryland, L.M., Bernard, S.L., and Gorham, J.R.: A Clinical Guide to the Pet Ferret. The Compendium on Continuing Education, Vol. 5, pp. 25–32. Lawrenceville, NJ, Veterinary Learning Systems, 1983.)

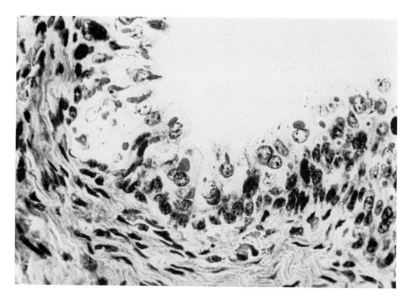

Fig. 11–7. Bladder mucosa depicting intracytoplasmic inclusion bodies in epithelium (trichrome stain; × 400). (Ryland, L.M., Bernard, S.L., and Gorham, J.R.: A Clinical Guide to the Pet Ferret. The Compendium on Continuing Education, Vol. 5, pp. 25–32. Lawrenceville, NJ, Veterinary Learning Systems, 1983.)

attenuated CDV that produced mild disease without encephalitis or mortality. Lymphocytopenia was noted at 5 to 30 DPI in all lymphocyte subpopulations. Transformation of lymphocytes by phytohemagglutinin, concanavalin A, and pokeweed mitogen is depressed at 5 DPI, lowest at 8 to 11 DPI, and returns to normal at 23 to 30 DPI. Macrophage migration inhibitory factor production by lymphocytes decreases at 7 to 14 DPI but is normal at 21 DPI (see Chap. 7 for further details).

Diagnosis. A presumptive diagnosis can be made, based on the typical signs. A fluorescent antibody (FA) test may be performed on a blood smear; this may be positive for antigen before the onset of fever.[27] The FA test can rapidly confirm a clinical diagnosis of distemper, therefore assisting in controlling epizootics. Histopathology also offers rapid confirmation of the diagnosis. The ferret inoculation test, traditionally performed by injecting susceptible ferrets with suspected CDV-infected secretions or tissue suspensions,

requires at least 10 days for diagnosis (for test animals to show signs of CDV infection), and requires susceptible ferrets and isolation facilities. Ferret alveolar macrophage cultures can also be inoculated with suspect material, and intracytoplasmic inclusions observed within 1 or 2 days.

Treatment and Prevention. High-titer antidistemper serum will protect experimental ferrets if administered before exposure, but the procedure is impractical in a clinical setting. Supportive therapy is unjustified. Euthanasia is always recommended for pet, laboratory, or commercially reared ferrets.

Distemper may be prevented by vaccination with a modified live vaccine virus of chicken embryo tissue culture origin (CETCO) by either subcutaneous, intramuscular, or even jet injection.[30] Kits from CDV-immune dams are vaccinated at 8 to 10 weeks of age, and again at 10 to 12 weeks. Kits from unvaccinated dams should be immunized initially at the earlier age of 4 to 6 weeks.[31] Ferrets should be revaccinated every 2 to 3 years for optimum protection.

Modified live CDV vaccines of ferret cell culture origin should never be used, because they are not attenuated for ferrets. In fact, some canine CDV vaccines may be contraindicated for ferrets. Four female black-footed ferrets died of vaccine-induced canine distemper after they were captured to establish a breeding program, and vaccinated with 2-ml (rather than the manufacturer's recommended 1-ml) doses of CETCO virus.[32] Inactivated distemper vaccine is not recommended for ferrets, because the resultant immunity is uncertain.

If an outbreak occurs on a commercial breeding farm, owners should remove and euthanize all clinically affected ferrets, and should immediately vaccinate ferrets that appear to be healthy. High-titer modified live virus vaccines protect ferrets against virulent challenge within 48 hours after vaccination.[33] After distemper virus became established experimentally in totally susceptible ferrets housed in individual cages, vaccination of 50 to 90% of the survivors failed to stop the outbreak.[34] Conversely, it was difficult to initiate an outbreak if 70% or more of the ferrets were immune to the disease at the time distemper virus was introduced by means of index ferrets inoculated experimentally with the virus.[34] Aerosol vaccines can control ferret and mink epizootics within 2 weeks.[23, 35] All equipment should be disinfected, and ferrets prevented from contact with fomites. Ranchers should quarantine and vaccinate new additions to the colony prior to introducing them to the resident population.

FELINE PANLEUKOPENIA

Ferrets are not susceptible either to feline panleukopenia virus (FPV) or to canine parvovirus type 2 (CPV2) under natural conditions. Kilham and associates[36] inoculated one group of ferret fetuses directly with virulent FPV 2 to 3 weeks before term. In another group of pregnant ferrets, the jills were inoculated IV with virulent FPV at different times from 18 to 35 days of gestation. Most of the fetuses inoculated directly had cerebellar lesion when killed from 2 weeks before to 1 day after birth. One fetus (in a litter of three) from a dam that had been inoculated IV had severe cerebellar disease when killed at 1 day of age, indicating the possibility of virulent virus penetrating the placental barrier. None of the dams in either group experienced clinical disease.[36]

Conversely, pregnant ferrets inoculated IP at different intervals throughout gestation with an attenuated (vaccine) FPV had no adverse effects on the dams, kits, litter size, or kit development.[37] When kits were inoculated IP at 1 to 2 days of age, however, they exhibited signs of cerebellar ataxia 6 to 7 weeks after exposure. Gross and histologic lesions of cerebellar hypoplasia accompanied the motor dysfunction shown by the kits. Interestingly, the inoculation of 3-day-old ferret kits resulted in no clinical signs or lesions.[37]

In a serologic survey in Finland, Veijalainen[38] found that 442 adult ferrets lacked serum antibody to canine parvovirus, mink enteritis virus, or feline parvovirus. Parrish and co-workers[39] found that adult ferrets were refractory to clinical illness when inoculated IP with virulent CPV2, FPV, MEV, or racoon parvovirus (RPV). However, feline panleukopenia virus and RPV isolates replicated in ferrets, but disease or microscopic lesions were not observed.

INFLUENZA VIRUS

Influenza in humans causes various respiratory symptoms, depending on the strain of virus and on the host resistance and immune status.

Types A and B of the virus are included in the class Orthomyxoviridae, and are widespread in the human population.

Ferrets have been used as animal models to study the disease since 1933, when Smith and colleagues[40] in their classic experiments on the isolation of influenza virus, demonstrated that the disease was transmitted experimentally to ferrets by intranasal inoculation of throat washings from humans suffering from influenza.

Epizootiology and Control. Epidemics of worldwide proportion occur with some frequency in humans, particularly in the winter months in the northern hemisphere and in the summer months in the southern hemisphere. Records of influenza epizootics were also documented in ferrets, but less frequently, occurring at times when there were localized outbreaks of the disease throughout the country (i.e., England and Canada).[41,42] It is probable that in these cases, as well as in those that go unreported, personnel introduce the infection into susceptible ferret colonies. It was also shown that the virus can be readily transmitted from ferret to ferret by way of aerosolized droplets containing infective virus particles. Experimental studies show that infected animals are subsequently resistant to reinfection with the same strain of influenza virus when challenged 5 weeks after primary infection.[43]

A number of vaccines have been used with varying degrees of success to protect ferrets against experimental challenge with influenza virus. Because the clinical disease in ferrets is relatively benign, however, and because of wide antigenic variation of the virus in humans, it is not recommended to vaccinate ferrets to confer short-term immunity to specific strains of the virus. Control of the disease must therefore rely on preventing exposure of susceptible ferrets to persons shedding the virus while actively infected. In colony management, it is advisable for all personnel to wear face masks when entering the animal room, and disposable gloves when handling the ferrets. The

disease can also be transmitted from ferrets to humans.[44]

Many studies have been performed to elucidate the mechanism of immunity in ferrets challenged experimentally with virulent, attenuated, or killed virus. Local and humoral immune mechanisms were demonstrated, as well as the protective effect of the pyrexia induced by the disease.[45,46] Influenza infection does not depress cell-mediated immunity.[47,48]

Clinical Signs and Pathology. Ferrets naturally infected with influenza have bouts of sneezing accompanied by a mucoserous nasal discharge, which produces noticeable crusting around the nares.[42] Conjunctiva are inflamed and a mucopurulent discharge is present, as well as photophobia. Animals are lethargic, and ferrets occasionally develop unilateral otitis. Clinical disease is present for 7 to 14 days. Experimentally, the infection causes a sharp biphasic febrile response, an increase in serum hemagglutination-inhibition (HI) antibody, an increase in protein in nasal washings, virus to be excreted in normal washings for several days, and transient occurrence of nasal HI and neutralizing antibody.[43,49] Interferon in turbinates, an increase in the erythrocyte sedimentation rate, and an increase in the polymorphonuclear leukocyte:lymphocyte ratio are also seen in ferrets inoculated experimentally with influenza virus types A, A_2, and B. Increased numbers of leukocytes in the nasal washings are also seen.[50,51] Occasional deaths have been attributed to the disease[42]; Lancefield group C hemolytic streptococci were isolated from the lungs.

The exudative phase of the disease is noted by an increase in nasal leukocytes 2 to 7 days after infection.[49] There is necrosis of the nasal mucosa and enhanced permeability of nasal capillaries as a consequence of inflammation. Reduction in nasal patency because of inflammatory edema is seen early in the infection, as measured by nasal air flow resistance.[52] In a quantitative study of viral replication, influenza virus localized and grew significantly only in nasal mucosa after inoculation of the virus directly into the bloodstream, and predominantly in the nasal mucosa of ferrets inoculated intranasally. The lung and trachea also become infected if the virus is inoculated intranasally.[53]

Diagnosis. The diagnosis of influenza in the ferret is based on clinical signs, isolation of the virus from nasal secretions, and demonstration of rising HI antibody titer from analysis of acute and convalescent serum samples.

Treatment. Various compounds, including pharmacologically active agents used to treat rhinitis in humans, can be used to diminish nasal congestion.[54, 55]

Experimentally, the efficacy of amantadine hydrochloride was demonstrated when administered in aerosol form twice daily (6 mg/kg). The drug had no toxic side effects, and consistently reduced the febrile response and shedding of influenza virus without suppressing the immune response.[56] Parenteral use of the same drug at doses of 100 mg/kg twice daily had no beneficial effect against influenza infection, and was toxic to the ferret. Ribavarin, another antiviral compound, was shown to inhibit in vitro[57] replication of influenza virus, as well as to have marked antiviral activity in ferrets.[58] Ferrets given ribavarin, 100 mg/kg/day, administered from day 1 through day 5 postinfection with influenza virus, showed a reduced temperature response, lower levels of nasal wash protein, and reduced virus excretion when compared to control animals.[58] Lower HI antibody was produced in treated animals and local nasal wash antibody could not be detected, indicating an immunosuppressive effect in ferrets treated with the ribavarin, 100 mg/kg. Smaller doses of

the drug (10 or 30 mg/kg/day) were not immunosuppressive, but had no antiviral activity in the ferret.

Reye's syndrome (RS), marked by encephalopathy and fatty visceral changes, was first diagnosed in human infants in 1963 and has been implicated to occur in association with viral infections, particularly those caused by influenza and varicella-zoster viruses. Epidemiologic studies have failed to establish a specific cofactor, but most children with RS have in common the ingestion of aspirin during the syndrome.[59] Influenza infection in concert with the administration of salicylates in ferrets, however, does not produce RS in the ferret.[60] Nevertheless, the use of an arginine-deficient diet, in addition to influenza virus infection, is being used in an experimental model of RS in ferrets (see Chap. 5, Nutrition).

RABIES VIRUS

The rabies virus is a member of the rhabdovirus group, and causes an acute, almost invariably fatal, disease in many mammalian hosts.

Epizootiology and Control. There were several cases (six since 1980) of ferret rabies reported in the United States in 1954, 1978, 1981, 1982, and 1985.[61–63] Poor or no histories were available concerning whether the ferrets were exposed to rabies or previously vaccinated with MLV rabies vaccine. The American Veterinary Medical Association counsels against keeping ferrets as companion animals because of their potential to transmit rabies to humans and attack human infants. The Centers for Disease Control (CDC) state, however, that ferrets are less likely to be exposed to rabies than are other domestic or wild pets. Preventing ferrets from having contact with wild animals decreases the likelihood of rabies exposure. Currently, there are no licensed rabies vaccines for use in ferrets. At the insistence of some owners pet ferrets have been given inactivated rabies vaccine. According to the CDC, ferrets that bite or may otherwise expose a human to rabies must be killed, and their brains submitted for rabies examination.[63]

Clinical Signs and Pathology. The signs observed in experimentally infected ferrets include anxiety, lethargy, and occasional posterior paresis. Survival or mortality, or the time at which death occurred, is directly related to the amount of virus administered IM.[64]

Although ferrets have been experimentally infected with rabies virus,[64,65] very little is known about the pathogenesis of the disease in ferrets. Investigators found that ferrets inoculated IM with virulent rabies virus do not secrete the virus in their saliva.[64] Survivors (11 of 40 died) had low levels of neutralizing antibodies.

In another experiment, each of ten ferrets was fed one rabies-infected mouse, but the ferrets failed to become infected. Serum samples obtained from six of the ferrets 3 months after oral challenge with the virus were negative for neutralizing antibodies.[65]

Diagnosis. Affected ferrets should be sacrificed and brain tissue submitted for laboratory confirmation by virus isolation or by specific fluorescent antibody staining of infected tissue. Distemper may occasionally evoke central nervous system signs, but may be ruled out if the history includes exposure to a rabid animal.

Treatment. Rabies is not a treatable disease. Rabies-suspect animals must be held in strict quarantine. If rabies is diagnosed clinically the animal is euthanized, and the brain should be immediately delivered to local public health officials. Confirmed rabies is a reportable disease, and appropriate authorities must be notified.

RESPIRATORY SYNCYTIAL VIRUS

The virus was first isolated in 1956 from a chimpanzee with upper respiratory infection.[66] It is now recognized as a universal cause of respiratory infection in humans.[67] Clinical symptoms are most pronounced in infants less than 6 months of age, when bronchiolitis and interstitial pneumonia are sometimes diagnosed.[68] Although the disease in ferrets is not recognized clinically, the ferret has been used experimentally to study the pathogenesis of respiratory syncytial virus (RSV).

Epizootiology and Control. RSV is taxonomically (all currently classified as paramyxoviruses) similar to influenza and canine distemper virus, but it is not known whether vaccination with CDV and/or antibody titer to influenza virus confers partial or total immunity to RSV. Humoral antibody response (IgG) following experimental infection in infant ferrets was detected in 10 of 54 animals using a 50% plaque reduction neutralization test.[69]

Ferrets, like humans, show a definite age dependence of viral replication in the lung; high titers of the virus are demonstrated in ferrets 0 to 3 days of age, whereas no pulmonary viral replication is detected when ferrets are infected experimentally at 28 days of age. Nasal tissue will replicate the virus regardless of the age of the ferret.[69] Age dependence of RSV growth in ferret lung was substantiated in tissue culture experiments.[70]

The virus can infect ferrets naturally. An apparent infection was demonstrated by seroconversion of a ferret mother during an experimental study of RSV in infant ferrets.[69] Clinical signs were not observed. Infant ferrets are protected from RSV infection if they are nursed by previously infected jills.[71]

Clinical Signs and Pathology. Although the virus replicates in both nasal and pulmonary tissues, clinical manifestations are not noted. In the infant ferret, RSV inoculated experimentally intranasally produces a mild rhinitis, consisting of mild focal desquamation of epithelial cells with occasional polymorphonuclear cell infiltrate.[69] Foci of atelectasis of the lung are also observed in experimentally infected animals, but not in a control ferret examined similarly (see Chap. 17, Viral Research Models).

ROTAVIRUS

Rotavirus belongs to the family *Reoviridae*; the term is derived from the wheel-like ultrastructure of the virus. The virus is unique because of its genome, double-stranded RNA.[72]

Partial characterization of a rotavirus isolated from 2- to 3-week-old ferrets indicates that it is a member of the "atypical" rotavirus group (Fig. 11–8).[73] These viruses cause diarrhea in infants as well as in a number of animals, including calves, piglets, lambs, and rats. The atypical rotaviruses have not been cultivated successfully in cell culture, despite extensive efforts. These rotaviruses lack a rotavirus common antigen and have a different RNA electrophoretic pattern, consisting of 11 dsRNA bands observed in polyacrylamide gel electrophoresis of viral nucleic acid (Fig. 11–9).[73]

Epizootiology and Control. Rotavirus can establish enzootic infections within breeding colonies of several species of animals. This infection was recently diagnosed in the United States at a large commercial ferret breeding colony, and is referred to as "ferret kit disease."[74] Also, in Finland, an outbreak killed thousands of ferret kits, and the mortality rate approached 100%.[74] Rotavirus was isolated from kits dying during the outbreak.[75]

In the piglet, lactogenic immunity plays a key role in protection against the virus. This may also be true in the ferret kit. A limited oral vaccination trial in pri-

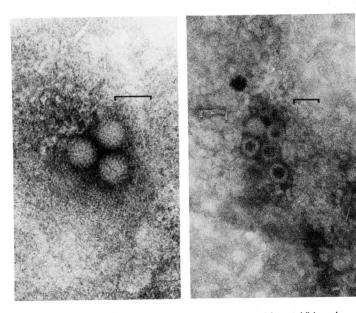

Fig. 11–8. Morphology of rotavirus particles observed in diarrheic neonatal ferret. Virions have evident hexagonal cores (*right*), but their morphologic details are obscured due to their association with intestinal contents. (Phosphotungstic acid stain; bar = 100 nm). (Torres-Medina, A.: Isolation of atypical rotavirus causing diarrhea in neonatal ferrets. Lab. Anim. Sci., *37*:167, 1987.)

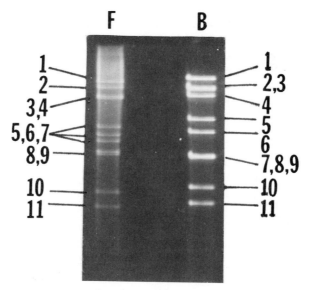

Fig. 11–9. Rotavirus dsRNA electrophenotype of ferret rotavirus (*F*) and bovine NCDV rotavirus (*B*). Migration is from top to bottom. The 11 segments of ferret rotavirus were arranged in four groups of four, three, two, and two gene segments, while those of the reference bovine group A rotavirus were arranged in groups of four, two, three, and two gene segments. (Torres-Medina, A.: Isolation of atypical rotavirus causing diarrhea in neonatal ferrets. Lab. Anim. Sci., 37:167, 1987.)

miparous jills was attempted at a ferret breeding farm. Results indicate that this procedure was not effective, however, and may not be feasible until the virus can be propagated in sufficient amounts in cell cultures.[73]

The disease was reproduced in 2- to 3-week old ferret kits by oral inoculation of bacteria-free fecal homogenates from ferret kits suffering from diarrhea.[73] Prevalence of the disease in ferrets is presently unknown because of the absence of reliable serologic tests. Experimental production of diarrhea was possible only with one fecal sample obtained from a field case, even though all inoculates used in unsuccessful challenges contained rotavirus. In addition, there were no fatalities and no microscopic intestinal lesions observed in kits infected experimentally.[73]

Clinical Signs and Pathology. The clinical disease occurs in 2- to 6-week-old ferret kits. When the jill stops grooming the kit, the diarrhea becomes evident. Diarrheic feces are noted in the perineal area (Fig. 11–10), and in severe cases stain the animal's hair and soil the nesting material. Mortality may be high in certain litters.[74,76]

Gross lesions are limited to the gastrointestinal tract. Fecal soiling of the hair is produced by yellowish-green liquid or mucoid feces, which also may distend the terminal colon. Subtle histologic lesions, if present, occur in the small intestine, and consist of villous atrophy and vacuolation of villar epithelial cells. In other species of animals, fuchsinophilic intracytoplasmic inclusion bodies were described in the villar epithelium early in the course of the disease.[77]

Treatment and Prevention. Although rotavirus is considered to be the primary etiologic agent, secondary bacteria may play a significant role in the severity of the diarrhea. Oral gentamicin (2 mg/lb) and ampicillin (10 mg/lb) administered IM for 5 days is sometimes effective in reducing morbidity and mortality rates within affected litters. Because oral gen-

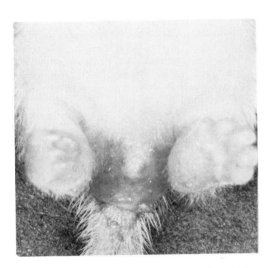

Fig. 11–10. Neonatal ferret with perianal scabbing and irritation attributed to rotavirus-associated diarrhea.

tamicin is not absorbed by the gastrointestinal tract, renal toxicity is avoided. If the kits resume feeding the mortality rate is reduced significantly. Affected kits can be supplemented with kitten milk replacer, administered by a plastic dropper.

Diagnosis. The characteristic virions are readily visualized in ultracentrifuged deposits of clarified fecal suspensions using direct electron microscopic examination, following negative staining.[72] Unfortunately, the ferret rotavirus does not react with commercially available enzyme immunoassays—Rotazyme and Dekto tests.[73]

CHLAMYDIA

In 1938 investigators isolated a chlamydial agent from ferrets inoculated with throat washings of humans infected with influenza virus.[78] The chlamydia induces pneumonitis in ferrets challenged with the agent intranasally. In mice, inoculated intraperitoneally or intracerebrally, the agent produces a meningoencephalitis as well as pneumonitis. A variable pneumonia occurs in ferrets infected nasally. Lung lobes are firm, plum-colored, and edematous. Histologically, bronchiolar epithelia may be hyperplastic, with exudate in the lumen. The alveolar walls are edematous, and densely infiltrated with large mononuclear cells. The alveolar spaces are distended, with the cellular exudate primarily composed of mononuclear cells, with occasional polymorphonuclear cells.[78] Subsequent to these findings the ferret chlamydial agent was used in numerous experimental studies.[79] It remains controversial, however, whether the chlamydia originated from ferrets or humans. The strain is available for study from the American Type Culture Collection Committee.

REFERENCES

1. Porter, D.D., Larsen, A.E., and Porter, H.G.: Aleutian disease of mink. Adv. Immunol., *29:* 261, 1980.
2. Porter, D.D.: Aleutian disease: A persistent parvovirus infection of mink with a maximal but infective host of humoral response. Prog. Med. Virol., 33:42, 1986.
3. Ohshima, K., Shen, D.T., Henson, J.B., and Gorham, J.R.: Comparison of the lesions of Aleutian disease in mink and hypergammaglobulinemia in ferrets. Am. J. Vet. Res., *39:* 653, 1978.
4. Ingram, D.G., and Cho, H.J.: Aleutian disease in mink: Virology, immunology and pathogenesis. J. Rheumatol., 1:74, 1974.
5. Porter, D.D., and Larsen, A.E.: Mink parvovirus infections. *In* CRC Handbook of Parvoviruses. Boca Raton, FL, CRC Press, 1986.
6. Porter, H.G., Porter, D.D., and Larsen, A.E.: Aleutian disease in ferrets. Infect. Immunol., *36:*379, 1982.
7. Kenyon, A.J., Magnano, T., Helmboldt, C.F., and Buko, L.: Aleutian disease in the ferret. J. Am. Vet. Med. Assoc., 149:920, 1966.

8. Kenyon, A.J., Howard, E., and Buko, L.: Hypergammaglobulinemia in ferrets with lymphoproliferative lesions (Aleutian disease). Am. J. Vet. Res., 28:1167, 1967.

9. Daoust, P.Y., and Hunter, D.B.: Spontaneous Aleutian disease in ferrets. Can. Vet. J., 19:133, 1978.

10. Kenyon, A.J., Helboldt, C.F., and Nielson, S.W.: Experimental transmission of Aleutian disease with urine. Am. J. Vet. Res., 24:1066, 1963.

11. Shen, D.T., Leendertsen, L.W., and Gorham, J.R.: Evaluation of chemical disinfectants for Aleutian disease virus of mink. Am. J. Vet. Res., 42:838, 1981.

12. Cho, H.J., and Greenfield, J.: Eradication of Aleutian disease of mink by eliminating positive counterimmunoelectrophoresis reactors. J. Clin. Microbiol., 7:18, 1978.

13. Diseases of the ferret. Surveillance, 11:28, 1984.

14. Kenyon, A.L., Kenyon, B., and Hahn, E.C.: Protides of the mustelidae: Immunoresponse of mustelids to Aleutian mink disease virus. Am. J. Vet. Res., 39:1011, 1978.

15. McGuire, T.C., et al.: Aleutian disease of mink: Detection of large quantities of complement-fixing antibody to viral antigen. J. Immunol., 107:1481, 1971.

16. Cho, H.J., and Ingram, D.C.: Antigen and antibody in Aleutian disease in mink. Precipitation reaction by agar-gel electrophoresis. J. Immunol., 108:555, 1973.

17. Porter, D.D., Porter, H.G., Larsen, A.E., and Bloom, M.E.: Restricted viral antibody specificity in many ferrets infected with the Aleutian disease parvovirus. Arch. Virol. (In press).

18. Porter, D.D., Larsen, A.E., and Cox, N.A.: Isolation of infectious bovine rhinotracheitis virus in Mustelidae. J. Clin. Microbiol., 1:112, 1975.

19. Shen, D.T., and Gorham, J.R.: Survival of pathogenic distemper virus at 5°C and 25°C. Vet. Med./Small Anim. Clin., 75:69, 1980.

20. Gorham, J.R., and Brandly, C.A.: The transmission of distemper among ferrets and mink. Am. Vet. Med. Assoc., 90:129, 1953.

21. Shen, D.T., Gorham, J.R., and Pedersen, V.: Viruria in dogs infected with canine distemper. Vet. Med./Small Anim. Clin., 76:1175, 1981.

22. Krakowka, S., Hoover, E.A., Koestner, A., and Ketring, K.: Experimental and naturally occurring transmission of canine distemper virus. Am. J. Vet. Res., 38:919, 1977.

23. Hagen, K.W., Goto, H., and Gorham, J.R.: Distemper vaccine in pregnant ferrets and mink. Res. Vet. Sci., 11:458, 1970.

24. Budd, J.: Distemper. *In* Infectious Diseases of Wild Mammals, Part 1: Viral Diseases. 2nd ed. Edited by J.W. Davis, L.H. Karstad, and D.O. Trainer. Ames, IA, Iowa State University Press, 1981.

25. Crook, E., Gorham, J.R., and McNutt, S.H.: Experimental distemper in mink and ferrets. I. Pathogenesis. Am. J. Vet. Res., 19:955, 1958.

26. Crook, E., and McNutt, S.H.: Experimental distemper in mink and ferrets. III. Appearance and significance of histopathological changes. Am. J. Vet. Res., 20:378, 1959.

27. Liu, C., and Coffin, D.L.: Studies on canine distemper by means of fluorescein-labeled antibody: I. The pathogenesis, pathology and diagnosis of the disease in experimentally infected ferrets. Virology, 3:115, 1957.

28. Kauffman, C.A.: Distemper virus infection in ferrets: Effect on cell-mediated immunity. Clin. Res., 29:228A, 1981.

29. Kauffman, C.A., Bergman, A.G., and O'Connor, R.P.: Distemper virus infection in ferrets: An animal model of measles-induced immunosuppression. Clin. Exp. Immunol., 47:617, 1982.

30. Shen, D.T., Gorham, J.R., Ryland, L.M., and Strating, A.: Using jet injection to vaccinate mink and ferrets against canine distemper, mink virus enteritis, and botulism, type C. Vet. Med./Small Anim. Clin., 76:856, 1981.

31. Ott, R.L., and Gorham, J.R.: The response of newborn and young ferrets to intranasal administration with egg-adapted distemper virus. Am. J. Vet. Res., 16:571, 1955.

32. Carpenter, J.W., Appel, M.J.G., Erickson, R.C., and Novilla, M.N.: Fatal vaccine-induced canine distemper virus infection in black-footed ferrets. J. Am. Vet. Med. Assoc., 169:961, 1976.

33. Baker, G.A., Leader, R.W., and Gorham, J.R.: Immune response of ferrets to vaccination with egg-adapted distemper virus. 1. Time of development of resistance to virulent distemper virus. Vet. Med., 47:463, 1952.

34. Kelker, D.: The effect of immunes on the spread of distemper in small ferret populations. Comput. Biol. Med., 10:53, 1980.

35. Hansen, M., and Lund, E.: Prophylactic, postinfectious and neonatal vaccination against canine distemper in mink. Nord. Vet. Med., 28: 585, 1976.

36. Kilham, L., Margolis, G., and Colby, E.D.: Congenital infections of cats and ferrets by feline panleukopenia virus manifested by cerebellar hypoplasia. Lab. Invest., 17:465, 1967.

37. Duenwald, J.C., Holland, J.M., Gorham, J.R., and Ott, R.L.: Feline panleukopenia: Experimental cerebellar hypoplasia produced in neonatal ferrets with live virus vaccine. Res. Vet. Sci., 12:394, 1971.

38. Veijalainen, P.: A serological survey of enteric parvovirus infections in Finnish fur-bearing animals. Acta Vet. Scand., 27:159, 1986.

39. Parrish, C.R., Leathers, C.W., Pearson, R.C., and Gorham, J.R.: Comparisons of canine parvovirus, feline panleukopenia, raccoon parvovirus and mink enteritis virus and their pathogenicity for mink and ferrets. Am. J. Vet. Res., 48:1429, 1987.

40. Smith, W., Andrews, C.H., and Laidlow, P.O.: The virus obtained from influenza patients. Lancet, 2:66, 1933.

41. Fisher, J.W., and Scott, P.: An epizootic of influenza A in a ferret colony. Can. J. Publ. Health, 35:364, 1944.

42. Bell, F.R., and Dudgeon, J.A.: An epizootic of influenza in a ferret colony. J. Comp. Pathol., 58:167, 1948.

43. Potter, C.W., et al.: Immunity to influenza in ferrets. I. Response to live and killed virus. Br. J. Exp. Pathol., 53:153, 1972.

44. Smith, W., and Stuart-Harris, C.H.: Influenza infection of man from the ferret. Lancet, 2i:121, 1936.

45. Toms, G.L., et al.: The relation of pyrexia and nasal inflammatory response to virus levels in nasal washings of ferrets infected with influenza viruses of differing virulence. Br. J. Exp. Pathol., 58:444, 1977.

46. McLaren, C., Butchko, G.M.: Regional T- and B-cell responses in influenza-infected ferrets. Infect. Immunol., 22:189, 1978.

47. Kauffman, C.A., Schiff, G.M., Phair, J.P.: Influenza in ferrets and guinea pigs: Effect on cell-mediated immunity. Infect. Immunol., 19:547, 1978.

48. Potter, C.W., et al.: Immunity to influenza in ferrets: IX. Delayed hypersensitivity following infection or immunization with A2/Hong Kong virus. Microbiros., 10A:7, 1974.

49. Haff, R.F., Schriver, P.W., and Stewart, R.C.: Pathogenesis of influenza in ferrets: Nasal manifestation of disease. Br. J. Exp. Pathol., 47:435, 1966.

50. Pinto, C.A., Itaff, R.F., and Stewart, R.C.: Pathogenesis of and recovery from respiratory syncytial and influenza infection in ferrets. Arch. Gesamte Virusforsch., 26:225, 1969.

51. Sweet, C., et al.: The local origin of the febrile response induced in ferrets during respiratory infection with a virulent influenza virus. Br. J. Exp. Pathol., 60:300, 1979.

52. Wardell, J.R., Familiar, R.G., and Haff, R.F.: A technique for measuring nasal airway resistance in ferrets. J. Allergy, 40:100, 1967.

53. Basarab, O., and Smith, H.: Quantitative studies on the tissue localization of influenza virus in ferrets after intranasal and intravenous or extracordial inoculation. Br. J. Exp. Pathol., 50:612, 1969.

54. Haff, R.F.: Symptomatic therapy of influenza rhinitis in ferrets by topical application of compounds. J. Allergy, 45:163, 1971.

55. Haff, R.F., and Pinto, C.A.: Nasal decongestant action of aspirin in influenza-infected ferrets. Life Sci. (Pt. 1), 12:9, 1973.

56. Fenton, R.J., Bessell, C., Spilling, C.R., and Potter, C.W.: The effects of per oral or local aerosol administration of 1-aminoadamantane hydrochloride (amantadine hydrochloride) on influenza infections of the ferret. J. Antimicrob. Chemother., 3:463, 1977.

57. Sidwell, R.W., et al.: Broad-spectrum antiviral activity of vivazole: Iß-D-ribofuranosyl 1-1,2,4-triazole-3-carboxamide. Science, 177:705, 1972.

58. Fenton, R.J., and Potter, C.W.: Dose-response activity of ribavirin against influenza virus infection in ferrets. J. Antimicrob. Chemother., 3:263, 1977.

59. Linnemann, C.C., Jr., et al.: Reye's syndrome: Epidemiologic and viral studies 1963–1974. Am. J. Epidemiol., 101:517, 1975.

60. Linnemann, C.C., Jr., et al.: Salicylate intoxication and influenza in ferrets. Pediatr. Res., 13:44, 1979.

61. Centers for Disease Control: Viral diseases: Pet ferrets and rabies. In Rabies Surveillance, Annual Summary. Washington, D.C., U.S. Department of Health and Human Services, 1980.

62. Centers for Disease Control: Viral diseases: Pet ferrets and rabies. In Rabies Surveillance, Annual Summary. Washington, D.C., U.S. Department of Health and Human Services, 1983.

63. Centers for Disease Control: Viral diseases: Pet ferrets and rabies. In Rabies Surveillance, Annual Summary. Washington, D.C., U.S. Department of Health and Human Services, 1986.

64. Blancou, J., Aubert, M.F.A., and Artois, M.: Rage experimentale du furet (*Mustela (putorius) furo*). Rev. Med. Vet., 133:553, 1982.

65. Bell, J.F., and Moore, G.J.: Susceptibility of carnivora to rabies virus administered orally. Am. J. Epidemiol., 93:176, 1971.

66. Morris, J.A., Blount, R.E., Jr., and Savage, R.E.: Recovery of cytopathogenic agent from chimpanzees with coryza. Proc. Soc. Exp. Biol. Med., 92:544, 1956.

67. Kim, H.W., et al.: Epidemiology of respiratory syncytial virus infection in Washington, D.C. I. Importance of the virus in different respiratory tract disease syndromes and temporal distribution of infection. Am. J. Epidemiol., 98:216, 1973.

68. Parrott, R.H., et al.: Epidemiology of respiratory syncytial virus infection in Washington, D.C. II. Infection and disease with respect to age, immunologic status, race and sex. Am. J. Epidemiol., 98:289, 1973.

69. Prince, G.A., and Porter, D.D.: The pathogenesis of respiratory syncytial virus infection in infant ferrets. Am. J. Pathol., 82:337, 1976.

70. Porter, D.D., Mark, K.B., and Prince, G.A.: The age dependency of respiratory syncytial virus growth in ferret lung can be shown in organ monolayer cultures. Clin. Immunol. Pathol., 15:415, 1980.

71. Suffin, S.C., Prince, G.A., Mark, K.B., and Porter, D.D.: Immunoprophylaxis of respiratory syncytial virus infection in the infant ferret. J. Immunol., 123:10, 1979.

72. Fenner, F., and White, D.O.: Medical Virology. 2nd ed. New York, Academic Press, 1976.

73. Torres-Medina, A.: Isolation of atypical rotovirus causing diarrhea in neonatal ferrets. Lab. Anim. Sci., 37:167, 1987.

74. Bernard, S.L., Gorham, J.R., and Ryland, L.M.: Biology and diseases of ferrets. *In* Laboratory Animal Medicine. Edited by J.G. Fox, B.J. Cohen, and F.M. Loew. New York, Academic Press, 1984.

75. Veijalainen, P.: Unpublished observation, 1983.

76. Marshall Farms: Personal communication, 1987.

77. Jacoby, R.O., and Fox, J.G.: Biology and diseases of mice. *In* Biology and Diseases of Mice. Edited by J.G. Fox, B.C. Cohen, and F.M. Loew. New York, Academic Press, 1984.

78. Francis, T., and Magill, T.P.: An unidentified virus producing acute meningitis and pneumonitis in experimental animals. J. Exp. Med., 68:147, 1938.

79. Storz, J.: Chlamydia and Chlamydia-Induced Diseases. Springfield, IL, Charles C Thomas, 1971.

chapter 12

PARASITIC DISEASES

J. G. Fox

PROTOZOAN INFECTIONS

Ferrets may suffer from various protozoan infectious disorders, including cocciodiosis, pneumocystic pneumonia, cryptosporidiosis, and *Giardia*.

COCCIDIOSIS

Intestinal invasion by three distinct species of the order Coccidia has been described in the ferret.[1] The pathogenicity of coccidia in the ferret is unknown; it may be a self-limiting disease in otherwise healthy animals. In certain cases, however, animals may develop diarrhea and tenesmus. *Coccidia sp.* in the ferret may produce a chronic carrier state, so reinfection is also a possibility.

Isospora

Ferrets are susceptible to *Isospora* infection, and oocytes can be observed in fecal flotations. Treatment of infected ferrets is by oral administration of sulfonamides. In one report, ferrets shedding *Isospora* oocysts were successfully treated with oral sulfamethazine.[2] In cats (and presumably ferrets) with symptomatic infections, triple sulfonamides (sulfamethazine, sulfamerazine, sulfadiazine) are administered orally at a dose of 50 mg/kg bid. Sulfadiazine-trimethoprim (30–60 mg/kg orally) in divided doses can also be used for 1 to 3 weeks. Prevention is based on heat sterilization of cages and utensils.

Toxoplasma

The ferret, like many animal species, can become infected with *Toxoplasma gondii*, and serve as an intermediate host. *Toxoplasma gondii* is an intracellular coccidian parasite belonging to the subphylum Sporozoa, and is closely related to Isospora.

Epizootiology and Control. In Laidlaw's work on distemper 150 English ferrets were examined histologically for toxoplasma; 12 were infected. All ferrets were strictly isolated from one another.[4] Another study isolated *Toxoplasma* by in vivo passage of brain tissue in mice, harvested from a ferret and from two ferret-polecat hybrids.[5] Morphologically, biologically, and serologically, the Mustelid toxoplasmas were indistinguishable from those isolated from rabbits in England.[5] A case of chronic toxoplasmosis in a ferret from South Africa was diagnosed.[6] Infection in ferrets, as in other carnivores, is probably a result of eating food contaminated with the infective stage of the toxoplasma oocyte shed in cat feces or of eating toxoplasma encysted in raw meat.[7] The worldwide distribution of cats and the susceptibility of the ferret to the disease indicate that it probably occurs wherever infected cat feces contaminate ferret food or ferrets have access to uncooked meat. Cats, the definitive host, excrete the oocytes for approximately 10 days after infection; the oocytes become infective 1 to

5 days later, depending on environmental conditions. To prevent infection of ferrets maintained in zoos, all wild Felidae should be maintained in a separate building apart from other animals.[7]

Recently, approximately 30% of 750 neonatal ferrets being raised for fur production, died without clinical signs. Multifocal necrosis associated with toxoplasma-like organisms were observed in lung, heart, and liver. The presence of the organism in 1-day-old kits suggested congenital infection.[10] Similar congenitally acquired toxoplasma infections have been described in stunted mink.[11] It is also known that goats and other laboratory animals infected with toxoplasma can transmit toxoplasmosis congenitally to their offspring over successive generations; the adult females do not appear to experience reinfection, change in antibody status, or clinical illness.[12] This may also be applicable in the ferret; however, experimental studies are needed to confirm this hypothesis.

Diagnosis. Determination of toxoplasma infection and previous exposure to the organism are based on immunologic methods, including the Sabin Feldman dye test, ELISA, complement fixation, and hemagglutination assays. Histologic examination or animal inoculation is also used to establish a diagnosis.[8] (Fig. 12–1).

Clinical Signs. Although not studied in any detail, it is presumed that the ferret, like the dog and cat, suffers clinical manifestations of systemic toxoplasmosis. Signs are dependent on organ involvement.

Treatment. Pyrimethamine (30 mg/100 g in food) plus sulfonamides (e.g., sulfadiazine 60 mg/100 ml drinking water or 60 mg/100 g in food) are two drugs of choice in treating toxoplasmosis.[9] Alternate therapy consists of a combination of sulfadiazine at an oral dose of 15 mg/kg/day divided four times daily and pyri-

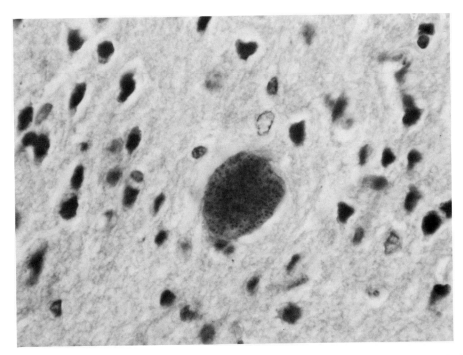

Fig. 12–1. Toxoplasmosis cyst in brain of ferret (H & E stain; × 750). (Armed Forces Institute of Pathology. Accession files. Washington, D.C.)

methamine (0.5–1 mg/kg/day orally). The drugs are directed against the tachyzoites, and act synergistically by blocking the metabolic pathway involving p-amino-benzoic acid and the folic-folinic acid cycle. These drugs, however, do not destroy the cyst stage. Folinic acid and baker's yeast are used as dietary supplements if treatment with these drugs is prolonged. Because folic acid is necessary for hematopoiesis, monitoring of bone marrow activity is essential.

Sarcocystis

Sarcocystis muris infection occurs as cysts in the muscles of mice, wild Norway rats, and black rats. The elongated cysts of S. muris have a thin smooth wall, are not compartmented, and are several millimeters long. Transmission to ferrets was demonstrated experimentally by ingestion of *Sarcocystis muris*-infected mice[13]; or presumably by eating food contaminated by fecal oocysts. In two experimentally infected ferrets, 7 days after ingestion of the S. muris-infected mice, the animals shed sporocysts in their feces that were indistinguishable from those of S. muris. Mice receiving 70 of these sporocysts developed cysts of S. muris in their musculature 4 months postinfection.[13] Cysts compatible with those of *Sarcocytsis muris* were diagnosed in ferret skeletal and cardiac muscles. (Fig. 12–2).[6] In the intestinal form, the oocytes may be confused with those of *Isospora*.

Unsuccessful attempts to establish infection and complete the life cycle of avian sarcocysts, *Sarcocystis rileyi*, were reported using ferrets fed duck muscle infected with sarcocysts, as well as dogs, coyotes, mink, cats, and rats.[2] All feeding experiments failed to produce an oocyst-sporocyst infection. Naturally occurring sarcosporidiosis in ferrets is probably asymptomatic, and is not routinely treated.

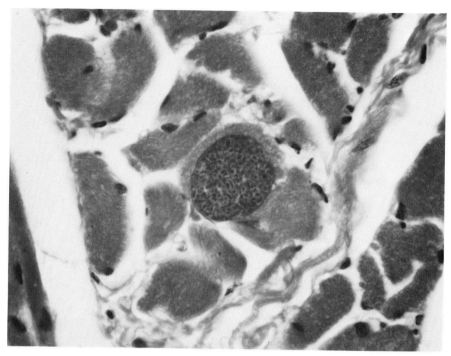

Fig. 12–2. Sarcosporidosis cyst in skeletal muscle of ferret (H & E stain; × 750). (Armed Forces Institute of Pathology. Accession files. Washington, D.C.)

PNEUMOCYSTIC PNEUMONIA

Pneumocystis carinii, a protozoan parasite, inhabits the lungs as a commensal in various domestic and laboratory animals. Its significance as a pathogen is recognized in hosts (both animal, and human) who are immunocompromised, either by immunosuppressive drugs or by infectious agents that compromise the immune system.[14,15] Rats treated with corticosteroids, and nude athymic mice are used in experimental studies of this organism.[9,16] More recently, the ferret was used to study *P. carinii* pneumonia.[18] Ferrets were immunosuppressed by long-term administration of cortisone acetate 10 to 20 mg/kg subcutaneously for 9 to 10 weeks. Microscopically, *P. carinii* was observed in all eleven treated animals, producing extensive disease in six of the ferrets. Histologically, lesions consist of interstitial pnemonitis, focal mononuclear cell infiltrates, and abundant cysts and trophozoites focally distributed, which are clearly demonstrable using Gomori's methenamine silver nitrate (GMS) and Giemsa stains (Fig. 12–3). Although abundant trophozoites were readily seen using these stains and paraffin-embedded thick sections, fine detail was best demonstrated in thin, l-μ plastic sections.[18]

The ferret, like humans, is resistant to body weight loss by corticosteroids. Stokes and colleagues[15] also noted that the ferret appears to be relatively susceptible to corticosteroid-induced *Pneumocystis carinii* pneumonia. Pneumocystic pneumonia should, therefore, be considered in a differential diagnosis in ferrets on long-term steroid therapy or in ferrets suffering from hyperadrenocorticism. Diagnosis of the disease in the ferret can be accomplished by bronchoalveolar lavage, by demonstration of the trophozoites in the aspirated bronchoalveolar fluid. This parasite was also diagnosed histologically

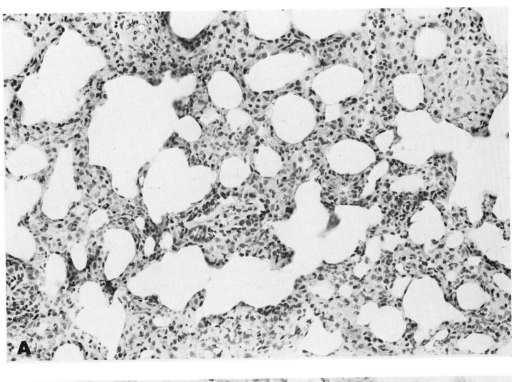

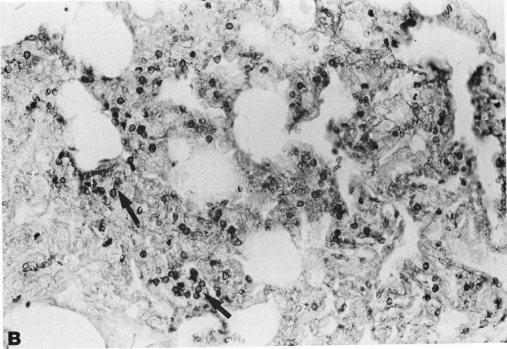

Fig. 12–3. *A,* Interstitial pneumonia in a ferret infected with *Pneumocystis carinii* (H & E stain; × 300). *B,* Trophozoites of *P. carinii* (*arrows*) focally distributed in lung of ferret immunosuppressed with cortisone GMS stain; × 600). (Stokes, D.C. et al.: Experimental *Pneumocystis carinii* pneumonia in the ferret. Br. J. Exp. Pathol., *68:*267, 1987.)

in the lung of a ferret experimentally infected with influenza virus.[6]

Treatment with oral trimethoprim-sulfamethoxazole appears to be effective against *P. carinii* pneumonia in ferrets, as it is in humans and rats.[18,19]

CRYPTOSPORIDIOSIS

Cryptosporidiosis, once considered an infrequent, inconsequential protozoan infection in mammals and reptiles, is gaining recognition as a significant enteric disease. It is reported to cause enteritis and diarrhea in calves, lambs (as well as other neonatal animals), and recently humans.[20] Chronic infections can also occur in immunocompromised hosts. The disease is caused by organisms of the genus *Cryptosporidium*, in the subclass Coccidiasina.

Epizootiology and Control. The disease was diagnosed in asymptomatic weanling ferrets and ferrets maintained on long-term corticosteroid therapy.[21] The life cycle is similar to that of other true coccidia. Infection is by ingestion of fecal oocysts or by autoinfective thin-walled oocysts released into the intestinal lumen, with reinitiation of the endogenous life cycle.[22,23] Because the oocysts passed in feces are resistant to disinfectants they can survive for long periods of time and remain infectious. Also, the parasite is believed to cross species barriers readily. Feeding raw meat products to ferrets in a commercial setting may result in infections of ferrets with *Cryptosporidia* from cattle. Studies indicate that calves and companion animals are potential sources of infection for humans.[22,23] Ferrets may therefore serve as another reservoir for infection in humans. Infection may be seasonal, occurring more frequently in the warmer, moist months of the year.

Diagnosis. Diagnosis is based on identification of cryptosporidian oocysts, measuring 4 to 6 μm in fecal specimens. Diagnostic procedures include using Sheather's sugar flotation and viewing either with bright field microscopy or phase contrast, the use of carbol fuchsin negative staining, or modified acid staining of a fecal smear. The oocysts must be differentiated from yeast spores.

Clinical Signs and Pathology. To date, ferrets with cryptosporidiosis have been asymptomatic. The disease in humans and young ruminants and piglets, however, can cause diarrhea and malabsorption with intestinal villous atrophy, fusion, and blunting.[20] In ferrets, a mild eosinophilic infiltrate is noted in intestinal sections infected with the organism (Figs. 12–4 and 12–5). Other enteric pathogens

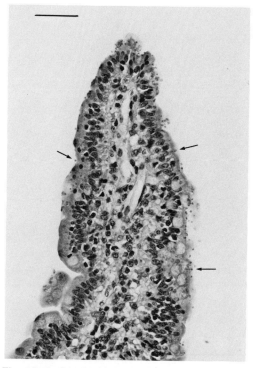

Fig. 12–4. Small intestine of ferret with numerous cryptosporidia (*arrows*) associated with the brush border of the villi (H & E stain; — = 35 μm). (Rehg, J.E., Gigliotti, F., and Stokes, D.C.: Cryptosporidiosis in ferrets. Lab. Anim. Sci., *38*:155–158, 1988.)

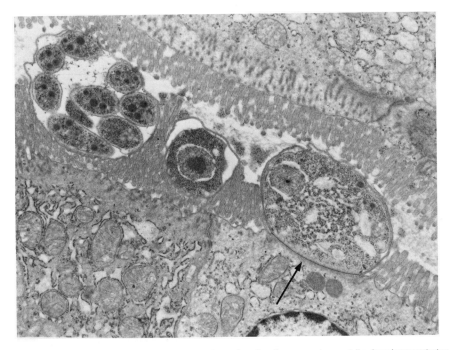

Fig. 12–5. Electron micrograph of ferret small intestine, showing three cryptosporidia development stages. Two abut the microvillous tips of a villous enterocyte. The other is attached to the microvillous surface of a villous epithelial cell. Shown (from right to left) are schizont with merozoites, early trophozoite, and late trophozoite. The late trophozoite shows the characteristic attachment zone (*arrow*) of cryptosporidia (magnification, × 19,000). (Rehg, J.E., Gigliotti, F., and Stokes, D.C.: Cryptosporidiosis in ferrets. Lab. Anim. Sci., *38*:155–158, 1988.)

causing concurrent infections must also be considered, as well as management practices, before arriving at a diagnosis of primary cryptosporidia-induced diarrhea.

Treatment. Drugs are ineffective in treatment or prophylaxis, even though over 50 have been tried.[24] Fortunately, in uncompromised hosts, the infection is self-limiting. Prevention of transmission to immunosuppressed hosts is obviously important.

GIARDIA

Giardia cysts have been noted in the feces of ferrets. Their pathogenicity in ferrets requires further study.

ECTOPARASITIC INFECTIONS

MITES

Ferrets can be infested with two types, ear mites and sarcoptic mites.

Ear mites

Ferrets, like the dog and cat, are susceptible to infestation with the ear mite *Otodectes cyanotis*.[25]

Epizootiology and Control. The mite is transmitted by contact with infected ferrets, dogs, or cats. Control is dependent on isolation and treatment of infected animals.

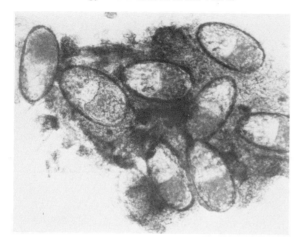

Fig. 12–6. Cluster of *Otodectes cyanotis* eggs from ear canal of ferret.

Clinical Signs. Affected ferrets may or may not show typical signs of otitis externa, such as scratching the ears or shaking of the head. Examination of the inner pinna, however, reveals the waxy brownish-black sebum often seen with ear mite infestation (Fig. 12–6). In a case of secondary otitis interna, a ferret was observed to be ataxic and circling.[26] Systemic antibiotic (chloramphenicol) and antiparasitic therapy resolves the infection and infestation. Ear mites may also be associated with mucormycosis (see Chap. 13).

Treatment. Ear mite medication, such as rotenone or pyrethrin preparations used to treat ear mites in cats or dogs, can be used to eradicate ear mites in ferrets. Two topical applications of the drug, 2 to 3 weeks apart, can be effective in eliminating the mite. In the pet ferret, treatment failure can result from the following: (1) the ferret resists treatment; (2) the small-diameter ear canal makes effective application of medication difficult; and (3) the ferret's body is not treated. Clients should be instructed accordingly; whole body treatment with a flea powder is recommended. A combination of thiabendazole, dexamethasone, and neomycin (Tresaderm) was used successfully to treat ear mites in pet ferrets.[27]

The experimental use of ivermectin to treat infected animals, 200–400 μg/lb, although a relatively high dose, appears to eradicate the infestation. Two treatments given at 14-day intervals may be needed. Marshall Farms, however, observed that 0.2 ml of 1% ivermectin given to jills at 2 to 4 weeks of gestation results in an abnormally high rate of congenital defects, such as cleft palates. They currently administer 0.1 ml of 1% ivermectin/jill at 4 weeks gestation, with no significant alteration of kit survival or increased frequency of congenital malformations.[28]

Diagnosis. The diagnosis is based on identifying various stages of the life cycle of the mite in scrapings of debris removed from the ferret's ear canal.

Sarcoptic Mites

The *Sarcoptes scabiei* mite was diagnosed in ferrets maintained for biomedical research.[29] The disease was reported to be common in feral ferrets in Europe.[30]

Epizootiology and Control. Transfer of the parasite is by direct contact with infected hosts and, to a lesser degree, by contact with infected bedding. A predator-prey relationship exists in nature, in which mite transfer appears to be facilitated between rabbits and ferrets, who often lie in the rabbit burrow for several hours after consuming the rabbit.[31] Control is based on treatment of infected hosts, decontamination of cages with appropriate insecticide, and destruction of all infested bedding.

Clinical Signs. Infestation with *Sarcoptes scabiei* may take two forms. In those animals in whom skin lesions predominate, focal to generalized alopecia with intense pruritus is often seen.[32] In the second form the sarcoptic lesions are confined to the feet and toes. The feet are swollen and inflamed, with numerous scabs, and if left untreated the ferret loses its claws. In earlier descriptions, the disease was referred to as foot rot.

Treatment. Treatment of affected digits consists of removing the diseased portion of the claw and debriding scabbed lesions after soaking the affected portions in warm water. Mites are eliminated by application of sulfa ointment or lime and sulfa dips and washes (30–32% calcium polysulfide.[29] Carbaryl (0.5%) shampoo applied weekly for 3 weeks effectively eliminated sarcoptic mange in one outbreak.[32] Organophosphates, carbamates, and ivermectin should be used cautiously in ferrets, because toxicity of these drugs in ferrets has not been determined. Pruritus can be treated with oral prednisone (2 mg/kg) and topical corticosteroids.

FLEAS

Ferrets can also be infested with fleas, of the species *Ctenocephalides*.[29, 32, 33]

Epizootiology and Control. Infested animals should be isolated, if possible, and treated with appropriate medication. The animal's environment, which contains flea eggs or fleas in various stages of development, should be treated with insecticide to destroy all stages of flea development.

Clinical Signs. Pruritus, scaly skin, and alopecia may be seen in affected animals, or animals may be asymptomatic.

Treatment. To be effective and long-lasting, flea control and treatment must consist of simultaneous treatment of the ferret as well as eradication of fleas from the premises. Because of the lengthy life cycle of the flea, residual chemicals (e.g., microencapsulated formulas of pyrethrins with synergists and Diazinon should be used.[34] Methoprene, or insect growth retardant, which prevents fourth instar larva metamorphosis, is also available for treatment of the environment. Treatment of infected ferrets is by flea shampoos or dips containing pyrethrins, lindane, or carbamates or by flea powders containing these same insecticides.[27] Flea collars to control fleas can be used, but with caution, because collars containing dichlorvos may have toxic effects.[35]

Diagnosis. The presumptive diagnosis is based on clinical signs and demonstration of flea excreta on the animal's pelage. Demonstration of the flea or of its larval stages confirms the diagnosis.

CUTANEOUS MYIASIS

Myiasis—maggot infestation—is caused by invasion of tissues or organs of the animal by dipterous larvae. A problem for commercial mink and ferret ranchers, and for pet owners who maintain ferrets outdoors, is flesh fly infestation. The flesh fly, *Wohlfahrtia vigil*, attacks mink kits when they are about 4 or 5 weeks old,[33] during the summer months.[36] The female deposits minute maggots on the face, neck, and flank of the kits, and the maggots bore into the skin. Kits become restless, whining, and anorectic. Considerable irritation results from attempted unsuccessful penetration of the larvae. Larvae in the subcutis produce small abscesslike lesions measuring 6 to 20 mm in diameter. The dam may remove the kits from the nest box, who may die from exposure, exhaustion, and emaciation. If there is early removal of larvae, with topical antibiotic and antiseptic treatment, recovery of infected animals is uneventful.[37]

Granulomatous masses and sinuses in the cervical region resulting from myiasis caused by the larval stage of *Hypoderma bovis* was also documented in ferrets.[38] *Cuterebra* larvae can also produce subdermal cysts in mustelids.[39]

TICKS

Ticks, along with mites, belong to the order Acarina. Ticks are occasionally found on ferrets used to hunt rabbits, or on ferrets allowed access to the outdoors. For example, in the British Isles, ferrets used for hunting are often infested with the tick *Ioxdes ricinus*. Ticks can be removed manually; care must be exercised to ensure that the mouth parts are removed from the ferrets skin.[40] It also must be remembered that ticks are significant vectors of various human diseases; proper care must be employed when handling ticks.

HELMINTHS

Because of the complex nature of their life cycles, migrations within their hosts, and apparent lack of clinical disease ascribed to most helminths in the ferret, these parasites, except for Dirofiliaria will be mentioned only briefly. Refer to parasitologic texts for a full description of these parasites and their pathogenicity on the host. Diagnostic procedures and treatment should follow guidelines established for cats and dogs.

INTESTINAL AND RESPIRATORY HELMINTHS

The list of internal helminths that may infect ferrets includes the following: nematodes; roundworms (*Toxascaris leonina* and *Toxocara cati*); hookworms (*Ancylostoma*); cestodes; tapeworms (*Mesocestoides, Ariotaenia procyonis,* and *Dipylidium caninum*); flukes; and lungworms (*Filarioides martis*). Occasionally, *Spiroptera nasicola* is found in the frontal sinus.[41] Clinical signs of intestinal parasitism in young ferrets are dull hair coat, pot belly, weight loss, and diarrhea. Diagnosis is confirmed by standard fecal flotation or by direct fecal smear. Treatment of intestinal parasites should be based on compounds designed for use in dogs and cats. Dichlorvos at the canine dosage of 12 to 15 mg/lb divided and administered over two or more days was recommended.[42] Oral mebendazole used at the recommended dog dosage also appears to be efficacious and safe.[40]

HEARTWORM INFESTATION

The heartworm, *Dirofilaria immitis*, a filarial nematode, can infect both domestic and wild carnivores, including the ferret. Ferrets are infected naturally with heartworms, and are experimentally susceptible to infection by *D. immitis, Brugia pahangi* (another filarial nematode), or both either by subcutaneous or intraperitoneal inoculation with larvae.[43,44]

Epizootiology and Control. The parasite is transmitted by and undergoes development in the mosquito. The disease in dogs has been reported throughout the United States, particularly in coastal areas, and in other parts of the world in which the mosquito, *Dirofilaria immitis,* and dog coexist. The parasite was first reported in ferrets commercially reared in New York and maintained in Newark,

Delaware, for 1 to 3 years.[43] Patent infections were also established experimentally in ferrets. They were subsequently diagnosed in pet ferrets from Florida, Louisiana, and Alabama by myself and others.[45–47] As pet ferrets become more popular, the disease will undoubtedly be encountered in many parts of the United States, as well as elsewhere. Control of the disease in ferrets, as in dogs, involves maintenance of ferrets indoors during the mosquito season; if the animal is kept outdoors, prophylactic anthelmintics should be used during this period.

Clinical Signs and Pathology. Ferrets present clinically with dyspnea, variable dehydration, lethargy, and pale mucous membranes. On thoracic auscultation the heart sounds are muffled, and radiographically an enlarged heart may be detected. Pulmonary congestion, pleural effusion, and/or ascites can be seen. Clinical signs may be vague, and only include anorexia and a protracted cough. Based on experimental studies and a review of the documented natural cases of the disease, it was postulated that adult *Dirofilaria immitis* infestation cannot be tolerated without lethal consequences. Cause of death is usually occlusion of major vessels by the adult *D. immitis*, with complicating features of congestion, hypoxia, and pulmonary edema.

Diagnosis. In naturally reported cases, as well as in experimental infections, microfilaremia is not a consistent finding. When demonstrated in blood smears the microfilaria measure 300 to 320 μ in length by 6 to 8 μ in width. They have tapered, cigar-shaped heads and straight tails, and move in a snakelike fashion. The ELISA test to diagnose occult infections may have promise, but data to indicate its usefulness is unavailable.

Treatment. Treatment is based on prevention. It is recommended that ferrets living in *Dirofilaria immitis* enzootic areas be given prophylactic diethylcarbamazine, applied daily in the feed at a dosage of 2.75 to 5.5 mg/kg.[45,48] Treatment in enzootic areas should commence 15 days prior to exposure to mosquitos, and extend 60 days after exposure has ceased. It was shown experimentally that ivermectin at a dosage of 0.1 mg/kg prevents the maturation of third-stage *D. immitis* larvae 2 days after inoculation into ferrets.[49] Newly formulated oral ivermectin for dogs, given once monthly, may therefore be of prophylactic value in ferrets.

Unfortunately, to date heartworm disease in the ferret has not been treated in any systematic fashion. Diagnosis should be guarded and if adulticide treatment is attempted, the regimen should follow the cat protocol. Thiacetarsamide sodium (Caprosolate) (0.22 ml/kg IV BID) is administered on 2 consecutive days, followed 4 to 6 weeks later by dithiazanine iodide (Dizan) 6 to 20 mg/kg orally until the ferret is negative for microfilaria (if positive initially).[50–52]

TRICHINOSIS

Several species of Mustelidae, including the wild ferret (*Mustela putorius*) were diagnosed as being infected with *Trichinella spiralis*.[53,54] Ferrets experimentally infected with larvae have adult worms recovered from the small intestine 4 and 7 days after oral inoculation with the larva.[55] Larvae subsequently became encysted in the ferret musculature, with the diaphragm becoming heavily parasitized. Infection of domestic ferrets could occur, therefore, if the ferrets are fed uncooked meat products infected with *Trichinella* larvae.

REFERENCES

1. Hoare, C.A.: The endogenous development of the coccidia of the ferret and the histopathological reaction of the infected intestinal villi. Ann. Trop. Med. Parasitol. *29*:111, 1935.
2. Drouin, T.E., and Mahrt, J.L.: The prevalence of *Sarcocystis* Lankester, 1882, in some bird species with notes on its life cycle. Can. J. Zool., *57*:1915, 1979.
3. Frenkel, J.K. et al.: Protozoan diseases. *In* Diseases of the Cat. Vol. I. Edited by J. Holzworth. Philadelphia, W.B. Saunders, 1987.
4. Coutelen, F.: The existence of a natural generalized toxoplasma of the ferret. A new toxoplasma *Toxoplasma laidlawi* n. sp. parasite of *Mustela (putorius) putorius* var. *furo.* C. R. Soc. Biol. Paris, *111*:284, 1932.
5. Lainson, R.: Symposium on toxoplasmosis. III. The demonstration of toxoplasma in animals, with particular reference to members of the Mustelidae. Trans. R. Soc. Trop. Med. Hyg., *51*:111, 1957.
6. Armed Forces Institute of Pathology: Accession files. Washington, D.C.
7. Dubey, J.P.: Toxoplasmosis. J. Am. Vet. Med. Assoc., *189*:166, 1986.
8. Dubey, J.P.: *Toxoplasma, Hammondia, Besnoitia, Sarcocystis,* and other tissue cyst-forming coccidia of man and animals. *In* Parasitic Protozoa. Edited by J.P. Kreier. New York, Academic Press, 1977.
9. Frenkel, J.K.: Protozoan diseases of laboratory animals. *In* Pathology of Protozoal and Helminthic Diseases, p. 319. Edited by R.A. Marcial-Rojas. Baltimore, Williams & Wilkins, 1971.
10. Thornton, R.N., and Cook, T.G.: A congenital Toxoplasma-like disease in ferrets (Mustela putorius furo). N.Z. Vet. J., *34*:31, 1986.
11. Fish, N.A.: Toxoplasmosis diagnosis by serological and cultural methods. Can. J. Public Health, *52*:107, 1961.
12. Dubey, J.P.: Repeat transplacental transfer of Toxoplasma gondii in goats. J. Am. Vet. Med. Assoc., *180*:1220, 1982.
13. Rommel, M.: The ferret *Putorius furo,* an additional final host of *Sarcocystis muris.* Z. Parasitenkd., *58*:187, 1979.
14. Hughes, W.T., and Smith, B.: Provocation of infection due to *Pneumocystis carinii* by cyclosporin A. J. Inf. Dis., *145*:767, 1982.
15. Farrow, B.R.H. et al.: Pneumocystis pneumonia in the dog. J. Comp. Pathol. *82*:447, 1972.
16. Frenkel, J.K., Good, J.T., and Schultz, S.A.: Latent pneumocystis infection in rats, relapse, and chemotherapy. Lab. Invest., *15*:1559, 1966.
17. Milder, J.E. et al.: Comparison of histological and immunological techniques for the detection of *Pneumocystis carinii* in rat bronchial lavage fluid. J. Clin. Microbiol., *2*:409, 1980.
18. Stokes, D.C. et al.: Experimental *Pneumocystis carinii* pneumonia in the ferret. Br. J. Exp. Pathol., *68*:267, 1987.
19. Hughes, W.T., McNabb, P.C., Makres, T.D., and Feldman, S.: Efficacy of trimethoprim and sulfamethoxazole in the prevention and treatment of *Pneumocystis carinii* pneumonitis. Antimicrob. Agents Chemother., *3*:289, 1974.
20. Current, W.L.: Cryptosporidiosis. J. Am. Vet. Med. Assoc., *187*:1334, 1985.
21. Rehg, J.E., Gigliotti, F., and Stokes, D.C.: Cryptosporidiosis in ferrets. Lab. Anim. Sci., *38*:155–158, 1988.
22. Tzipori, S.: Cryptosporidiosis in animals and humans. Microbiol. Rev. *47*:84, 1983.
23. Current, W.L. et al.: Human cryptosporidiosis in immunocompetent and immunodeficient persons: Studies of an outbreak and experimental transmission. N. Engl. J. Med., *308*:1252, 1983.
24. Jokipii, L., and Jokipii, A.M.: Cryptosporidiosis. *In* Infectious Diseases and Medical Microbiology, p. 931. 2nd Ed. Edited by A.I. Braude, C.E. Davis, and J. Fierer. Philadelphia. W.B. Saunders, 1986.
25. Sweatman, G.K.: Biology of *Otodectes cyanotis,* the ear canker of carnivores. Can. J. Zool., *36*:848, 1958.
26. Nie, I.A., and Pick, C.R.: Infestation of a colony of ferrets with ear mite (*Otodectes cyanotis*) and its control. J. Inst. Anim. Technol., *29*:63, 1978.
27. Randolph, R.W.: Preventative medical care for the pet ferret. *In* Current Veterinary Therapy, Vol. IX. Edited by R.W. Kirk. Philadelphia, W.B. Saunders, 1986.
28. Marshall Farms: Unpublished results, 1986.
29. Ryland, L.M., and Gorham, J.R.: The ferret and its diseases. J. Am. Vet. Med. Assoc., *173*:1154, 1978.
30. Warburton, C.: Sarcoptic scabies in man and animal. A critical survey of our present knowledge regarding the acari concerned. Parasitology, *1*:265, 1920.
31. Sweatman, G.K.: Mites and pentastomes. *In* Parasitic Diseases of Wild Mammals. Edited by J.W. Davis and R.C. Anderson. Ames, IA, Iowa State Press, 1973.
32. Ryland, L.M., Bernard, S.L., and Gorham, J.R.: A clinical guide to the pet ferret. Comp. Cont. Ed., *5*:25, 1983.

33. Kaufman, J., Schwartz, P., and Mero, K.: Pancreatic beta cell tumor in a ferret. J. Am. Vet. Med. Assoc., 185:998, 1984.

34. Muller, G.H., Kirk, R.W., and Scott, D.W.: Small Animal Dermatology, 3rd Ed. Philadelphia, W.B. Saunders, 1983.

35. Farrell, R.K., Bill, T.C., and Padgett, G.A.: Toxicity of flea collars. J. Am. Vet. Med. Assoc., 166:1054, 1975.

36. Gorham, J.R., Hagen, K.W., and Farrell, R.K.: Minks: Diseases and Parasites. Washington, D.C., U.S. Department of Agriculture, Agricultural Research Handbook No. 175, 1972.

37. Eschle, J.L., and DeFoliart, G.R.: Control of mink myiasis caused by the larvae of *Wohlfahrtia vigil*. J. Econ. Entomol., 58:529, 1965.

38. Skulski, G., and Symmers, W. St.C.: Actinomycosis and torulosis in the ferret. J. Comp. Pathol., 64:306, 1954.

39. Capelle, K.J.: Myiasis. *In* Parasitic Diseases of Wild Mammals. Edited by J.W. Davis and R.C. Anderson. Ames, IA, Iowa State Press, 1973.

40. Cooper, J.E.: Ferrets. *In* Manual of Exotic Pets. Edited by J.E. Cooper, M.F. Hutchison, and O.F. Jackson. Cheltenham, England, British Small Animal Veterinary Association, 1985.

41. Petrov, A.M.: Addition to the explanation of systematics of nematode parasites in the frontal sinus and lungs of the Mustelidae. Ann. Trop. Med. Parasitol. 22:259, 1928.

42. Corde, B.D., Moye, S.L., Nixon, C.R., and Smith, T.T.: Wildlife notebook: The ferret (*Mustela putorius furo*). Anim. Health Technol., 4:56, 1983.

43. Campbell, W.C., and Blair L.S.: *Dirofilaria immitis*: experimental infections in the ferret, *Mustela putorius furo*. J. Parasitol., 64:119, 1978.

44. Campbell, W.C., and Blair, L.S.: *Brugia pahangi* and *Dirofilaria immitis*: Experimental infections in the ferret (*Mustela putorius furo*). Exp. Parasitol., 47:327, 1979.

45. Parrott, T.Y., Greiner, E.C., and Parrott, J.D.: *Dirofilaria immitis* infection in three ferrets. J. Am. Vet. Med. Assoc., 184:582, 1984.

46. Moreland, A.F., Battles, A.H., and Nease, J.H.: Dirofilariasis in a ferret. J. Am. Vet. Med. Assoc., 188:864, 1986.

47. Miller, W.R., and Merton, D.A.: Dirofilariasis in a ferret. J. Am. Vet. Med. Assoc., 180:1103, 1982.

48. Kaufmann, P.H.: Procynidae and Mustelidae. *In* Zoo and Wild Animal Medicine. Edited by M.E. Fowler. Philadelphia, W.B. Saunders, 1984.

49. Blair, L.S., Williams, E., and Ewanciw, D.V.: Efficacy of ivermectin against third-stage *Dirofilaria immitis* larvae in ferrets and dogs. Res. Vet. Sci., 33:386, 1982.

50. Dillon, R.: Feline dirofilariasis. Vet. Clin. North. Am., 14:1185, 1984.

51. Swartz, A.: Two cases of feline heartworm disease. Feline Pract., 5:20, 1975.

52. Harpster, N.K.: The cardiovascular system. Chapter 18. *In* Diseases of the Cat. Volume 1. Edited by J. Holzworth. Philadelphia, W.B. Saunders, 1987.

53. Merkushev, A.V.: Trichinosis in the Union of Soviet Socialist Republics. *In* Trichinosis in Man and Animals. Edited by S.E. Gould. Springfield, IL, Charles C Thomas, 1970.

54. Cironeanu, I.: Trichinellosis in domestic and wild animals in Rumania. *In* Trichinellosis. Edited by C.W. Kim. New York, Educational Publishers, 1974.

55. Campbell, W.C., Blair, L.S., Kung, F.Y., and Ewanciw, D.V.: Experimental *Trichinella spiralis* infection in the ferret (*Mustela putorius furo*). J. Helminthol. 56:55, 1982.

chapter 13

MYCOTIC DISEASES

J. G. Fox

SYSTEMIC FUNGAL INFECTIONS

Ferrets are susceptible to systemic infections caused by the fungi *Blastomyces*, Cryptococcus, and *Histoplasma*.

BLASTOMYCOSIS

This disease was recently reported in a ferret; the case had many of the same characteristics of the disease in dogs.[1] North American blastomycosis is a systemic fungal disease caused by *Blastomyces dermatitidis*, and infects primarily humans and dogs.[2,3] The disease was also reported in horses, cats, and sea lions. The fungus is dimorphic, and grows as a yeast in tissue and in enriched culture media at 37°C and as a mold at room temperature.

Epizootiology and Control. The disease occurs sporadically in both domestic animals and humans. The reservoir is probably soil, and the mode of transmission is most likely by inhalation of the conidia in spore-laden dust. The disease does not appear to be transmitted directly from animal to animal or from animal to human. This disease occurs most frequently in central and southeastern United States, Canada, Africa, and (rarely) in Latin America.[3] The low number of reported cases in humans and animals (including the ferret) suggests that mammalian hosts are relatively resistant to the disease. Animals housed outdoors with exposure to fungus-laden dust may be at a higher risk of infection.

Clinical Signs and Pathology. Systemic blastomycosis is most often a chronic granulomatous mycosis, primarily affecting the lungs. Cutaneous blastomycosis is also diagnosed and characterized by chronic ulcerated skin lesions, which spread slowly and peripherally. In the affected ferret, an ulcerated swelling on the metacarpal pad was noted.[1] Tissue imprint of the lesion demonstrated broad-based budding yeasts consistent with *Blastomyces dermatitidis*. The animal sneezed and coughed, and an enlarged spleen was palpated. Thoracic radiography revealed reticulonodular interstitial pneumonia, with focal consolidation of a portion of the lung, and pleural fluid. Radiographic findings were consistent with mycosis or neoplasia. Necropsy revealed bilateral diffuse granulomatous pneumonia, characterized by nodules throughout the lungs. Granulomatous pleuritis, meningoencephalitis, and splenitis were also noted.[1]

The disease described in the ferret represents the chronic respiratory form, with spread of the disease to other organs by way of blood or lymph.[1]

Diagnosis. Isolation of *Blastomyces dermatitidis* from cutaneous or lung aspirate confirms a diagnosis of the disease. Tissue imprints demonstrating the budding yeast provide a tentative diagnosis. The characteristic "snowstorm" interstitial changes seen in cases of canine blasto-

mycosis are also present in the ferret.[1,4] Agar immunodiffusion demonstrating circulating antibody titer to the organism may also be useful in establishing a clinical diagnosis of the disease.

Treatment. The treatment used in canines consists of amphotericin B at dosages of 0.25 to 1 mg/kg given intravenously for several treatments, until a total dosage of 0.7 to 25 mg/kg has been administered.[2,5,6] Treatment with ketoconazole (10–30 mg/kg) orally once daily for 60 days was also used successfully to treat the disease in dogs.[7] Initial treatment in the ferret with amphotericin B intravenously (0.5 mg in 1 ml 5% dextrose) every other day for a calculated dosage of 0.8 mg amphotericin B/kg was instituted, supplemented with ketoconazole, 5 mg orally. Blood urea nitrogen (BUN) levels were monitored, and fluid given subcutaneously as needed. Because the first treatment of amphotericin B caused anorexia, pyrexia, and azotemia, the dosage was reduced to 0.25 mg (0.4 mg/kg) to be given intravenously as often as BUN level values permitted; this regime was established according to the clinical appearance of the animal, and was instituted approximately 1 week after the first treatment. The animal responded by resolution of the ulcer in the forepad and regression of primary lesions. Because of inaccessible veins, intravenous amphotericin had to be discontinued, and subcutaneous amphotericin was given every other day. Two weeks after initiation of subcutaneous treatment, however, the ferret relapsed and was euthanized.

Blastomycosis treatment in ferrets obviously requires further study. It is recommended that jugular catheterization may aid in effective treatment with amphotericin, monitoring of BUN values, and provision of fluid therapy; intraperitoneal injections may be attempted.[1] Increasing the oral dose of ketoconazole dosage to 30 mg/kg/day in the ferret may increase its efficacy in treating blastomycosis.

CRYPTOCOCCOSIS

Three cases of cryptococcosis have been described in the ferret. The disease is caused by *Cryptococcus neoformans* and usually presents clinically as a subacute or chronic meningoencephalitis, with occasional involvement of other organs.

Epizootiology and Control. The organism is present universally, and is often found in the soil. *Cryptococcus neoformans* growth is enhanced by creatinine, which is found in the excreta of pigeons and of certain other birds. It is probable that one ferret used to control rodents in an aviary was infected from pigeon excreta present in the environment. Control therefore includes minimizing contact with soil contaminated with the feces of pigeons and other birds. As noted in another ferret, susceptibility to the disease is increased during corticosteroid therapy or when the animal is immunosuppressed.

Clinical Signs. A mature albino male ferret (case 1) was found dead by its owner in England.[8] No clinical signs prior to its death had been noted.

Cryptococcosis was also diagnosed at necropsy in a 3-year-old male (case 2) suffering from cardiomyopathy. The animal was examined because of posterior paralysis and listlessness. Neurologic examination revealed hyperaphia of L2 and L3 and decreased sensation and slow withdrawal of the hind limbs.[9] A diagnosis of intervertebral disc disease was made; the ferret was treated with dexamethasone for 1 month. The ferret's condition improved markedly for 1 month, but it was examined at another veterinary clinic because of serous nasal discharge and moderate dyspnea. Therapy with antibiotics was instituted for 5 days, but the animal's condition worsened and it became anorectic. Cardiomegaly and pulmonary edema were diagnosed by thoracic radiography and electrocardiography. Fu-

rosemide (1 mg/kg), cephalexin (10 mg/kg), digitalis (0.0025 mg/kg), and oxygen were administered, but the animal died the following day.

In case 3, reported from Australia, a 3-year-old ferret was purchased by an owner of an aviary to control wild mice.[10] Pigeons also were commonly attracted to the aviary. Initially, the ferret appeared to work effectively as a "mouser," but after several weeks the mouse population again increased. The ferret was given to a ferreter, who noticed the animal had a nasal discharge and was inactive; it died 3 weeks later.

Pathology. In case 1 the serosal surfaces of adhered abdominal organs were covered with a colorless, jellylike material that was easily removed from the underlying serosa. White nodules were present on the serosa of the intestine, in the parenchyma of the spleen, and in mesenteric lymph nodes and spleen. Histologically, masses of yeastlike organisms compatible with cryptococci, 10 μ in diameter and surrounded by a mucoid capsule, were observed in the jellylike material adhering to the abdominal organs. Identical organisms were present in the cytoplasm of macrophages and multinucleated giant cells, which formed tuberclelike granulomata and corresponded to the nodules seen on the small intestine at necropsy.

Histologic examination of case 2, with cardiomegaly, indicated changes in the heart, lung, and liver compatible with congestive cardiomyopathy and associated congestive heart failure.[9] A marked diffuse lymphocytic meningeal infiltrate involved the cerebral and cerebellar meninges. A moderate number of yeastlike budding organisms were seen in the inflamed meninges, compatible in size and shape to those of *Cryptococcus neoformans* (Figs. 13–1 and 13–2). Histologic examination of pneumonic lungs in case 3 revealed thick-walled budding yeasts, compatible with those of *C. neoformans*.

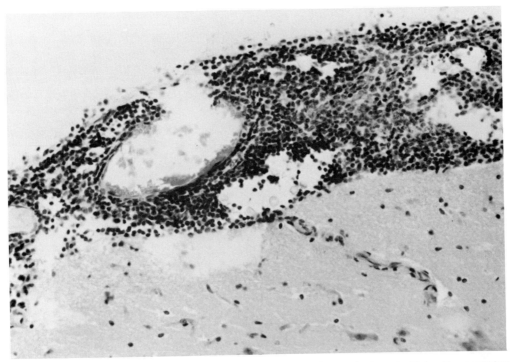

Fig. 13–1. Photomicrograph illustrating marked diffuse nonsuppurative cerebral meningitis in a 3-year-old ferret (H & E stain; × 20). (Greenlee, P.G., and Stephens, E.: Meningeal cryptococcosis and congestive cardiomyopathy in a ferret. J. Am. Vet. Med. Assoc., *184*:840, 1984.)

Treatment. To date, in ferret cryptococcosis, the diagnosis has been made postmortem, and treatment was not attempted. In other companion animals, treatment with amphotericin B is sometimes used. In the cat, a dosage of 0.15 to 1.0 mg/kg, dissolved in 5 to 20 ml 5% dextrose and water, and given rapidly IV, three times weekly for 2 to 4 months, is used. The drug is nephrotoxic, and caution must be exercised to ensure proper hydration and monitoring of kidney function during the treatment period; antiemetics also may be needed.

Diagnosis. If cryptococcal meningitis is suspected, microscopic examination of the cerebral spinal fluid, mixed with India ink, allows visualization of encapsulated budding forms of the fungus. Diagnosis is confirmed by cultural isolation of the organism or by histopathology.

HISTOPLASMOSIS

The disease is infectious, but not contagious, and is caused by an intracellular organism, *Histoplasma capsulatum.*

Epizootiology and Control. In the one recorded case, the ferret was used to hunt rabbits and rats.[11] Its diet consisted of dog food, table scraps, and rabbit heads. The organism usually infects the host by the respiratory route, and exposure to aerosolized dust containing the organism is a probable mechanism of infection.

The disease in carnivores, particularly in the dog, is more commonly diagnosed in the central part of the United States, in which the organism is commonly isolated from the soil. Interestingly, the one recorded case of histoplasmosis was diagnosed in a ferret used for hunting in Illinois.[11] Ferrets maintained in outdoor

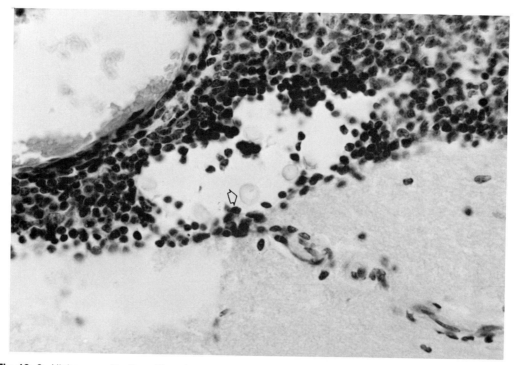

Fig. 13–2. Higher magnification of that shown in Figure 13–1, depicting a typical organism, *C. neoformans,* with a distinct capsule (*arrow*) (H & E stain; × 200). (Greenlee, P.G., and Stephens, E.: Meningeal cryptococcosis and congestive cardiomyopathy in a ferret. J. Am. Vet. Med. Assoc., *184*:840, 1984.)

enclosures, and those used for hunting where the animal enters burrows in pursuit of prey, would more likely become infected with this disease. "Epidemics" of histoplasmosis arise from infected hosts sharing the same environment.

Clinical Signs and Pathology. The ferret with histoplasma presented with severe abdominal pain, marked splenomegaly, and subnormal temperature.[11] In humans benign histoplasmosis may become acute and present clinically as pneumonitis, lymphadenopathy, anorexia, and weight loss. In dogs with disseminated disease there is weight loss, hepatomegaly, splenomegaly, pneumonia, ascites, and generalized lymphadenopathy.

Diagnosis. Biopsy of affected tissue and demonstration of organisms by special stains, periodic acid-Schiff (PAS), or Bauer's or Gridly's fungus method helps to establish a diagnosis. Culturing of the organism from infected tissues provides a definitive diagnosis.

SUPERFICIAL MYCOSES

In the ferret, these include ringworm and mucormycosis.

MUCORMYCOSIS

Otitis media is associated with primary otitis externa infection with *Otodectes cyanotis* and with secondary fungal infection by *Absidia corymbifera (ramosa).* Mucormycosis is an opportunistic mycotic infection caused by a number of mold species of the order Mucorales. The disease was reported in ferrets raised for fur in New Zealand.[12]

Epizootiology and Control. The prevalence in New Zealand ferret farms is reportedly common; on four farms, the infection rate ranged from 0.3 to 30%. *Absidia corymbifera*, a thermotolerant saprophyte, is not normally found in ferret ears but is widespread in the environment. Control of the infection relies on regular examination of the ears and on aggressive therapy to eliminate ear mites. Moldy litter (hay and straw) should be avoided. Regular disinfection of ferret cages is also required. Antibiotic therapy instituted for suspected bacterial otitis externa may predispose these animals to secondary fungal infection.

Clinical Signs. Scratching and irritation of the external auditory canal, indicative of mite infestation, is observed together with brown granular debris containing ear mites and fungal hyphae. Clinically the animals can present with depression and lethargy. Torticollis, with the affected side of the head turned toward the body, loss of balance, circling, and prostration are occasionally observed.

Diagnosis and Pathology. Diagnosis is based on the demonstration of ear mites and *Absidia* hyphae in the external auditory canal. Aspiration biopsy of regional lymph nodes, and the presence of *Absidia* in histopathologic tissue section, in addition to positive culture, helps to confirm a diagnosis. Necrosis and granulomatous inflammation of the petrous temporal bone, along with granulomatous meningoencephalitis, are sometimes present. Focal lesions in the temporal and pyriform lobes of the cerebrum and adjacent areas of the cerebellum and brain stems are also seen.[12]

DERMATOMYCOSES

The most common causative agents of ringworm in domestic animals are *Microsporum canis* and *Trichophyton*

mentagrophytes. The dermatophytes are grouped taxonomically as related fungi that have an affinity for cornified epidermis, hair, horn, nails, and feathers.[13]

Epizootiology and Control. Dermatophytes are distributed worldwide, with some species more commonly reported in certain geographic areas. In an outbreak of ringworm in mink, cats were allowed to sleep in nest box bedding stored for mink kits. The cats were suffering from clinical cases of ringworm. Cats may also have been involved in an outbreak of ringworm in a ferret colony.[14]

Dermatophytes are usually spread from animal to animal by direct contact, or indirectly by contaminated fomites. Concentration of ferrets in limited housing also enhances the probability of the spread of infection.

Control of infection depends on removal of infected animals from the premises and disinfection or destruction of all contaminated bedding, caging, and other potentially contaminated materials.

Transmission of dermatophytes from animals to humans is a well-known and serious public health concern. Ferrets with ringworm therefore present a zoonotic risk, and care should be exercised by personnel who handle infected animals.[15]

Clinical Signs. Younger animals are at higher risk to develop clinical disease. Lesions appear as circumscribed areas of alopecia and inflammation distributed on all areas of the skin. The skin is thickened, inflamed, and covered by scaly crusts.

Diagnosis. Presumptive diagnosis is based on suspicious skin lesions that begin as small papules and spread peripherally, leaving scaly inflamed areas of alopecia. Examination of the lesion under ultraviolet light (Wood's lamp) for yellow-green fluorescence is helpful in diagnosing infections caused by *Microsporum canis*. *Trichophyton* species do not fluoresce.

Microscopic examination of skin scrapings containing scales and hair, using 10% potassium hydroxide, shows characteristic arthrospores. Definitive diagnosis requires culture of the fungus.

Treatment. Clinical signs may regress without treatment. Griseofulvin, 25 mg/kg given orally, however, also results in remission of clinical signs of ringworm in the ferret.[14]

REFERENCES

1. Lenhard, A.: Blastomycosis in a ferret. J. Am. Vet. Med. Assoc., *186*:70, 1985.
2. Legendre, A.M., et al.: Canine blastomycosis: A review of 47 clinical cases. J. Am. Vet. Med. Assoc., *178*:1163, 1981.
3. Benensen, A.S. (ed.): Control of Communicable Diseases in Man. 13th ed. Washington, DC, American Public Health Association, 1981.
4. Walker, M.A.: Thoracic blastomycosis: A review of its radiographic manifestations in 40 dogs. Vet. Radiol., *22*:22, 1981.
5. Ausherman, R.J.: Treatment of blastomycosis and histoplasmosis in the dog. J. Am. Vet. Med. Assoc. *163*:1048, 1973.
6. Kaufmann, A.F., Kaplan, W., and Kraft, D.E.: Filamentous forms of *Ajellomyces (Blastomyces) dermatitidis* in a dog. Vet. Pathol., *16*:271, 1979.
7. Dunbar, M., Jr., et al: Treatment of canine blastomycosis with ketoconazole. J. Am. Vet. Med. Assoc., *182*:156, 1983.
8. Skulski, G., and Symmers, W.St.C.: Actinomycosis and torulosis in the ferret. J. Comp. Pathol., *64*:306, 1954.
9. Greenlee, P.G., and Stephens, E.: Meningeal cryptococcosis and congestive cardiomyopathy in a ferret. J. Am. Vet. Med. Assoc., *184*:840, 1984.
10. Lewington, J.H.: Isolation of *Cryptococcus neoformans* from a ferret. Aust. Vet. J., *58*:124, 1982.
11. Levine, N.D., Dunlop, G.L., and Graham, R.: An intracellular parasite in ferret. Cornell Vet., *28*:249, 1938.
12. Diseases of the fitch. Surveillance, *11*:28, 1984.
13. Rebell, G., and Taplin, D.: Dermatophytes. Their Recognition and Identification. Miami, University of Miami Press, 1970.
14. Hagen, K.W., and Gorham, J.R.: Dermatomycoses in fur animals: Chinchilla, ferret, mink and rabbit. Vet. Med. Small Anim. Clin., *67*:43, 1972.
15. Fox, J.G., Newcomer, C.E., and Rozmiarek, H.: Selected zoonoses and other health hazards. *In* Laboratory Animal Medicine. Edited by J.G. Fox, B.J. Cohen, and F.M. Loew. New York, Academic Press, 1984.

chapter 14

SYSTEMIC DISEASES

J. G. Fox

GASTROINTESTINAL TRACT

In the ferret, gastrointestinal tract disorders include dental malformations, periodontal disease, gingival hyperplasia, salivary mucocele, esophageal perforation, gastritis-gastric ulcers, bloat syndrome, ingestion of foreign bodies, infiltrates in the liver, and accessory gallbladders.

DENTAL MALFORMATIONS

Supernumerary deciduous incisors were recorded on a frequent basis in albino ferrets,[1,2] as were supernumerary permanent incisors in polecats and ferret-polecat hybrids.[3] Andrews and colleagues[4] noted ferrets with less than the usual six incisors in the upper jaw, including incisors with distal bifurcations.

Biting and gnawing behavior often results in broken or worn canines. If the dental pulp is exposed, corrective dental procedures such as root canal or surgical removal of the tooth should be undertaken. Deciduous canines may have to be removed by manual extraction if excessive tartar accumulates at the junction with the permanent canines. Usually, however, the deciduous tooth is removed during the normal process of eating hard food.

PERIODONTAL DISEASE

Periodontal disease in ferrets, as in many other animal species including humans, occurs with regularity and in ferrets is associated with the feeding of moist or semimoist diets. Experimentally, it was found that ferrets fed a bread-meat-milk diet developed periodontal disease clinically, and histologically had calculus formation on the teeth.[5,6] Calculi contained calcium and phosphorus in the form of hydroxyapatite. The benefit of feeding rib bones to remove dental tartar was noted.[5,6] Diets for ferrets should therefore in part include a dry pelleted feed. If necessary, preventive dental care such as teeth cleaning should be done; this procedure is performed, of course, under general anesthesia.[5,6]

GINGIVAL HYPERPLASIA

Occasionally ferrets suffer from idiopathic epilepsy, which requires administration of medication to control seizures. Diphenylhydantoin is occasionally used for this purpose to control seizures in dogs, cats, and humans. Diphenylhydantoin has a side effect of producing gingival hyperplasia, but the exact cause of how this occurs is unknown. Gingival hyperplasia is also produced in ferrets using this drug at a dosage of 40 mg/kg daily administered over a period of 6 months.[7] Similar results were documented in cats, dog and human.[8] Diphenylhydantoin-induced gingival hyperplasia in ferrets produces unorganized proliferation of connective tissue and epithelium, with inflammatory edematous lesions and leukocyte infiltration.

Care should therefore be exercised if this drug is to be administered on a chronic basis to the ferret.

SALIVARY MUCOCELE

Salivary mucoceles are accumulations of saliva extravasated from the salivary glands or ducts, which are located in the neck. A ranula is a mucocele beneath the tongue. Pharyngeal mucoceles, although less common, develop in the pharyngeal area and may cause obstruction of the trachea and pharyngeal area. Mucoceles located in the buccal commissure were diagnosed in two ferrets.[9]

Clinical Signs and Diagnosis. The mucocele is diagnosed by its anatomic and subcutaneous location, and by its appearance as a cystlike structure. Aspiration of the contents reveals a clear viscous fluid consisting of amorphous material and occasional red blood cells. Sialography or injection of dye directly into the cyst may help to locate the origin of the saliva that has collected in the cyst.

Treatment. Linear incision in the medial wall and removal of the extravasated saliva resulted in successful marsupialization of the mass in one ferret, but similar treatment in the second ferret did not have a satisfactory result—there were two recurrences of the mucocele. A wide circular incision using a biopsy punch in the medial wall, however, did produce remission and disappearance of the mucocele.[9] In the canine, treatment often relies on removal of the sublingual and mandibular salivary glands from the affected portion of the head or neck.[10] Knowledge of the superficial anatomic structure of the head and neck is necessary in case surgical removal of the glands is indicated (see Chap. 2).

ESOPHAGEAL PERFORATION

This condition was reported in a ferret maintained on a diet of dead rats.[4] It was postulated that sharp edges of bone present in rat carcasses perforated the esophagus. Other ferrets were diagnosed as having abscesses located in the neck and mandible area, suggestive of actinomycosis or lumpy jaw (see Chap. 10 for further description).

GASTRITIS-GASTRIC ULCERS

Gastric ulcers in ferrets were first observed in 1972 in ferrets maintained in England,[11] and similarly documented in 1976 and 1979.[4] The ulcers were attributed to undefined environmental stress. Extensive hemorrhage of the gastrointestinal tract was observed in three other ferrets, but the cause was not determined. Gastric disease was also described in ferrets in the United States and New Zealand.[12, 13]

Clinical Signs. Gastritis and ulcer disease in the ferret may be asymptomatic, or may be accompanied by vague signs of abdominal distress. Occasionally animals will vomit and have halitosis. If bleeding occurs there may be blood in the vomitus, or melena may be present. Causes of gastritis in humans and animals can result from various factors, including the following:[13, 14]

1. Ulcerogenic agents: aspirin, indomethacin, flunixin, phenylbutazone, bile salts, pancreatic juice, hypertonic solutions, alcohols, certain heavy metals, acetazolamide, urea
2. Stress factors: shock, trauma, severe illness, environmental stress
3. Gastric ischemia
4. Bile reflux
5. Neurologic disease
6. Metabolic disease: renal failure, liver disease, adrenocortical insufficiency, gastric outflow obstruction
7. Gastric hyperacidity: systemic mastocytosis, gastrinoma
8. *Campylobacter*-like organisms

Treatment. Treatment or control of ulcers in ferrets has not been described. With the recent discovery of *Campylobacter pylori* as a purported cause of acute gastritis and possibly ulcers in humans, antimicrobials and bismuth preparations are being used to treat suspected infectious gastritis.[15] Because *Campylobacter*-like organisms were also isolated from inflamed gastric mucosa in ferrets, the use of antibiotics may be indicated. Further investigations are warranted, however, to determine whether or not this organism can cause gastritis and/or ulcers in ferrets.[13, 16] In humans, *C. pylori* is treated with a combination of amoxicillin or other antibiotics and an antisecretory preparation, bismuth subsalicylate. Encouraging results have been documented.[15] If this regimen is contemplated in the ferret, a dose of 20 mg/kg amoxicillin orally once daily and 0.25 ml/kg bismuth subsalicylate orally every 4 to 6 hours is recommended for 7 to 10 days. The ferret should be watched closely for nausea or vomiting, although in our experience vomiting has not been a problem with amoxicillin treatment in the ferret. Erythromycin treatment may be attempted, but recent experience in treating *C. pylori* gastritis in humans indicates that relapse rates are high with erythromycin therapy. Systemic antacids such as cimetidine are indicated if serious gastric or duodenal bleeding is suspected because of erosive gastritis. The dosage of cimetidine in the ferret is similar to that for the dog and cat, 5 to 10 mg/kg orally three or four times daily.

Pathology. Recently, *Campylobacter*-like organisms (CLO) associated with gastric ulcer disease in the ferret were documented (see Chap. 10, *Campylobacter*-like organisms).[16] Circular depressed ulcers are found on the fundus and antrum of the stomach (Fig. 14–1). In addition, I have observed a chronic atrophic gastritis in

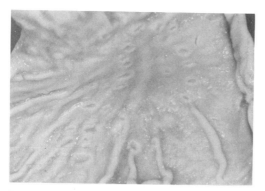

Fig. 14–1. Diffuse circular ulcers in the stomach of a ferret, particularly prominent in the fundus and antrum.

ferrets, with hyperplastic regenerative changes that are quite similar to those described in humans.

Using Warthin-Starry stain, *Campylobacter*-like organisms were noted below the mucous layers and on the surface of epithelium in some ferrets with severe gastritis. These are also visualized by electron microscopy in association with disrupted microvilli.[13] Histologically, chronic ulcers are fibrotic, with infiltrates of macrophages and lymphocytes in the disrupted hyperplastic lamina propria and submucosa (Fig. 14–2).

Ferrets commonly have lymphoid aggregates of various sizes in the lamina propria and submucosa in the region of the pyloric antrum, extending into the proximal duodenum. It is not known whether these infiltrates are produced by local antigenic stimulation or are a normal component of ferret gastric mucosa.[13]

BLOAT SYNDROME

The etiology of this condition is unknown, but it may be associated with overeating and the production of excessive gas caused by the proliferation of *Clostridium welchii* in stomach ingesta.[12]

Epizootiology and Control. The prevalence is variable, but the disease was recorded on ferret farms in New Zealand in which the incidence varied from 6 to 50%. Overeating after prolonged fasting of over 24 hours appears to be a predisposing factor. Also, sudden changes in diet, particularly inclusion of cereal into the dietary regime or nonhygienic food preparations, increases the likelihood of bloat and excessive food in the gastric lumen. Avoidance of predisposing factors markedly reduces the incidence of the disease.

Clinical Signs. The disease often occurs in weanling animals and is noted by acute gastric distension, dyspnea, and cyanosis. Clinical signs appear $\frac{1}{2}$ to 4 hours after feedings. Animals are often found dead, with marked abdominal distension.[12]

Pathology. Grossly, the stomach is distended with food and gas. Subcutaneous emphysema with little or no putrefaction is also present. *Clostridium welchii*, an anaerobic gas-forming microorganism, is sometimes isolated from the gastric contents in bloated ferrets.[12] The pathophysiologic mechanism of gastric dilatation-volvulus in dogs (and presumably ferrets) consists of gastric wall ischemia and circulatory shock resulting from pressure occlusion of the caudal vena cava and portal vein.[17]

Treatment. Parenteral smooth muscle relaxants were used with some success in cases diagnosed before signs became severe.[12] In ferrets, as in dogs with gastric dilatation, the immediate treatment consists of decompression of the distended stomach, which dramatically improves cardiac output by relieving the venous occlusion. The procedure is performed by passage of an orogastric tube (no. 4 French), using a speculum and physical restraint. If this fails, a gastrocentesis is performed. The site of entry is the right flank caudal to the costal arch.[18] Shock therapy is also instituted, including administration of balanced electrolyte solu-

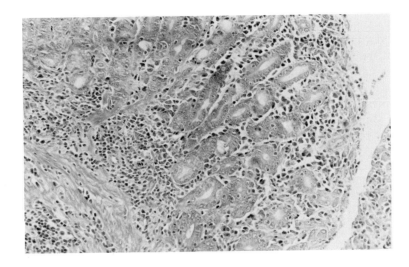

Fig. 14–2. Chronic gastritis. The mucosa are infiltrated with a moderate amount of lymphoplasmacytic infiltrate throughout the lamina propria, extending through the muscularis mucosa (H & E stain; × 150).

tions (90 ml/kg every 30 minutes) until the patient is stabilized. A nonsteroidal drug such as flunixin meglumine (1 mg/kg) is used to prevent the prostaglandin-mediated hypotension noted in endotoxemia. It is not known whether gastropexy is required to prevent the recurrence of the condition in ferrets.

FOREIGN BODIES

If ferrets are fed rodents or chicken parts, or if they kill and eat feral rodents present in their environment, bones or intact skulls may become lodged and cause intestinal or gastric occlusion. Occlusion of the gastrointestinal tract by ingestion of foam rubber caused death in two ferrets.[19] Similarly, if animals are on corticosteroid therapy, pica may result in ingestion of foreign objects and produce gastrointestinal obstruction or irritation. Pet ferrets are also very prone to ingestion of various foreign bodies. Supportive therapy and surgery may be necessary

to remove these foreign objects. If poisoning is suspected—for example, by a rodenticide—and an emetic is required, apomorphine (0.7 mg/kg) subcutaneously or ipecac (2.2–6.6 ml of 7% ipecac in glycerin syrup) given orally can be used to induce vomiting.

INFILTRATES IN THE LIVER

Clinically, normal ferrets often have periportal lymphocytic infiltrates in the liver. A minimal amount of infiltrate may be normal. It is suspected, however, that some ferrets with this lesion may have a subclinical infection with Aleutian disease (see Chap. 11).

ACCESSORY GALLBLADDER

Accessory gallbladders were diagnosed in two ferrets.[4] Neither clinical signs nor functional deficits caused by this abnormality were documented.[4]

GENITOURINARY SYSTEM

In a ferret colony maintained for research in Cambridge, England, diseases reported at necropsy included uterine infection, urinary calculi, and ovarian tumors.[20, 21] Unfortunately, clinical signs and treatments of the disorders were not discussed in these reports. Clinical diagnosis and management of these diseases would presumably be the same as in the dog or cat.

PYELONEPHRITIS

Pyelonephritis was encountered in ferrets maintained in our laboratory, and diagnosed at necropsy by others.[11] Infections of the kidney, in our experience, are associated with ascending urinary infections (with or without calculi), or septicemia. Hemolytic *Escherichia coli* is often isolated from diseased kidneys and incriminated as the etiologic agent (Fig. 14–3). Other enterobacteria present in fecal flora can also cause infection of the urinary tract, similar to urinary tract infections in other species.

Diagnosis. The condition is diagnosed by the presence of blood, leukocytes, renal tubular or white blood cell casts and bacteria in urine collected by sterile techniques. It must be differentiated from lower urinary infections, which is sometimes difficult. Acute onset may be noted clinically by anorexia, fever, and depression.

Treatment. Supportive fluid therapy is essential because the animals are often anorexic and have reduced fluid intake. Broad-spectrum antibiotics are indicated to treat the infection. Use of parenteral gentamycin (5 mg/kg once daily) and ampicillin (10 mg/kg twice daily) to treat urinary tract infections, including pyelonephritis, is often successful. Treatment for 7 to 10 days is essential.

CYSTIC KIDNEYS

Cystic kidneys were observed at necropsy in 5 of 50 animals. The cysts had a maximum diameter of 3 mm, and were located in the juxtamedullary region.[4] We have also frequently diagnosed kidney cysts in ferrets. Clinical signs are not associated with these lesions, which are presumed to be congenital in origin (Fig. 14–4).

Recently, polycystic kidneys were diagnosed at postmortem in a 3-year-old pet ferret.[22] The animal was presented

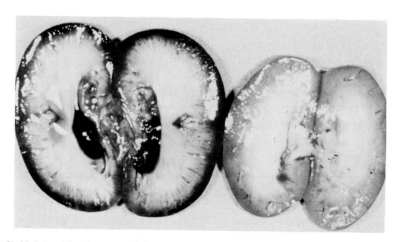

Fig. 14–3. Unilateral involvement of the left kidney with pyelonephritis and renal vein thrombus.

with a history of multiple seizures over the preceding 12 months. Radiographically, the abdomen had a diffuse ground-glass appearance indicative of peritoneal effusion. The animal was euthanized and necropsied. Fluid was present in the abdomen, and both kidneys were enlarged, with multiple cysts present in the cortex and medulla. Histologically, the kidney contained cystic spaces of various sizes lined with cuboidal epithelium. There was fibrosis of intervening renal tissue, with multifocal infiltration of lymphocytes. Renal cysts may be developmental, hereditary, or acquired.[23] Kidney cysts in ferrets most frequently appear in the absence of other concurrent abnormalities, making a hereditary etiology unlikely.[22]

Bilateral multiple cortical cysts must be distinguished from those of polycystic disease. Cortical renal cysts usually have an irregular distribution, versus the diffuse involvement in polycystic disease. Also, polycystic disease usually produces cysts in other organs, particularly the liver, in which cystic bile ducts are often present. Family history and renal function are also important in distinguishing renal cortical cysts from those of polycystic disease.

In the pet ferret, the relationship between seizures and renal disease could not be firmly established. The episodes of seizures may have been caused by uremic encephalopathy, but the brain was unavailable for examination.[24]

CHRONIC INTERSTITIAL NEPHRITIS

Ferrets, like dogs and cats, can suffer from chronic interstitial nephritis. Older pet ferrets are susceptible to the disease. Clinical signs and prognosis are similar to those described for the dog and cat. Polydipsia and polyuria may be observed in advanced cases, as well as weight loss. Clinically, ferrets can also present with

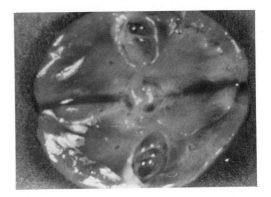

Fig. 14–4. Multiple cysts in the kidney of a ferret.

signs compatible with those of glomerulonephropathy; in some cases this is caused by Aleutian disease (see Chap. 11).

UROLITHIASIS

This disease is reported commonly in ferrets and, like pyelonephritis, can occasionally be seen with bacterial urinary infections.[25]

Diagnosis. The condition is diagnosed clinically by frequent urination, licking of the genital area, difficult urination, and occasionally complete urinary blockage in male ferrets. Urethral calculi can be encountered secondary to the bacterial infection. Red blood cells, leukocytes, and urinary crystals also are noted on urinalysis.

Treatment. Treatment is generally the same as that for cats suffering from feline urolithiasis syndrome. Patency of the urinary system is required to prevent electrolyte imbalance and uremia. Difficulty may be encountered, however, in catheterizing male ferrets because of the os penis. Sedation or anesthesia is routinely required, and urethrostomy may be necessary. Transcutaneous centesis of the bladder to relieve bladder distension can be used as a temporary measure. Antibiotics and urinary acidifiers may also be used. Renal function must be monitored closely. Salting of food may be used to increase fluid intake. Dietary management may also be similar to that used to treat the disease in cats—for example, reduction of the amount of ash in the diet. It is not known whether ferrets are susceptible to herpesvirus-induced urolithiasis, as suggested in cats.[26]

URINARY CALCULI

The disease was described in ferrets,[25] and also occurs frequently in another mustelid, the mink.[27,28]

Prevalence and Control. In one study, which reviewed 43 necropsies on ferrets dying from various causes, 6 (14%) of the animals were found to have urinary calculi.[25] Renal calculi up to 0.8 cm in diameter were found in three cases, and cystic calculi up to 1.5 cm in diameter were noted in four cases. Similar cases were observed in ferrets maintained in our colony (Fig. 14–5). Two of the calculi were composed of magnesium ammonium phosphate (struvite), which is formed in alkaline urine and is often considered to be produced by urea-splitting bacteria.[29] Urinary acidifiers are therefore recommended in treatment of these calculi as well as treatment of the underlying bacterial infection. In cats, however, di-

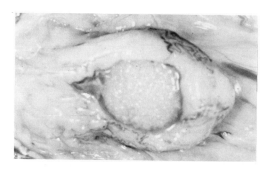

Fig. 14–5. Single large struvite calculus filling the lumen of the bladder.

etary ingredients are increasingly cited as contributing significantly to urolithiasis and calculi formation. Because many ferrets are maintained on commercial cat rations, it is conceivable that diets and mineral metabolism that predispose cats to urolithiasis may also have the same effect in ferrets.[30]

ACCESSORY URINARY BLADDER

A ferret with an accessory urinary bladder was observed clinically, and the diagnosis confirmed at necropsy. On abdominal palpation a 1- to 2-cm cystic structure was palpated in the posterior part of the abdomen. The saclike structure had a lumen that communicated with the lumen of the normal bladder.[31]

ENDOCRINE SYSTEM

Endocrine disorders in the ferret include hyperadrenocorticism, insulinoma, and diabetes mellitus.

HYPERADRENOCORTICISM (CUSHING'S SYNDROME)

This disease is caused by functional adrenal adenoma, carcinoma, or pituitary tumor (causing bilateral adrenocortical hyperplasia), each of which results in excessive production of glucocorticoids by the adrenal cortex. Hyperadrenocorticism was reported recently in the ferret.[32] The disease has many of the same clinical and clinicopathologic features as those described for Cushing's syndrome in dog and humans.[33,34]

Clinical Signs and Pathology. Ferrets with the disease have progressive hair loss, signs of weakness, muscle atrophy, polydipsia, and polyuria. In the case reported, the ferret had striking bilateral symmetric hair loss over 80% of the body (Fig. 14–6). The alopecia extended from the neck to the tip of the tail, but did not involve the head or extremities. The skin is thin, and the abdominal vessels may be prominent, as well as superficial abrasions.[32] Ferrets suffering from the disease have increased susceptibility to infectious diseases, and may have pneumonia or septicemia.

Pathologic lesions are either adrenocortical adenoma or carcinoma; the contralateral adrenal is atrophied. The disease can also be caused by a pituitary tumor. Lymph nodes have lymphocyte depletion; skin and muscle mass are atrophied. Hair follicles are sparse, and collagen in the skin is irregularly arranged. Other organs may have inflammatory changes caused by secondary microbial infection.

Diagnosis. An evaluation of clinicopathologic data is helpful in establishing a diagnosis. Significant lymphopenia and eosinopenia are attributed to elevated glucocorticoid levels. This phenomenon, seen in the ferret, is well documented in Cushing's syndrome in humans and dogs.

ACTH stimulation and the dexamethasone suppression response are used to evaluate the response of the pituitary and adrenal glands in dogs tentatively diagnosed as having hyperadrenocorticism, and appears to be useful in ferrets with the disease (see Chap. 7). Twenty-four hour urine-free cortisol is a sensitive and specific screening test for Cushing's syndrome in human patients, and perhaps could be used in ferrets. The use of this test, however, requires housing the ferret in a metabolism cage.

Treatment and Prognosis. Long-term prognosis and treatment modalities in the ferret with hyperadrenocorticism are unknown. Adrenal or pituitary tumors can be removed surgically.[33–35] Medical treatment with *o,p'*-DDD (mitotane) may be attempted.[34]

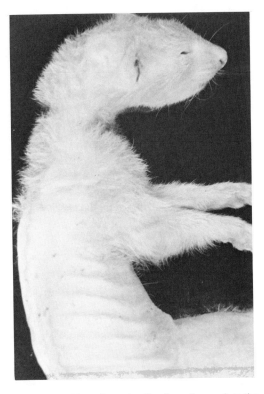

Fig. 14–6. Alopecia, extending from the neck to the tip of the tail in a ferret with hyperadrenocorticism.

The ferret should be evaluated prior to treatment to confirm the presence of hyperadrenocorticism, to differentiate bilateral adrenocortical hyperplasia from adrenal tumor, and to recognize primary or secondary conditions (e.g., possible hypothyroidism, diabetes mellitus, microbial infections, CNS dysfunction, and degenerative changes resulting from excessive glucocorticoid production).[36]

PANCREATIC INSULIN-SECRETING TUMOR (INSULINOMA)

The term is used to describe a functional tumor of the beta cells of the islets of Langerhans, which produce excessive quantities of insulin. This disease was described in eight ferrets,[37–39] and I have observed an additional case.

Clinical Signs and Pathology. The increased surge of insulin results in increased mobilization of glucose into cells, resulting in hypoglycemia and neurologic dysfunction. Neurologic signs are characteristically intermittent, except in late stages of the disease, in which the hypoglycemia is nearly constant. Stimuli such as exercise, excitement, and eating may precipitate seizures. Other related signs may be generalized weakness, apparent hindlimb weakness, generalized muscle twitching, and a syndrome of disorientation and apparent blindness.[40] Prolonged or severe hypoglycemia may cause brain damage as a result of hypoxia.

Beta cell carcinoma was recently reported in a 0.8-kg 6-year-old castrated male ferret and in a 7-year-old neutered female ferret.[37,38] The ferrets were examined because of weakness, ataxia, and dehydration and, in the second ferret, seizures. Hypoglycemia was detected, and the male ferret responded favorably to corticosteroids, fluid therapy, and oral glucose. The female ferret responded for 2 weeks to 50% glucose solution orally, but relapsed and was euthanized at the request of her owner.

In another series, insulin-secreting tumors were found in six ferrets, 5 to 6 years of age. Clinical signs in five animals consisted of episodes of generalized weakness, severe lethargy and weakness, and hypersalivation, but neither focal nor grand mal seizures were observed.[41] Surgical laparotomy revealed multiple pancreatic nodules in four of the ferrets and a single nodule in the remaining two, with no signs of metastasis. The tumors were removed in all ferrets, and histopathologic diagnosis revealed islet cell hyperplasia and adenoma, with transition to invasive carcinoma. One ferret died postoperatively.

Diagnosis. Plasma insulin levels can now be determined in many commercial laboratories. Unfortunately, fasting immunoreactive insulin (IRI) concentrations in normal ferrets have not been determined. In fasting hypoglycemia in the dog resulting from other causes, the plasma IRI concentration is usually normal or below normal, whereas it is usually normal or above normal in dogs with insulinoma.[41] It is also helpful to measure the amended insulin:glucose ratio (AIGR).* In one case the AIGR was 362.5, whereas in the second case it was calculated to infinity (given a fasting glucose level of 30). This was strongly suggestive of insulinoma in both cases.[42]

The differential diagnosis in ferrets with CNS signs must include epilepsy, rabies, distemper, listeriosis, severe liver disease, CNS tumor, lead poisoning, hypoparathyroidism, spinal disease, and hypoadrenocorticism. There are also other causes (not as well recognized) that should be included in the differential diagnosis if hypoglycemia is seen in ferrets:[40,43]

1. Functional hypoglycemia (no recognizable lesion): neonatal hypoglycemia; starvation
2. Hepatic enzyme deficiencies: Von Gierke's disease (glycogen storage disease, type I); Cori's disease (glycogen storage disease, type III); other enzyme defects
3. Exogenous agents: insulin excess; sulfonylurea administration; ethanol; salicylate ingestion; propranolol
4. Bacterial shock
5. Organic hypoglycemia (recognizable lesion): severe hepatic disease; adrenocortical insufficiency; renal failure; cardiac disease-induced hypoglycemia; extrapancreatic tumor-induced hypoglycemia; hyperinsulinism secondary to islet cell tumor of the pancreas

Treatment. Surgical removal of the tumor is the treatment of choice. In dogs (and perhaps ferrets), however, this is often only a palliative measure, because the malignancy of this tumor is high and early metastasis is common. Also, the tumor is sometimes not visible grossly.

$$* \text{ AIGR} = \frac{\text{serum insulin } (\mu l/ml) \times 100}{\text{plasma glucose (mg/dl)} - 30}$$

Postoperative monitoring and supportive care are indicated, including fluid and antibiotic therapy. Pancreatic function tests and glucose and BUN levels should be monitored.[44,45] In one ferret, a 5-mm nodule on the pancreas was discovered by exploratory laparotomy and excised. Histopathologic findings confirmed a pancreatic beta cell tumor (see Chap. 15, Neoplasia in Ferrets). The animal continued to be hypoglycemic but was sent home on oral therapy, including prednisolone (0.2 mg twice daily) and diazoxide (5 mg twice daily) as insulin antagonists. Frequent meals also helped to prevent weakness and collapse in one ferret.[37] In another five ferrets who were followed clinically after removal of islet cell nodules, all remained hypoglycemic and hyperinsulinemic postoperatively. All ferrets required prednisone (1.25 mg once or twice daily) and diazoxide (2.5–5 mg twice daily) to control clinical signs. One ferret with progressive clinical signs was euthanized 9 months after surgery; necropsy revealed metastasis of the islet cell tumor to regional lymph nodes and the liver.[39]

DIABETES MELLITUS

Diabetes mellitus is a complex metabolic disease characterized by hyperglycemia and glycosuria. It is described as a naturally occurring entity in humans and in various domestic and wild animals. Numerous animal models of diabetes mellitus were studied in an attempt to understand this common disease process.[46,47] Although the disease was not reported in the domestic ferret, it was diagnosed clinically.[48] Also, a case of diabetes mellitus was described in the black-footed North American ferret, *Mustela nigripes*.[49]

Clinical Signs and Diagnosis. Weight loss, polyphagia, polydipsia, and polyuria were observed in a 5-year-old, wild-caught, male black-footed ferret.[49] In addition, urinalysis indicated glycosuria and ketonuria. Blood chemistry analysis revealed hyperglycemia (724 mg/100 ml), an elevated serum glutamic-oxaloacetic transaminase (SGOT) level (780 U/L), and increased lactic dehydrogenase (2739 U).

Treatment. The objectives of treatment are to maintain the animal in a symptom-free state, and active. Attention is given to the animal's diet, body weight, activity and, if necessary, use of insulin.[50] In the case of the ferret mentioned above, it was given a maintenance diet in constant amounts. Water and food consumption, urine production, and urine glucose, ketones, pH, and protein levels were recorded daily. Because of the difficulty in obtaining blood samples, CBC, blood glucose, and BUN levels could not be monitored on a regular basis. Insulin therapy (2–3 U daily) maintained the animal for a 3-month period before its condition deteriorated. The animal's health was also compromised from a metastatic adenocarcinoma of the sweat gland in the perineal area, glomerulonephritis, and arteriosclerosis. Anorexia and dehydration developed, and the animal died in spite of intensive therapy. Prognosis in ferrets with diabetic mellitus should be guarded until further studies determine the insulin requirements of normal and diabetic ferrets.

Recently, a 4-year-old 1110-g male pet ferret was diagnosed as having diabetes mellitus.[50] The animal had polyuria and polydipsia. Although the animal was on 5 U of NPH Insulin, there were periods of hyperglycemia and ketosis. The cause of insulin resistance has not been determined. Clearly, more reports of diabetes mellitus in ferrets will be forthcoming, and will allow a better understanding of treatment modalities for this disease.

Pathology. In the diabetic black-footed ferret, special histologic stains of the pancreas indicated an adequate number of beta granules in the islets of Langerhans. It was speculated that the diabetes was caused by a lack of release of synthesized insulin or by diminished effectiveness of the secreted insulin.[49] For a more detailed description of the pathology of diabetes mellitus in animals, refer to other texts on veterinary pathology.[51,52]

LYMPHATIC SYSTEM

Lymphatic disorders in the ferret include enzootic malignant granulomatosis and idiopathic hypersplenism.

ENZOOTIC MALIGNANT GRANULOMATOSIS

This disease was described only once in the European literature. Its etiology is unknown.[53]

Epizootiology and Control. During a period extending from January 1948 to January 1951, 142 of 1227 ferrets examined were diagnosed as having the disease. The ferrets were being used in Denmark to study various viral diseases. Prior to the outbreak, the breeding colony had not experienced significant mortality for a number of years. The disease affected animals 6 months to 1 year of age.[53] Bacterial examination of lesions, including culture for *Mycobacterium* (as well as for other infectious agents), was consistently negative. Transmission studies using ferrets, mink, mice, guinea pigs, and rabbits were equally unrewarding.

Clinical Signs. In some cases the affected ferrets had protracted loss of appetite, weight loss, and eventual cachexia, leading to death. Many animals, however, had no clinical signs, and the disease was diagnosed at necropsy in ferrets used for other experiments.

Diagnosis. Because the etiology of the disease is unknown, diagnosis is based on gross and histopathologic findings. Grossly, nodules of varying size, from several millimeters to 2 cm, with a consistency from fibrous to fleshy, were found in mesenteric lymph nodes, peripheral lymph nodes and, less frequently, in other organs. Histologically, tissue was composed of granulation tissue with areas of connective tissues, blood vessels, lymphocytes, lymphoblastic cells, plasma cells, polymorphonuclear cells, histiocytes, fibroblasts, and large epithelioid cells. Giant cells were absent. The lesions suggested infectious granuloma produced by an intestinal route to the mesenteric lymph nodes and to other organs, most frequently the spleen and liver. Because infectious etiologies were not demonstrated, however, the disorder was classified as enzootic malignant granulomatosis of unknown etiology.

Treatment. Methods of treatment and prevention are unknown.

IDIOPATHIC HYPERSPLENISM

Hypersplenism is a term used to denote splenomegaly associated with cytopenia that reverses after splenectomy.[54,55] The bone marrow is normal or hypercellular.

Idiopathic hypersplenism was recently reported in a 3-year-old spayed female ferret.[58] The ferret had a palpable abdominal mass, polyphagia, polydipsia, and polyuria. She also had weight loss, flea infestation, pale and slightly icteric mucous membranes, and lethargy. Clinical pathologic examination revealed pancytopenia with regenerative anemia; the red blood cell volume (PCV) fluctuated between 12 and 18% (normal, 42–61%), and the platelet count was markedly lowered, from 10,000 to 38,000/μl, determined on days 4 and 7 after hospital admission. The mass was found to be an enlarged spleen by radiography. Whole blood transfusion (10 ml) did not alter the PCV. Because the pancytopenia persisted despite supportive therapy, tetracycline (25 mg/kg orally, twice daily), and prednisolone acetate (2.2 mg/kg, subcutaneously), the spleen was removed surgically. After splenectomy, the ferret's PCV, leukocyte count, and platelet count increased, and her general health improved. The spleen was grossly enlarged, 25 cm long (normal, 6–8 cm) and turgid. Microscopically, the spleen retained normal architecture with foci of necrosis. Extramedullary hematopoiesis was marked, but there was no evidence of myelopoiesis or megakaryocytopoiesis. Mesenteric lymph nodes examined histologically were normal. The ferret remained healthy 20 months after splenectomy.

To determine whether removal of an enlarged spleen reverses pancytopenia, methods that demonstrate splenic hypersequestration must be used; these include increased splenic uptake of chromium-labeled RBC or epinephrine-induced splenic contractions followed by an exaggerated rise in PCV.[55,56] Differential diagnosis in idiopathic hypersplenism in ferrets includes lymphosarcoma or other neoplasms of the spleen, autoimmune hemolytic anemia, Aleutian disease, estrogen-induced pancytopenia, and bacterial sepsis. Enlarged spleens, and splenic rupture causing death, were cited in ferrets with lymphosarcoma.[57,58]

RESPIRATORY AND CARDIOVASCULAR SYSTEMS

In addition to other disorders mentioned previously in conjunction with the respiratory and cardiovascular systems, the ferret may suffer from subpleural histiocytosis and cardiomyopathy.

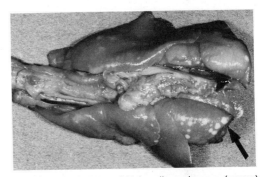

Fig. 14–7. Multiple whitish-yellow plaques (*arrow*) extending above the surface of the lobe of a ferret lung.

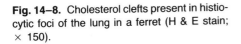

Fig. 14–8. Cholesterol clefts present in histiocytic foci of the lung in a ferret (H & E stain; × 150).

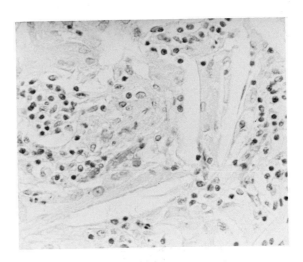

SUBPLEURAL HISTIOCYTOSIS

Small yellow to white foci can be observed in the lungs of ferrets at necropsy (Fig. 14–7). Histologically, these are subpleural emphysematous lesions with macrophages occluding alveoli.[11] Subpleural histiocytosis, described grossly as pale grey subpleural plaques, was also observed in control ferrets and in ferrets administered estrogen.[59] We have also observed this condition in ferrets, and histologically have seen cholesterollike clefts in portions of the involved lung (Fig. 14–8). The etiology of the condition is unknown.

CARDIOMYOPATHY

Cardiomyopathies are usually defined as myocardial diseases of unknown etiology, although secondary cardiomyopa-

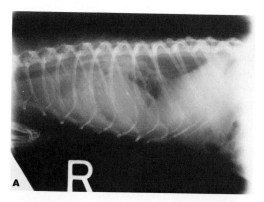

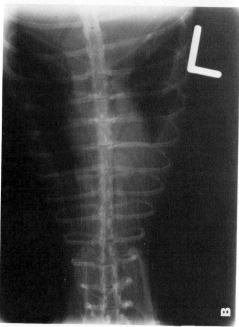

Fig. 14–9. Lateral (*A*) and ventrodorsal (*B*) thoracic radiographs reveal severe bilateral pleural effusion and cardiomegaly. (Lipman, N., and Fox, J.G.: Clinical, functional, and pathologic changes associated with a case of dilatative cardiomyopathy in a ferret. Lab. Anim. Sci., *37*:210, 1987.)

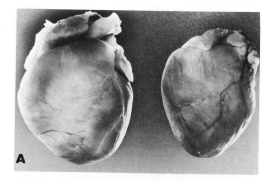

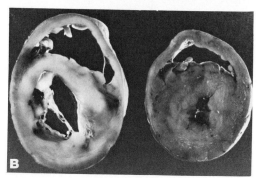

Fig. 14–10. *A* and *B*, Heart from a ferret with cardiomyopathy on the left and from a ferret of the same sex and similar age and body weight on the right. These are formalin-fixed specimens. The intact heart on the left is larger and has a rounded profile. In cross section, both ventricles are dilated and the ventricular free walls and interventricular septum are thin in the heart on the left as compared with the heart on the right. The pale areas in the myocardium of the heart on the left correspond to areas of fibrosis found on histologic examination. (Lipman, N., and Fox, J.G.: Clinical, functional, and pathologic changes associated with a case of dilatative cardiomyopathy in a ferret. Lab. Anim. Sci., *37*:210, 1987.)

thies are often associated with infectious agents, particularly viruses.[60,61] Primary cardiomyopathies, those with undefined etiologies, are further classified according to their functional, anatomic, and pathophysiologic characteristics. Dilatative cardiomyopathy is increasingly recognized as a cause of congestive heart failure in the ferret, as well as in other species.[62-64]

Clinical Signs and Diagnosis. Ferrets presenting with cardiomyopathy have weight loss and lethargy of several months duration, despite adequate dietary intake. Radiographically, an enlarged globoid cardiac silhouette, signs of pleural effusion, pulmonary congestion, and edema are observed (Fig. 14–9). The animal is often dyspneic, and fatigues easily after exercising.[62,63] Hepatomegaly and splenomegaly are usually present on abdominal palpation. Echocardiographic findings commonly include dilatation of all four cardiac chambers, decrease in cardiac output, fractional shortening, and contractility. Electrocardiograms can indicate either a bradycardia or tachycardia, premature complexes, tall and wide QRS complexes, and ST segment depression.[60,61,65]

Treatment. Furosemide (2.5–4 mg/kg IM twice daily) and digoxin elixir (0.01 mg/kg orally twice daily) were used in ferrets with cardiomyopathy to decrease pulmonary edema and to improve cardiac function. Digoxin was increased gradually until a serum level of 1.3 mg/ml was reached 10 days after initiation of treatment.[63] Clinical improvement may or may not be observed. Treatment failure in other species with severe congestive heart failure is common; in our experience with ferrets, this idiopathic primary cardiomyopathy treatment is palliative with a fairly rapid clinical course, and prognosis is guarded to poor. Differential diagnosis includes congestive heart failure caused by *Dirofilaria immitis*.

Pathology. Gross observation reveals dilated ventricles and atria, with thin interventricular septum and ventricular free walls (Fig. 14–10). Hydrothorax is a common finding, with fluid volume often in excess of 100 ml (a clear serosanguinous fluid). On cytologic examination, the fluid contains few inflammatory and red blood cells. The liver is firm, dark red, and slightly enlarged. Ascites may or may not be present. Histologically, multifocal myocardial degeneration, necrosis, and fibrosis are common findings.[66] These lesions are seen in atria, ventricles, and the interventricular septum. Muscle fibers have loss of striation, of staining intensity, and of fibers. Mild to moderate infiltration of macrophages, lymphocytes, plasma cells, and occasional polymorphonuclear cells are seen in areas of myocardial necrosis and degeneration.

NERVOUS SYSTEM

Disorders of the nervous system in the ferret include Creutzfeldt-Jakob disease, cataracts, idiopathic seizures and ataxia, and posterior paralysis.

CREUTZFELDT-JAKOB DISEASE

Four diseases are classified as slow onset virus spongiform encephalopathies: scrapie in sheep, transmissible mink encephalopathy (TME), and kuru and Creutzfeldt-Jakob disease (CJD) in humans. CJD is transmissible to animals in the laboratory, and TME is experimentally infectious to albino ferrets (see Chap. 17).[67] Ferrets may recover from the clinical disease, although the brain remains infectious to mink.

A tenuous association with ferret contact and development of CJD in humans was proposed.[68,69] In one case, a 63-year-old man was bitten on the thumb by a feral ferret who had been taken home as a pet. Approximately 2 years later the man died of histologically proven CJD after a 6-month history of typical CJD symptoms. The clinically normal ferret was killed and submitted for necropsy and histologic examination. No spongiform changes were noted in the brain, although a lymphocytic infiltrate around several capillaries and a leptomeningeal vein were observed. Frozen brain was inoculated into four different species of monkeys and a cat. As of this writing, the surviving animals were asymptomatic and the two dead animals had no spongiform encephalopathy.[69]

In an additional 41 human cases with histologically confirmed CJD, two kept ferrets. One, a woman who died in 1971, had a husband who kept ferrets from 1943 to 1956 and from 1960 to 1965; her chief contact with the ferrets was washing their food dishes. In the second case, a 67-year-old man who died in 1975 of CJD had used ferrets for rabbiting as a young man and had kept ferrets from 1950 to 1955. A third probable case of CJD was a 61-year-old man who had kept ferrets for many years and allowed a pet ferret to roam freely underneath his shirt. He had had no contact with ferrets for 10 years prior to his death. Their source as a reservoir for infection of CJD, however, is not proven, nor is there further documentation in the literature associating ferret ownership with CJD in humans.

CATARACTS

There are a number of causes of cataracts in humans and domestic animals, including metabolic, hereditary, congenital, infectious, and traumatic etiologies. Juvenile cataracts were reported in ferrets.[70] They may be congenital or hereditary in origin. In one breeding colony, the incidence in juvenile animals was estimated at 0.5%.[71] Another colony of ferrets used for biomedical research also had a low incidence of cataracts. Five cases of unilateral cataracts were reported, which caused blindness in the affected eye and, according to the authors, interfered with the animals' ability to eat from a bowl. Another ferret was diagnosed as having bilateral cataracts. Possible etiologies were not discussed.[4] A case of bilateral cataracts in a pet ferret was also reported.[72] The cataracts appeared to involve both the nucleus and cortex of the lens. Repeated urinalysis and clinical examination indicated the animal was not diabetic.

IDIOPATHIC SEIZURES AND ATAXIA

Occasionally ferrets have seizures of undetermined etiology. A neurologic syndrome of suspected viral etiology was recently described in ferrets. Signs included pyrexia (41.7–43.4°C), tremor, and ataxia. The animals recovered after supportive therapy.[73]

Seizures and ataxia were reported in a 3-year-old male neutered ferret. The animal was diagnosed as having bilateral polycystic kidneys. The CNS signs may have been caused by uremic encephalopathy. Unfortunately, the brain was unavailable for examination.[74] Differential diagnoses would include rabies, listeriosis, distemper, fungal encephalitis, toxoplasmosis, insulinoma, and hypoadrenocorticism.

POSTERIOR PARALYSIS

Occasionally ferrets present with posterior paralysis accompanied by incontinence. Posterior paralysis has several causes, including hemivertebrae, vertebral fractures, intervertebral disc diseases,[75] hematomyelia associated with prolonged estrus,[59,76] or myelitis caused by fungal infections or *Mycobacterium*.[64,77] Detailed clinical examination, clinical pathology, radiography, and response to supportive therapy will confirm the diagnosis. The condition may recur, and long-term prognosis is guarded if the spinal cord is severely damaged. The posterior ataxia and weakness seen in distemper must be distinguished from the clinical entities listed above. Also, a posterior paralysis and weakness were associated with a demyelinating disease in ferrets raised in New Zealand; the disease was linked to Aleutian disease, but definitive studies were not performed[14] (see Chap. 11).

CONGENITAL MALFORMATION STUDIES

In 1985, McLain and associates[78] compiled demographic information on ferrets from a commercial breeding farm.

Although litter size was found to be greater in young primiparous females (10.3 ± 0.2) than in older third parity females (8.1 ± 0.1), the rate of congenital malformations was higher for females of low previous parity (0–2) than for females with 3 or more pregnancies. The overall rate of congenital malformations was low (1%), 24-hour neonatal mortality was 7%, and mortality from birth to weaning was 20%. In two other studies[79,80] the incidence of congenital malformations was reported as 3%. The most common defects seen in the three studies were cleft palate, cranioschisis, anencephaly (and exencephaly), neuroschisis, meningocele, spina bifida, gastroschisis, corneal dermoids, cryptorchidism, anuria, and amelia. Albino and pigmented ferrets did not differ in the occurrence of congenital malformations.

REFERENCES

1. Berkovitz, B.K.B.: Supernumerary deciduous incisors and the order of eruption of the incisor teeth in the albino ferret. J. Zool., 155:445, 1968.
2. Berkovitz, B.K.B., and Thomson, P.: Observations on the etiology of supernumerary upper incisors of the albino ferret (*Mustela putorius*). Arch. Oral Biol., 18:457, 1973.
3. Bateman, J.A.: Supernumerary deciduous teeth in mustelids. Mammal Rev., 1:81, 1970.
4. Andrews, P.L.R., Illman, O., and Mellersh, A.: Some observations of anatomical abnormalities and disease states in a population of 350 ferrets (*Mustela furo*). Z. Versuchstierkd., 21:346, 1979.
5. King, J.D., and Glover, R.E.: The relative effects of dietary constituents and other factors upon calculus and gingival disease in the ferret. J. Pathol. Bacteriol., 57:353, 1945.
6. King, J.D., Rowles, S.L., Thewlis, J., and Little, K.: Chemical and x-ray examination of deposits removed from the teeth of golden hamsters and ferrets. J. Dent. Res., 34:650, 1955.
7. Steinberg, A.D., Alvarez, J.A., and Jeffay, H.: Lack of relationship between the degree of induced hyperplasia and the concentration of diphenylhydantoin in various tissues of ferrets. J. Dent. Res., 51:657, 1972.
8. Moore, P.A., Smudski, J.K.W., and Hopper, S.: Diphenylhydantoin-induced gingival hyperplasia in ferrets; a precautionary note. J. Dent. Res., 58:1812, 1979.
9. Bauck, L.B.: Salivary mucocele in two ferrets. Mod. Vet. Pract., 66:337, 1985.
10. O'Brien, J.A., and Harvey, C.E.: Diseases of the upper airway. In Textbook of Veterinary Internal Medicine, Chap. 39. 2nd ed. Edited by S.J. Ettinger. Philadelphia, W.B. Saunders, 1983.
11. Hammond, J., Jr., and Chesterman, F.C.: The ferret. In The Universities Federation for Animal Welfare Handbook on the Care and Management of Laboratory Animals, p. 345. London, Churchill Livingstone, 1972.
12. Diseases of the fitch. Surveillance, 11:28, 1984.
13. Fox, J.G., Goad, M.E.P., and Hotaling, L.I.: Gastric ulcers in ferrets. Lab. Anim. Sci., 36:562, 1986.

14. Twedt, D.C.: Gastric ulcers. *In* Current Veterinary Therapy VIII. Edited by R.W. Kirk. Philadelphia, W.B. Saunders, 1983.

15. Goodwin, C.S., Armstrong, J.A., and Marshall, B.J.: *Campylobacter pyloridis*, gastritis and peptic ulceration. J. Clin. Pathol., *39*:353, 1986.

16. Fox, J.G., Edrise, B.M., Cabot, E.B., et al.: Campylobacter-like organisms isolated from gastric mucosa of ferrets. Am. J. Vet. Res., *47*:236, 1986.

17. Orton, E.C., and Muir, W.W.: Hemodynamics during experimental gastric dilatation-volvulus in dogs. Am. J. Vet. Res., *44*:1512, 1983.

18. Orton, E.C.: Gastric dilatation-volvulus. *In* Current Veterinary Therapy IX. Edited by R.W. Kirk. Philadelphia, W.B. Saunders, 1986.

19. Kunstyr, I.: Lethal occlusion of the gastrointestinal tract in ferrets (*Mustela putorius furo*) due to aberrant voracity. Z. Versuchstierkd., *24*: 231, 1982.

20. Hammond, J., Jr.: Ferret mortality on a pellet diet. J. Anim. Tech. Assoc., *12*:35, 1971.

21. Hammond, J., Jr.: The ferret as a research animal. Carnivore Genet. Newsletter, 6:126, 1969.

22. Dillberger, J.E.: Polycystic kidneys in a ferret. J. Am. Vet. Med. Assoc., *186*:74, 1985.

23. Bernstein, J.: A classification of renal cysts. *In* Cystic Diseases of the Kidney. Edited by K. Gardner. New York, John Wiley & Sons, 1976.

24. Wolf, A.M.: Canine uremic encephalopathy. J. Am. Anim. Hosp. Assoc., *16*:735, 1980.

25. Nguyen, H.T., Moreland, A.F., and Shields, R.P.: Urolithiasis in ferrets (*Mustela putorius*). Lab. Anim. Sci., *29*:243, 1979.

26. Fabricant, C.G.: Feline urolithiasis. *In* Diseases of the Cat. Vol. 1. Edited by J. Holzworth. Philadelphia, W.B. Saunders, 1987.

27. Nielsen, I.M.: Urolithiasis in mink. Pathology, bacteriology and experimental production. J. Urol., *75*:602, 1956.

28. Leoschke, W.L., Zekria, E., and Elvchjem, C.A.: Composition of urinary calculi from mink. Proc. Soc. Exp. Biol. Med., *80*:291, 1952.

29. Griffith, D.P.: Struvite stones. Kidney Int., *13*: 372, 1978.

30. O'Donnell, J.A., and Hayes, K.C.: Nutrition and nutritional disorders. *In* Diseases of the Cat. Edited by J. Holy. Philadelphia, W.B. Saunders, 1987.

31. Fox, J.G., Lipman, N., Murphy, J.C., and Goad, M.P.: Unpublished observations, 1987.

32. Fox, J.G., et al.: Hyperadrenocorticism in a ferret. J. Am. Vet. Med. Assoc., *191*:343, 1987.

33. Carpenter, P.C.: Cushing's syndrome: Update of diagnosis and management. Clin. Proc., *61*: 49, 1986.

34. Feldman, E.C.: The adrenal cortex. *In* Textbook of Veterinary Internal Medicine. Vol. 2. 2nd ed. Edited by S.J. Ettinger. Philadelphia, W.B. Saunders, 1983.

35. Owens, J.M., and Drucker, W.D.: Hyperadrenocorticism in the dog: Canine Cushing's syndrome. Vet. Clin. North Amer., *7*:583, 1977.

36. Schechter, R.D.: Hyperadrenocorticism. *In* Current Veterinary Therapy, VI. Edited by R.W. Kirk. Philadelphia, W.B. Saunders, 1977.

37. Kauffman, J., Schwarz, P., and Mero, K.: Pancreatic beta cell tumor in a ferret. J. Am. Vet. Med. Assoc., *185*:998, 1984.

38. Luttgen, P.J., Storts, R.W., Rogers, K.S., and Morton, L.D.: Insulinoma in a ferret. J. Am. Vet. Med. Assoc., *189*:920, 1986.

39. Quesenberry, K.E., Peterson, M.E., Moroff, S.D., and Scarelli, T.D.: Pancreatic insulin-secreting tumor in the ferret (abstract). *In* Proceedings of the Fifth Annual Veterinary Medical Forum. San Diego, American College of Veterinary Internal Medicine, 1987.

40. Leifer, C.E.: Hypoglycemia. *In* Current Veterinary Therapy, IX. Edited by R.W. Kirk. Philadelphia, W.B. Saunders, 1986.

41. Johnson, R.K., and Atkins, C.E.: Hypoglycemia in the dog. *In* Current Veterinary Therapy, VI. Edited by R.W. Kirk. Philadelphia, W.B. Saunders, 1977.

42. Knowlen, G.G., and Schall, W.D.: The amended insulin-glucose ratio. Is it really better? J. Am. Vet. Med. Assoc., *185*:998, 1984.

43. Leifer, C.E., et al.: Hypoglycemia associated with non-islet cell tumor in 13 dogs. J. Am. Vet. Med. Assoc., *186*:53, 1985.

44. Leifer, C.E., Peterson, M.E., and Matus, R.E.: Insulin-secreting tumor. Diagnosis and medical and surgical management in 55 dogs. J. Am. Vet. Med. Assoc., *188*:60, 1986.

45. Mehlhaff, C.J., et al.: Insulin-producing islet cell neoplasms. Surgical considerations and general management in 35 dogs. J. Am. Anim. Hosp. Assoc., *21*:607, 1985.

46. Like, A.A.: Spontaneous diabetes in animals. *In* The Diabetic Pancreas. Edited by B.W. Volk, and K.F. Wellman. New York, Plenum Press, 1977.

47. Lage, A.L., Mordes, J.P., and Rossini, A.A.: Animal models of diabetes mellitus. Comp. Pathol. Bull., *12*:4, 1980.

48. Hillyer, E.V.: Unpublished observations, 1987.

49. Carpenter, J.W., and Novilla, M.N.: Diabetes mellitus in a black-footed ferret. J. Am. Vet. Med. Assoc., *171*:890, 1977.

50. Feldman, E.C.: Diabetes mellitus. *In* Current Veterinary Therapy, VII. Edited by R.W. Kirk. Philadelphia, W.B. Saunders, 1980.

51. Smith, H.A., Jones, T.C., and Hunt, R.D.: Veterinary Pathology. 4th ed. Philadelphia, Lea & Febiger, 1972.

52. Jubb, K.V.F., and Kennedy, P.C.: Pathology of Domestic Animals. 3rd ed. New York, Academic Press, 1985.

53. Momberg-Jorgensen, H.C.: Enzootic malignant granulomatosis in ferrets. Acta Pathol., *29*:297, 1951.

54. Madewell, B.R., and Feldman, B.F.: Characterization of anemias associated with neoplasia in small animals. J. Am. Vet. Med. Assoc., *176*: 419, 1980.

55. Jacob, H.S.: Hypersplenism. *In* Hematology. Edited by W.J. Williams, et al. New York, McGraw-Hill, 1972.

56. Ferguson, D.C.: Idiopathic hypersplenism in a ferret. J. Am. Vet. Med. Assoc., *186*:693, 1985.

57. Smith, S.H., and Bishop, S.P.: Diagnostic exercise: Lymphoproliferative disorder in a ferret. Lab. Anim. Sci., *35*:291, 1985.

58. Fox, J.G., Lipman, N.S., and Murphy, J.C.: Lymphoma in the ferret. Lab. Anim. Sci., *36*:562, 1986.

59. Bernard, S.L., Leathers, C.W., Brobst, D.F., and Gorham, J.R.: Estrogen-induced bone marrow depression in ferrets. Am. J. Vet. Res., *44*:657, 1983.

60. Dodge, H.T., and Kennedy, J.W.: Cardiac output, cardiac performance, hypertrophy, dilatation, valvular disease, ischemic heart disease, and pericardial disease. *In* Pathological Physiology Mechanisms of Disease. Edited by W.A. Sodeman, and T.M. Sodeman. Philadelphia, W.B. Saunders, 1979.

61. Tilley, L.P., Liu, S., and Fox, P.R.: Myocardial disease. *In* Textbook of Veterinary Internal Medicine. Edited by S.J. Ettinger. Philadelphia, W.B. Saunders, 1983.

62. Ensley, P.K., and Van Winkle, T.: Treatment of congestive heart failure in a ferret. J. Zoo Anim. Med., *13*:23, 1982.

63. Lipman, N., and Fox, J.G.: Clinical, functional, and pathologic changes associated with a case of dilatative cardiomyopathy in a ferret. Lab. Anim. Sci., *37*:210, 1987.

64. Greenlee, P.G., and Stephens, E.: Meningeal cryptococcosis and congestive cardiomyopathy in a ferret. J. Am. Vet. Med. Assoc., *184*:840, 1984.

65. Fox, P.R.: Feline myocardial diseases. *In* Current Veterinary Therapy. Vol. 8. Edited by R.W. Kirk. Philadelphia, W.B. Saunders, 1983.

66. Goad, B., and Fox, J.G.: Unpublished observations, 1986.

67. Marsh, R.F., et al.: A preliminary report on the experimental host range of the transmissible mink encephalopathy agent. J. Infect. Dis., *120*: 713, 1969.

68. Matthews, W.B.: Epidemiology of Creutzfeldt-Jakob disease in England and Wales. J. Neurol. Neurosurg. Psychiatr., *38*:210, 1975.

69. Matthews, W.B., Campbell, M., Hughes, J.T., and Tomlinson, A.H.: Creutzfeldt-Jakob disease and ferrets. Lancet, *2*:828, 1979.

70. Ryland, L.M., and Gorham, J.R.: The ferret and its diseases. J. Am. Vet. Med. Assoc., *173*:1154, 1978.

71. Gorham, J.R.: Personal communication, 1979.

72. Utroska, B., and Austin, W.L.: Bilateral cataracts in a ferret. Vet. Med. Small Anim. Clin., *74*:1176, 1979.

73. Niemi, S.M., Newcomer, C.E., and Fox, J.G.: Neurological syndrome in the ferret (*Mustela putorius furo*). Vet. Rec., *114*:455, 1984.

74. Dillberger, J.E.: Polycystic kidneys in a ferret. J. Am. Vet. Med. Assoc., *186*:74, 1985.

75. Frederick, M.A.: Intervertebral disc syndrome in a domestic ferret. Vet. Med. Small Anim. Clin., *76*:835, 1981.

76. Sherrill, A., and Gorham, J.R.: Bone marrow hypoplasia associated with estrus in ferrets. Lab. Anim. Sci., *35*:280, 1985.

77. Symmers, W.St.C., and Thomson, A.P.D.: Observations on tuberculosis in the ferret (*Mustela furo* L.). J. Comp. Pathol. Therap., *63*:20, 1953.

78. McLain, D.E., et al.: Congenital malformations and variations in reproductive performance in the ferret: Effects of maternal age, color and parity. Lab. Anim. Sci., *35*:251, 1985.

79. Willis, L.S., and Barrow, M.V.: The ferret (*Mustela putorius furo* L.) as a laboratory animal. Lab. Anim. Sci., *21*:712, 1971.

80. Rowlands, I.L.W.: The ferret. *In* Universities Federation of Animal Welfare Handbook on the Care and Management of Laboratory Animals. 3rd ed. London, Baillière, Tindall and Cox, 1967.

chapter 15

NEOPLASIA IN FERRETS

M. E. P. Goad

J. G. Fox

Reports of tumors in domestic and non-domestic ferrets have been increasing since the first published case by Figgs in 1944.[1] As more ferrets are used in biomedical research and are owned as pets, more tumors will be observed in this species. Currently, there are fewer than 30 review articles or single case reports on ferret tumors. To determine tumor prevalence in ferrets more accurately, tumors that are diagnosed clinically and confirmed histologically should be reported.

Tumors in ferrets were observed in animals as young as 1 year old. Most reports are seen in adult ferrets older than 2 years of age. Reports totaled 161 tumors in limited studies of cases from the literature and from the following research institutions and veterinary colleges:

Angell Memorial Animal Hospital (AMAH)
Animal Medical Center (AMC)
Armed Forces Institute of Pathology (AFIP)
Auburn University
Colorado State University (CSU)
Cornell University
Iowa State University (ISU)
Kansas State University (KSU)
Louisiana State University (LSU)
Massachusetts Institute of Technology (MIT)

Mississippi State University (MSU)
Ohio State University (OSU)
University of Illinois (UI)
University of Tennessee (UT)
Washington State University (WSU)
Western College of Veterinary Medicine (WCVM)

Most of these animals were pet ferrets, but some were research animals. Tumors were infrequently induced experimentally in laboratory ferrets. Tumors in these animals are predominantly seen in ferrets kept for more than 1 year or with transplanted tumors.[2]

Primary neoplasms in ferrets were reported in every system except the cardiovascular, respiratory, and nervous systems.

Of 161 reported ferret tumors, 37 (23%) were lymphosarcomas. Lymphosarcoma is the most commonly observed neoplasm of the ferret. The second most common site of tumors is the reproductive tract, but this includes 20 cases of leiomyomas in a single group of ferrets.[3] The third most common system with tumors is the skin. Of 161 tumors reported, 30 were of the skin or subcutaneous tissues.

LYMPHOID AND HEMATOPOIETIC TUMORS

Lymphosarcoma is the most common tumor reported in the ferret (Table 15-1). The types and locations of lymphosarco-

TABLE 15–1. LYMPHOID-HEMATOPOIETIC TUMORS OF FERRETS

Tumor	Type/Site	Number of Animals	Reference
Lymphosarcoma	Undetermined/disseminated	7	AFIP, Cornell, Fox et al.,[4] WCVM[6]
	Undetermined/liver	1	Andrews et al.[5]
	Undetermined/thymus and liver	1	AFIP
	Undetermined/abdomen	2	Auburn, OSU
	Undetermined/mesenteric lymph nodes	1	ISU
	Undetermined/lymph nodes	1	Smith and Bishop[6]
	Undetermined/leukemic, disseminated	2	AFIP, Kenyon and Williams[7]
	Undetermined/leukemic	1	UI
	Lymphocytic/leukemic	1	Altman and Lamborn[8]
	Lymphocytic and prolymphocytic/ leukemic	1	AFIP
	Lymphoblastic/disseminated	7	AFIP, AMAH, Symmers and Thomson,[9] WCVM
	Lymphoblastic/spleen	1	WCVM
Histiocytic	Disseminated	2	AFIP, Fox et al.[4]
Myeloma	Multiple	1	UT
	Plasma blast cell/disseminated	1	Yanoff[10]
	Plasma cell	1	Methiyapun et al.[11]
Megakaryocytic	Liver and spleen	1	AFIP
	Leukemic/disseminated	1	Chowdhury and Shillinger[12]
Myeloid	Granulocytic/spleen	1	AFIP
	Poorly differentiated/spleen	1	AFIP
Hemangiosarcoma	Spleen	2	WCVM
Total:		37	

mas in ferrets are similar to those seen in dogs and cats.[13] Because of restraints imposed by tissue collection and fixation and examination, lymphoid tumors in ferrets were classified nonspecifically, usually by histologic examination of tissues and blood samples. Current methods for determination of lymphosarcoma tumor types are much more specific than previously reported. These techniques include histochemical staining, fluorescent cell typing, ultrastructural examination, and monoclonal and other antibody reactions.

The lymphosarcomas described in ferrets include solid disseminated and leukemic types (Fig. 15–1). Specific diagnosis of cell types from morphology include lymphocytic, prolymphocytic, and lymphoblastic tumors.[9] Diagnosis of lymphosarcoma is based on history, clinical findings and, most importantly, cytology and histology of blood, tissue, and fluid aspirates, and solid tumors. Other

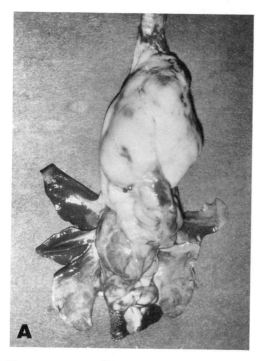

Fig. 15–1. Lymphosarcoma in a ferret with leukemia. The tumor in the cranial mediastinum caused marked dyspnea. *A,* Gross appearance of the cranial mediastinal tumor. Figure 15–1 continued on facing page.

techniques for detecting tumors include electrodiagnostics, radiography, and ultrasound.[14] Clinical signs in ferrets with lymphoid neoplasms are as varied as in other species. Signs and presentations depend on the organ most affected by the tumor.

The older classification of solid versus leukemic, and disseminated versus specific organ involvement, was also seen in affected ferrets.[7,8,13] The following organs were reported involved in disseminated cases: lymph nodes, spleen, thymus, liver, meninges, thoracic and abdominal cavities, and circulating blood. The most commonly involved single organs are the lymph nodes, spleen, and liver.[5]

Preliminary results from one investigator, using chemotherapy to treat lymphosarcomas in ferrets, are encouraging (Dr. Susan Brown, personal communication). In a series of 10 confirmed cases (via biopsy of lymph node or spleen), a regimen of prednisolone (2 mg/kg once daily), vincristine, and cyclophosphamide has resulted in long-term clinical improvement in 8 of 10 ferrets. Vincristine (0.75 mg/m^2, once weekly IV, for a maximum of 4 weeks) is administered using the following doses: 400 to 500 g, female = 0.05 mg; 1 kg, female = 0.07 mg; and 1.5 kg, male = 0.10 mg. Treatment is accomplished by anesthetizing the ferret with 3% isoflurane, inserting a 23-gauge butterfly catheter into the cephalic vein, and delivery of the drug preceded and followed by a 3-cc isotonic saline flush. In addition, 4 oral doses of cyclophosphamide (50 mg/m^2) are given during the first 4 weeks of treatment. Ferrets are monitored each week during treatment for possible toxicity by evaluation of hemograms. Ferrets are maintained on prednisolone for at least 3 months. More clinical studies are required to confirm these observations. For further discussions on chemotherapy for lymphosarcoma, the reader is referred to detailed assessment of this treatment modality in dogs and cats.[14a,b]

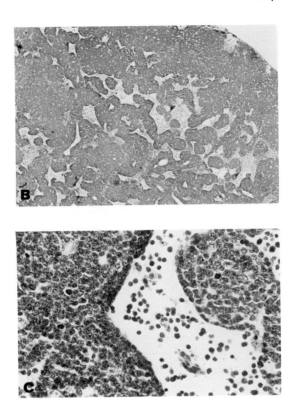

Fig. 15–1, *continued. B,* Tumor mass, lymph node. The tumor cells obliterated the normal architecture of affected lymph nodes. *C,* Tumor consisted of fairly uniform large lymphoblast-type cells.

Most cases of lymphosarcoma in ferrets are seen in adult animals (older than 2 years), and occur as individual cases.[4] Male and female animals and neutered animals are affected equally. Multiple cases from single households or institutions were observed.[4,15]

Potential causes of lymphosarcoma in the ferret, other than spontaneous occurrence, include ferret parvovirus (Aleutian disease virus) and a proposed ferret retrovirus.[15] Ferret parvovirus causes a persistent viral infection of the lymphoid tissues and subsequent interference with normal immune system functions. Over the prolonged course of the infection, the severe interference and stimulation of the immune system by persistent parvoviral infection may result in lymphoid tumors.[7,16]

Evidence exists to suggest a relationship between Aleutian disease and lymphosarcoma in ferrets. From three ferret ranches studied, seven ferrets developed monoclonal gammopathies typical of myelomas.[16] In another study, five of seven ferret kits infected with Aleutian disease virus developed monoclonal hypergammaglobulinemias, and one of these kits subsequently developed disseminated lymphosarcoma.[7]

Other lymphoid-hematopoietic neoplasms reported in ferrets include histiocytic tumors, plasma cell myelomas, megakaryocytic tumors, and granulocytic neoplasms.[10–12] Splenic hemangiosarcomas were also observed.

Therefore, ferrets appear to be most susceptible to lymphoid system tumors. More research should be done to elucidate the pathogenesis of this disease in ferrets. A ferret retrovirus will probably be demonstrated.

REPRODUCTIVE TRACT TUMORS

The second most reported group of tumors in the ferret are those of the reproductive system. Of 136 tumors, 35 were in this organ system (Table 15–2). Ovar-

ian tumors are the most common. Leiomyomas of the ovary were observed in 21 ferrets, and several of these were bilateral. Of these leiomyomas, 20 were from ferrets at a single source.[3] These 20 ferrets may have been exposed to a pre-

TABLE 15–2. REPRODUCTIVE TRACT TUMORS OF FERRETS

Tumor	Site	Number of Animals	Reference
Leiomyoma	Ovary	21*	Cotchin,[3] AFIP
	Uterus	1	Cornell
Theca cell	Ovary	2	Chesterman and Pomerance,[17] AFIP
Fibromyoma	Ovary	1	Chesterman and Pomerance[17]
Fibromatoid	Ovary	1	Symmers and Thomson[9]
Granulosa cell	Ovary	1	AFIP
Undifferentiated	Ovary	1	Cornell
Carcinoma	Ovary	1	WCVM
Arrhenoblastoma	Ovary	1	AFIP
Papillary cystadenocarcinoma	Mammary gland	1	Carpenter, et al.[18]†
Sertoli's cell	Testis	2	AFIP, WCVM
Interstitial cell	Testis	2	WCVM
Total:		35	

* 20 cases from one source (Cotchin[3]).
† *Mustela nigripes,* black-footed ferret.

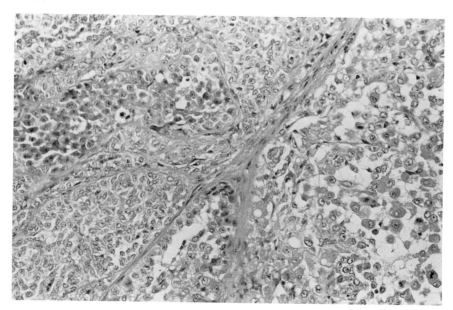

Fig. 15–2. Ferret testis. Sertoli's cell tumor (left of fibrous connective tissue) and interstitial cell tumor (right of fibrous tissue) in the same testis (H & E stain; × 100). (Courtesy of Western College of Veterinary Medicine, Canada.)

disposing factor. Other ovarian tumors reported include theca cell tumor, fibromyoma, granulosa cell tumor, arrhenoblastoma, and undifferentiated carcinoma.[9, 17]

Only one uterine tumor, a leiomyoma, was observed. One case of a mammary carcinoma was reported, but this was in a wild black-footed ferret (*Mustela nigripes*).[18] In male ferrets, Sertoli's cell and interstitial cell tumors of the testis were reported (Fig. 15–2). Clinical signs of ferrets with reproductive tumors may be absent, but are usually related to fertility problems.

SKIN AND SUBCUTANEOUS TUMORS

The third most common group of tumors in ferrets is seen in skin and subcutaneous tissues (Table 15–3). Of these, squamous cell carcinoma is the most reported tumor type.[19–21] The second most reported tumor is the poorly differentiated sebaceous gland adenocarcinoma.[9, 17, 22, 25] This tumor is described as a basisquamosebaceous adenocarcinoma, which has cells that appear as basal cells, squamous cells, and sebaceous cells (Fig. 15–3). All three cell types have characteristics of anaplasia. Individual adenocarcinomas of the sebaceous glands, perianal gland, and preputial gland were also observed.[24] Mast cell tumors are considered to be a common skin tumor in ferrets, but only one case was published and three reported.[23] Mast cell tumors may be single, multiple, or metastatic (Fig. 15–4).

Two myxosarcomas of the subcutis were reported; the other reported subcutaneous tumor was a myelosarcoma. Other re-

TABLE 15–3. SKIN AND SUBCUTANEOUS TUMORS OF FERRETS

Tumor	Site	Number of Animals	Reference
Squamous cell carcinoma	Trunk, forelegs, maxillary skin, disseminated	5	Engelbart and Strasser,[19] LSU, MIT, Olsen, et al.,[20] Zwicker and Carlton[21]
Basisquamosebaceous adenocarcinoma	Trunk, chin	4	Chesterman and Pomerance,[17] MIT, Symmers and Thomson[9, 22]
Mast cell	Hind leg	3	AFIP, Poonacha and Hutto,[23] WCVM
Myxosarcoma	Thorax, tail	2	Chesterman and Pomerance,[17] WCVM
Adenocarcinoma	Perianal gland	1	KSU, Carpenter and Novilla,[18]
	Sebaceous gland*	1	Miller, et al.[24]
	Prepuce	1	
Basal cell carcinoma	Cheek	1	WCVM
Neurofibrosarcoma	Eyelid	1	AFIP
Myelosarcoma	Subcutis	1	AFIP
Histiocytoma	Thorax	2	MIT, WCVM
Adenoma	Sebaceous gland	2	MIT, UI, Cornell
	Ear	1	
Basal cell	Hind leg	1	KSU
Hemangioma	Foreleg	1	WCVM
Neurofibroma	Neck	1	Andrews, et al.[5]
Undifferentiated or undetermined	Foot	2	CSU, Cornell
Total:		30	

* *Mustela nigripes,* black-footed ferret.

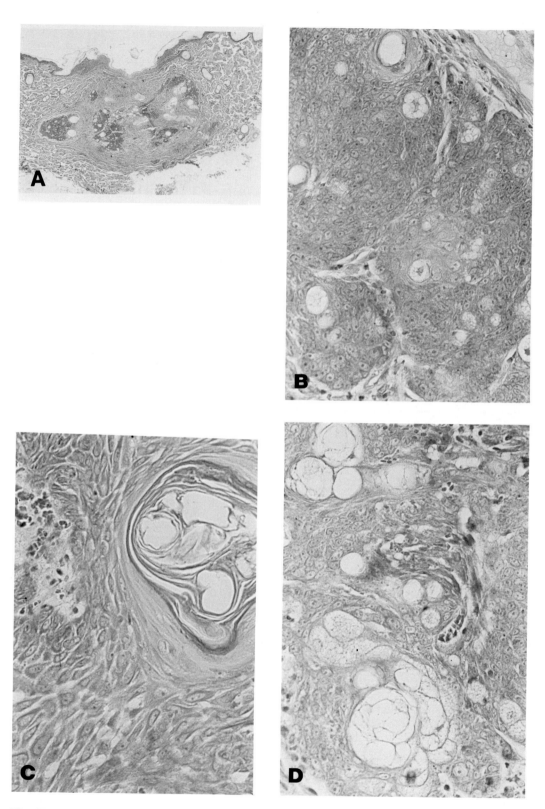

Fig. 15–3. A basosquamosebaceous adenocarcinoma. This tumor has histologic characteristics of all three tumor types—basal cell, sebaceous gland, and squamous cell carcinomas. *A,* Overview of the tumor. *B,* Basal cell component. *C,* Squamous cell component. *D,* Sebaceous cell component (H & E stain; × 100).

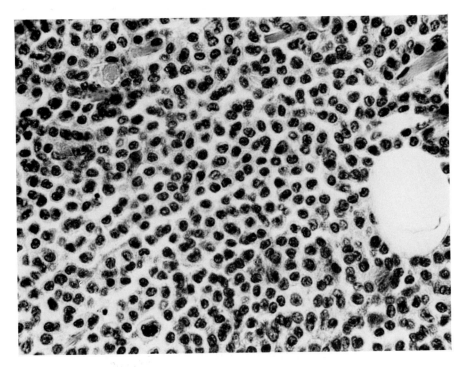

Fig. 15–4. Cutaneous mast cell tumor from a ferret (H & E stain; × 100). (Poonacha, K.B., and Hutto, V.L.: Cutaneous mastocytoma in a ferret. J. Am. Vet. Med. Assoc., *185*:442, 1984.)

ported skin tumors were basal cell carcinoma, neurofibrosarcoma, histiocytoma, sebaceous gland adenoma, basal cell tumor, hemangioma, neurofibroma, and undetermined tumors.[5]

GASTROINTESTINAL TRACT TUMORS

No reports of oral, esophageal, or gastric tumors in the ferret were made or published. The tumors reported were in the parenchymal organs, the liver, the pancreas, and the intestine (Table 15–4).

The liver is most often affected; 17 of 20 tumors were observed in the liver, and 2 in the pancreas. Most hepatic tumors reported are hemangiosarcomas, all

of which were seen in ferrets at the Western College of Veterinary Medicine in Canada (Fig. 15–5).[26] Four adenocarcinomas were seen, one in the liver, one in the bile duct, and two in the pancreas.[5,17] The large number of hepatic tumors reported, 17 of 155, may be related to the susceptibility of mustelids to hepatotoxins and hepatocarcinogens.[27,28] The intestinal tumor seen was in a 4- to 6-month-old male ferret with signs of lethargy, diarrhea, and anorexia.

ENDOCRINE TUMORS

Pancreatic islet cell tumors are the most commonly observed endocrine neoplasm in ferrets (Fig. 15–6 and Table 15–5).

TABLE 15–4. GASTROINTESTINAL TRACT TUMORS OF FERRETS

Tumor	Site	Number of Animals	Reference
Hemangiosarcoma	Liver	9	WCVM
Adenocarcinoma	Liver	1	Andrews, et al.[5]
	Pancreas	2	WCVM, Chesterman and Pomerance[17]
	Bile duct	1	UT
Hemangioma	Liver	2	WCVM
Undifferentiated	Liver, pancreas	1	UI
Hemangioma	Liver	2	WCVM
Hepatocellular adenoma	Liver	1	Cornell
Bile duct cystadenoma	Liver	1	Symmers and Thomson[9]
Adenoma	Pancreas	1	Cornell
Tumor	Intestine	1	MIT
Total:		22	

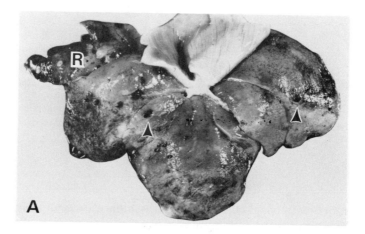

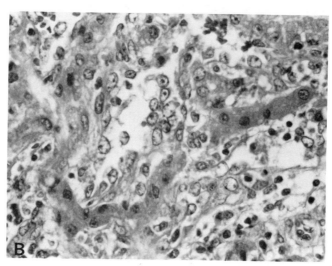

Fig. 15–5. Hepatic hemangiosarcoma. *A,* Grossly, the tumor is seen as hepatic foci (*arrowheads*). *B,* Histologically, the hemangiosarcoma has anaplastic vessels and fibrous connective tissue, H & E stain; × 100). (Courtesy of Dr. B. Cross.)

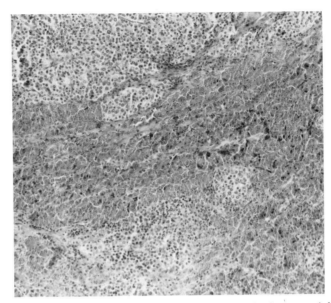

Fig. 15–6. Pancreas with B-cell adenocarcinoma. Neoplastic B-cells are in the upper left corner; normal pancreatic islets are in the lower right corner (H & E stain; × 25). (Courtesy of the Western College of Veterinary Medicine, Canada.)

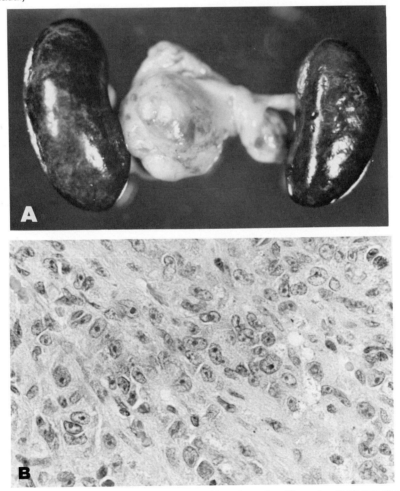

Fig. 15–7. Adrenocortical adenocarcinoma. *A,* Left adrenal is enlarged and irregular. *B,* Histologically, the cells are moderately anaplastic. The nuclei are pleomorphic, with prominent nucleoli (H & E stain; × 100).

TABLE 15–5. ENDOCRINE TUMORS OF FERRETS

Tumor	Site	Number of Animals	Reference
Insulinoma/beta cell	Pancreatic islets	13	AMC, CSU, ISU, MIT, UT, WCVM, Lumeij, et al.[29]
Adrenal adenocarcinoma	Adrenal cortex	2	Cornell,[4] MIT[5]
Islet cell adenocarcinoma	Pancreas	1	KSU
Adrenal	Adrenal cortex	1	Chesterman and Pomerance[17]
Total:		17	

Thirteen of 19 endocrine tumors were beta cell tumors, of which two were considered malignant.[30] The remaining three endocrine tumors were adrenocortical tumors (Fig. 15–7); two were considered malignant.[17,31]

Clinically, beta islet cell tumors cause episodic or persistent hypoglycemia and hyperinsulinemia. Signs can include depression, lethargy, stupor, and hypersalivation.[30] Seizures are usually not seen in ferrets, as they are in dogs and humans. Adrenocortical tumors cause signs and lesions in ferrets similar to those seen in dogs and cats. These changes include a neutrophilic leukocytosis with lymphopenia, bilateral alopecia, and pendulous abdomen (see Chap. 14).

ABDOMINAL TUMORS

Of ten abdominal tumors observed in ferrets, three were mesotheliomas (Fig. 15–8 and Table 15–6). All three were from ferrets brought to the Western College of Veterinary Medicine. Other presumed primary tumors found in the abdominal cavity were carcinoma, adenocarcinoma, and several anaplastic tumors.

MUSCULOSKELETAL TUMORS

Osteomas and three cases of chondroma were observed in ferrets (Table 15–7). Osteomas were described on the head, larynx, and vertebral body.[32] Tumors appear as focal periosteal proliferations that can be diagnosed radiographically (Fig. 15–9). Chondromas were seen in many locations, including the pharynx and tail. Chondromas must be differentiated from osteomas (Fig. 15–10). Another tumor reported in the ferret is the chordoma. Chordomas, tumors of notochord remnants, were seen on the tails of two ferrets. No muscle tumors were observed or reported in ferrets.

MISCELLANEOUS TUMORS

Other tumors observed or reported in ferrets (Table 15–8) include a renal papillary cystadenoma and a hemangioma.[9] An undifferentiated mediastinal tumor was also seen. Other organs or systems may have tumors, but pet owners may be reluctant to submit ferrets for complete necropsies, and laboratory ferrets may have only one system examined thoroughly.

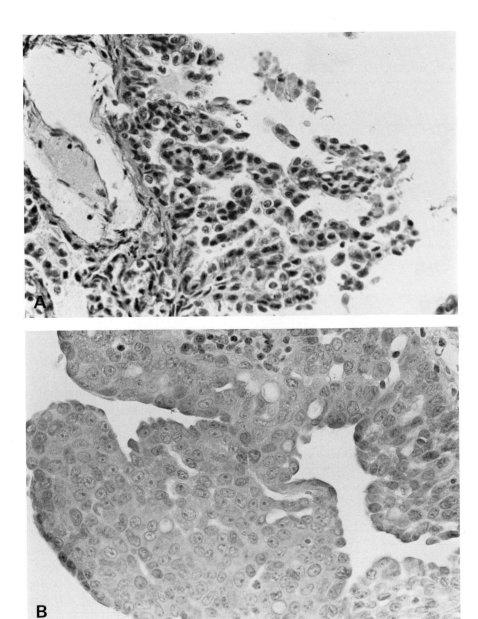

Fig. 15–8. Mesotheliomas from the abdomen of ferrets. *A,* This tumor extended along peritoneal surfaces (H & E stain; × 50). *B,* This more dense mesothelioma was seen in the thorax as well as in the abdomen (H & E stain; × 100). (Courtesy of the Western College of Veterinary Medicine, Canada.)

TABLE 15–6. ABDOMINAL TUMORS OF FERRETS

Tumor	Number of Animals	Reference
Mesothelioma	3	WCVM
Undifferentiated or undetermined	5	CSU, Cornell
Carcinoma	1	AFIP
Adenocarcinoma	1	WCVM
	—	
Total:	10	

TABLE 15–7. MUSCULOSKELETAL TUMORS OF FERRETS

Tumor	Site	Number of Animals	Reference
Osteoma	Vertebral body	1	UT
	Larynx	1	Jensen, et al.[32]
	Head	1	WSU
Chondroma	Intervertebral cartilage, caudal vertebrae	2	MIT, UT
Chordoma	Caudal vertebrae	2	MSU
Total:		7	

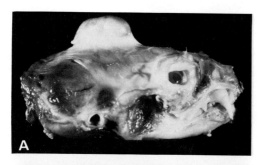

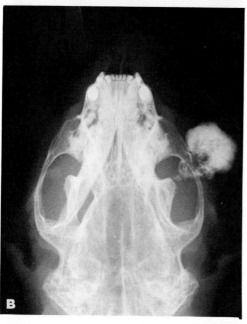

Fig. 15–9. Osteoma on the skull of a ferret. *A,* Osteoma on the parietal bone of an adult male. *B,* Radiograph of an osteoma ventral to the orbit. (*A,* Courtesy of Dr. D.P. Knowles; *B,* courtesy of Dr. W.A. Jensen.)

EXPERIMENTAL NEOPLASMS

Chemically induced tumors were not observed in ferrets. Newborn ferrets, however, are susceptible to polyoma virus. Harris and co-workers[1] injected Mill Hill polyoma virus into newborn ferrets and induced tumors. Injection of Rous sarcoma virus into ferrets did not induce tumor formation.[33]

Ferrets have been used for chemotherapeutic agent studies. Chemotherapeutic agents tested in ferrets include ethylenediamine platinum (II) malonate and the mitomycin derivative BMY-25282.[34,35] The platinum malonate caused some nephrotoxicity but less emesis in ferrets.[35] The mitomycin derivative produced depression and subsequent recovery of lymphocytes, neutrophils, and platelets; recovery was faster than that seen with motomycin C.[34]

A wide variety of neoplasms has been reported in ferrets. The most common tumors are lymphosarcomas, ovarian tumors, and skin tumors. Lymphosarcoma may be associated with infectious agents. The reported and observed number and variety of tumors in both laboratory and companion ferrets will increase as more ferrets are used in research, and as ferrets become more popular as pets. Clinical signs, presenting complaints, and treatment of ferret neoplasias are similar to those seen in cats and dogs.[36]

TABLE 15–8. MISCELLANEOUS TUMORS OF FERRETS

Tumor	Site	Number of Animals	Reference
Papillary cystadenoma	Kidney	1	Symmers and Thomson[9]
Hemangioma	Unknown	1	WCVM
Undifferentiated	Mediastinum	1	Auburn
Total:		3	

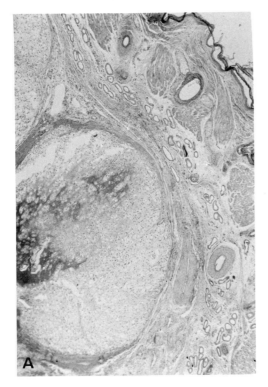 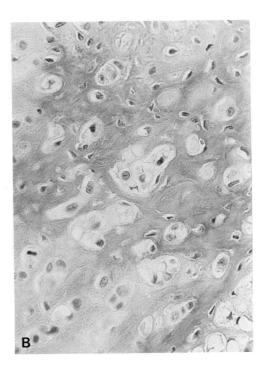

Fig. 15–10. *A,* Chondroma associated with a caudal vertebra. The tumor consists of cartilaginous foci around the vertebral body (H & E stain; × 25). *B,* Neoplastic chondrocytes in cartilaginous matrix (H & E stain; × 100).

REFERENCES

1. Figgs, F.H.J.: Naturally-occurring mustelid tumors. Cancer Res., 4:465, 1944.
2. Harris, R.J., Chesterman, F.C., and Negroni, G.: Induction of tumors in newborn ferrets with Mill Hill polyoma virus. Lancet, 1:788, 1961.
3. Cotchin, E.: Smooth muscle hyperplasia and neoplasia in the ovaries of domestic ferrets. J. Pathol., 130:163, 1980.
4. Fox, J.G., Lipman, N.S., and Murphy, J.C.: Lymphoma in the ferret. Lab. Anim. Sci., 36:562, 1986.

5. Andrews, P.L.R., Illman, O., and Mellersh, A.: Some observations of anatomical abnormalities and disease states in a population of 350 ferrets (*Mustela furo* L.). Z. Versuchstierkd., 21:346, 1979.

6. Smith, S.H., and Bishop, S.P.: Diagnostic exercise: Lymphoproliferative disorder in a ferret. Lab. Anim. Sci., 35:291, 1985.

7. Kenyon, A.J., and Williams, R.C., Jr.: Lymphatic leukemia associated with dysproteinemia in ferrets. Nature, 214:1022, 1967.

8. Altman, N.H., and Lamborn, P.B., Jr.: Lymphocytic leukemia in a ferret (*Mustela furo*). Vet. Pathol., 21:361, 1984.

9. Symmers, W.S.C., and Thomson, A.P.D.: Multiple carcinomata and focal mast-cell accumulations in the skin of a ferret (*Mustela furo* L.), with a note on other tumors in ferrets. J. Pathol. Bacteriol., 45:481, 1953.

10. Yanoff, S.R.: Malignant lymphoma in a ferret. Vet. Pathol., 21:95, 1984.

11. Methiyapun, S., and Myers, R.K.: Spontaneous plasma cell myeloma in a ferret. Vet. Pathol., 22:517, 1985.

12. Chowdhury, K.A., and Shillinger, R.B.: Spontaneous megakaryocytic myelosis in a four-year-old domestic ferret (*Mustela furo*). Vet. Pathol., 19:561, 1982.

13. Moulton, J.E.: Tumors in Domestic Animals. 2nd Ed. Berkeley, University of California Press, 1978.

14. Miller, C.W., Wingfield, W.E., and Boon, J.A.: Applications of ultrasound to veterinary diagnostics in a veterinary teaching hospital. I.S.A. Trans., 21:101, 1982.

14a. Owen, L.N.: Cancer chemotherapy and immunotherapy. *In* Veterinary Internal Medicine, Vol. 1. 2nd Ed. Edited by S.J. Ettinger. Philadelphia, W.B. Saunders, 1983.

14b. Theilen, G.H., and Madewell, B.R.: Veterinary Cancer Medicine. Philadelphia, Lea & Febiger, 1979.

15. Rodger, B.A.: Possibility of virally induced lymphoma in pet ferrets. Can. Vet. J., 24:237, 1980.

16. Kenyon, A.J., et al.: Monoclonal gamma-globulins in ferrets with lymphoproliferative lesions. Proc. Soc. Exp. Biol. Med., 123:510, 1966.

17. Chesterman, F.C., and Pomerance, A.: Spontaneous neoplasms in ferrets and polecats. J. Pathol. Bacteriol., 89:529, 1965.

18. Carpenter, J.W., Davidson, J.P., Novill, M.N., and Huang, J.C.M.: Metastatic papillary cystadenocarcinoma of the mammary gland in a black-footed ferret. J. Wildl. Dis. 16:587, 1980.

19. Engelbart, K., and Strasser, H.: Squamous carcinoma in the ferret. Blue Book, Vet. Profile, No. 11:28, 1966.

20. Olsen, G.H., Turk, M.A.M., and Foil, C.S.: Disseminated cutaneous squamous cell carcinoma in a ferret. J. Am. Vet. Med. Assoc., 186:702, 1985.

21. Zwicker, G.M., and Carlton, W.W.: Spontaneous squamous cell carcinoma in a ferret. J. Wildl. Dis., 10:213, 1974.

22. Symmers, W.S.C., and Thomson, A.P.D.: A spontaneous carcinoma of the skin of a ferret (*Mustela furo* L.). J. Pathol. Bacteriol., 62:229, 1950.

23. Poonacha, K.B., and Hutto, V.L.: Cutaneous mastocytoma in a ferret. J. Am. Vet. Med. Assoc., 185:442, 1984.

24. Miller, T.A., Denman, D.L., and Lewis, G.C., Jr.: Recurrent adenocarcinoma in a ferret. J. Am. Vet. Med. Assoc., 187:839, 1985.

25. Rewell, R.E.: Tumors reported in ferrets and polecats. Proc. Zool. Soc., 119:791, 1950.

26. Cross, B.M.: Hepatic vascular neoplasms in a colony of ferrets. Vet. Pathol., 24:94, 1987.

27. Carter, R.L., Percival, R.H., and Roe, F.J.: Exceptional sensitivity of mink to the hepatotoxic effects of dimethylnitrosamine. J. Pathol., 97: 79, 1969.

28. Koppang, N., and Rimeslatten, H.: Toxic and carcinogenic effects of nitrosodimethylamine in mink. Environmental N-nitroso compounds. I.A.R.C. Sci. Publ., 15:443, 1976.

29. Lumeij, J.T., et al.: Hypoglycemia due to a functional pancreatic islet cell tumor (insulinoma) in a ferret (*Mustela putorius furo*). Vet. Rec., 120:129, 1987.

30. Quesenberry, K.E., Peterson, M.E., Moroff, S.D., and Scanelli, T.D.: Pancreatic insulin-secreting tumor in the ferret. *In* Fifth Annual A.C.V.I.M. Proceedings. San Diego, 1987. (In press.)

31. Fox, J.G., Goad, M.E.P., Garibaldi, B.A., and Wiest, L.: Hyperadrenocorticism in a ferret. J. Am. Vet. Med. Assoc., 191:343, 1987.

32. Jensen, W.A., Myers, R.K., and Liu, C.-H.: Osteoma in a ferret. J. Am. Vet. Med. Assoc., 187:1375, 1985.

33. Harris, R.J., and Chesterman, F.C.: Growth of Rous sarcoma virus in rats, ferrets, and hamsters. Natl. Cancer Inst. Monogr., 17:321, 1964.

34. Bradner, W.T., et al.: Antitumor activity and toxicity in animals of BMY-25282, a new mitomycin derivative. Cancer Res., 45:6475, 1985.

35. Winograd, B., et al: Phase I study of ethylenediamine platinum (II) malonate (NSC 146068), a second-generation platinum analogue. Cancer Res., 46:2148, 1986.

36. Ryland, L.M., Bernard, S.L., and Gorham, J.R.: A clinical guide to the pet ferret. Compend. Cont. Educ. Pract. Vet., 5:25, 1983.

chapter 16

ANESTHESIA AND SURGERY

J. G. Fox

DRUG AND FLUID ADMINISTRATION

Fluids and medications may be given to ferrets by parenteral injection or oral inoculation.

PARENTERAL INJECTION

Subcutaneous injections can be given in the dorsal aspect of the neck. Care should be exercised, however, not to deposit the drug or fluid into the subcutaneous fat pad, because some drugs are poorly absorbed in lipid tissue. *Intraperitoneal* (IP) injections are given using a 21-gauge 1½-inch needle placed lateral and posteriorly to the umbilicus. *Intramuscular* (IM) injections are routinely administered on the lateral aspect in the muscle mass of the upper leg. *Percutaneous intravenous* (IV) injections can be given by way of the cephalic or jugular vein. This procedure may require sedation, local anesthesia, and a surgical skin incision over the jugular or cephalic vein for placement of a catheter for short-term drug or fluid administration. For prolonged IV therapy, a chronic indwelling catheter can be used (see later discussion on bleeding techniques).

ORAL INOCULATION

Ferrets can be given drugs or fluids orally with a rodent dosing needle and syringe or a plastic dispensing dropper (Fig. 16–1). Adults drink at about the rate of 10 ml/minute, up to 100 ml during a session.[1] Alternatively, a stomach tube with a diameter no larger than 5 mm can be inserted orally through a speculum. We routinely administer 50 ml orally to adult ferrets with no adverse results. During this procedure the animal is held on its back, with the head held securely. Sedation may be required during tube insertion because the animal may struggle or vomit. Proper placement of the tube is essential because the ferret lacks a cough reflex when its tracheal mucosa is mechanically stimulated, a reflex that would help to prevent the improper placement of the tube into its trachea.[2]

ORAL MEDICATION

Administering medication to ferrets in capsule or tablet form is difficult, because inexperienced personnel fear be-

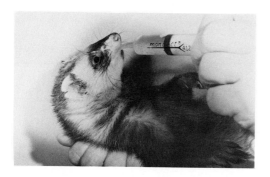

Fig. 16–1. Restraint of ferret being held on its back. The oral dosing is done by one individual.

ing bitten during the process. Therefore, when oral medication (capsule or tablet) is required, it is advisable to prepare the medication in powder form first (i.e., remove medicated powder from the capsule or pulverize the tablet). The medication can then be mixed in a vitamin supplement* and placed on an applicator stick. Ferrets will then readily ingest most of the common antimicrobial oral medications, as well as receive beneficial nutritional supplementation. Medication can be dispensed in tablet or capsule form with the supplement, and the owner or technician can effectively and safely deliver the drug.

ANESTHESIA

It is advisable that, during all surgical procedures, a circulating hot water mattress be placed under ferrets because they are susceptible to hypothermia during anesthesia.

PREANESTHETICS AND TRANQUILIZERS

Atropine sulfate is used as a preanesthetic to minimize possible cardiac arrhythmias caused by vagal stimulation and to limit bronchial, salivary, and gastrointestinal secretions during anesthesia. The dosage administered is 0.05 mg/kg, either IM or subcutaneous (SC).

Ketamine alone or in combination with xylazine, acepromazine, or diazepam can also be used as a tranquilizing agent or preanesthetic. Acepromazine, xylazine, diazepam, alphaxolone-alphadone, and fentanyl citrate-fluanisone can also be used individually as tranquilizers or pre-

---

* Nutrical–EVSCO Pharmaceutical Corp., Buena, NJ.

TABLE 16–1. TRANQUILIZERS, PREANESTHETICS, ANESTHETICS, AND ANALGESICS USED IN FERRETS

Drug	Dosage	Route
Tranquilizers		
Acepromazine	0.2–0.5 mg/kg	SC, IM
Xylazine	1.0 mg/kg	SC, IM
Diazepam	1.0–2.0 mg/kg	IM
Ketamine	10–20 mg/kg	IM
Preanesthetic (injectable)		
Atropine	0.05 mg/kg	SC, IM
Acepromazine	0.1–0.25 mg/kg	SC, IM
Alphaxolone-alphadone acetate	6–8 mg/kg	IM
Fentanyl citrate-fluanisone	0.3 ml/kg	IM
Anesthetic		
Ketamine	30–60 mg/kg	IM
Ketamine-xylazine	20–30 mg/kg	IM
(combination)	1–4 mg/kg	SC
Ketamine-diazepam	25–35 mg/kg	IM
(combination)	2–3 mg/kg	SC
Urethane	1.5 mg/kg	IP
Pentobarbital	30–36 mg/kg	IP
Alphaxolone-alphadolone acetate	12–15 mg/kg	IM
Inhalation		
Diethyl ether	15–20% induction	IH
(short procedures)	3.5% maintenance	
Isoflurane	1.5–3% maintenance	IH
Halothane*	3–3.5% induction	IH
	0.5–2.5% maintenance	
Methoxyflurane	1–3% induction	IH
Nitrous oxide	0.3–0.5% maintenance	IH
(given in equal pro-		
portions with O_2 as		
supplement to 2.5%		
halothane)		
Analgesics		
Aspirin†	200 mg/kg	PO
Phenylbutazone†	100 mg/kg	PO
Meperidine	4 mg/kg	IM
Fentanyl citrate-fluanisone	0.2 ml/kg	IM

* Do not use in open-drop method or bell jar, because of high concentrations achieved.
† May interfere with platelet function.

anesthetics (Table 16–1). If fentanyl citrate-fluanisone is used, its effects can be rapidly reversed, if necessary, by naloxone hydrochloride (0.04–1.0) mg/kg given IV, IM, or SC.[3]

NONBARBITURATE ANESTHETICS

Ferrets should be carefully evaluated to ascertain their health status before administration of anesthesia. Animals should be fasted overnight but allowed free access to water.

Ketamine and Ketamine Combinations

Ketamine is a nonbarbiturate with anesthetic and analgesic properties, but it lacks the pharmacologic ability to induce muscle relaxation.[4] Several investigators have used ketamine alone, or in combination with other drugs, to anesthetize ferrets as well as various other domestic and laboratory animals.[5-7]

Xylazine, a sedative and analgesic with muscle-relaxing properties, and diazepam, primarily used as a tranquilizer, are two compounds that are combined with ketamine for anesthesia. In a recent detailed and controlled study, ketamine (60 mg/kg), ketamine-xylazine (25 mg/kg ketamine, 2 mg/kg xylazine), and ketamine-diazepam (35 mg/kg ketamine, 3 mg/kg diazepam) were compared as anesthetic regimens in ferrets. Fifteen castrated males over 4 months of age were utilized; each weighed 0.6 to 1.2 kg.[6] The animals were randomized into three groups of five ferrets. Each group was rotated through the three anesthetic trials, allowing 1 week (or longer) between trials. For each of the three treatment groups, investigators measured heart rate, electrocardiograms before and after anesthesia, induction time, and reflex responses. Nonanesthetized heart rates of 250 (160–320) beats per minute (bpm) were recorded. Animals under ketamine or ketamine-diazepam had higher heart rates (30–50 bpm; range, 240–400) than unanesthetized ferrets, whereas the ketamine-xylazine combination produced lower heart rates as anesthesia progressed, reaching 150 bpm at 45 minutes and then returning to preanesthetic levels at about 60 minutes postinduction. Except for one ferret with premature ventricular contractions (PVCs), the ECG responses in unanesthetized animals showed a normal sinus rhythm (this ferret was excluded from further ECG analyses). Under ketamine or ketamine-diazepam anesthesia 79% (11 of 14) ferrets had a normal sinus rhythm, with only 21% (3 of 14) showing PVCs. Under ketamine-xylazine anesthesia, however, 36% (5 of 14) had PVCs and 64% (9 of 14) had normal sinus rhythms (see Fig. 7–4).

The induction time for all three regimens was 2 to 3 minutes. Reflex responses were also evaluated (Table 16–2). The authors concluded that the ketamine-xylazine combination produces acceptable analgesia, muscle relaxation, duration of anesthesia, and smooth recoveries.[6] Nevertheless, they cautioned that the animals should be closely monitored for cardiac arrhythmias. Atropine, normally used to control arrhythmias, was deliberately excluded from this study to isolate the effects of the primary drugs without interference from another pharmacologic agent. The other two regimens effectively immobilized the subjects, but muscle rigidity and incomplete analgesia were noted when ketamine was used alone and in combination with diazepam, respectively.[5] The ketamine-xylazine combination also produced excellent results in the cat, horse, and dog.[7]

This combination, however, as noted above, can have side effects such as bradycardia, hypotension, and long recovery periods. It was suggested that these effects result from central inhibition of α_2-adrenergic input into the cardiovascular system. Yohimbine, an α_2-adrenergic antagonist, when given in a dose of 0.5 mg/kg (1 mg/ml) IM 15 minutes after a combination of 25 mg/kg ketamine and 2 mg/kg xylazine, reverses the ketamine/xylazine-induced bradycardia and significantly reduces recovery time (by >50%). Thus, yohimbine may reverse anesthetic complications.[8]

These anesthetics, when used in doses to produce sedation, can also be supplemented with inhalation anesthetics, methoxyflurane, halothane, or isoflurane.

TABLE 16–2. INDUCTION TIME AND REFLEX RESPONSES OF FERRETS UNDER THREE ANESTHETIC REGIMENS

Response/Duration	Treatment Group A (Ketamine)	Treatment Group B (Ketamine-Xylazine)	Treatment Group C (Ketamine-Diazepam)
Induction time (min)	2.2	2.7	2.2
Loss of palpebral reflex	0/15*	12/15	0/15
Duration of loss (min)		33	
Loss of pain, toe	0/15	15/15	3/15
Duration of loss (min)		40	8
Loss of pain, abdomen	13/15	15/15	12/15
Duration of loss (min)	23	47	21
Paddling	13/15	0/15	14/15
Duration of paddling (min)	33		24
Righting reflex regained (min)	55	69	41

* Numerator, Number showing indicated condition; denominator, population in group.

(Moreland, A.F., and Glaser, C.: Evaluation of ketamine, ketamine-xylazine and ketamine-diazepam anesthesia in the ferret. Lab. Anim. Sci., *35:*287, 1985.

Urethane

Urethane has been used as an anesthetic for ferrets undergoing acute experiments. It provides a stable long-lasting anesthesia, but must be used with extreme caution because of its carcinogenic properties.[1]

BARBITURATE ANESTHESIA

Because it is difficult to perform venipuncture in ferrets, IP injections of pentobarbital at a dose of 30 to 35 mg/kg were used for anesthesia (see Table 16–1).[9, 10] IP injection of barbiturates, however, compromises the clinician's ability to maintain a correct level of anesthesia, and poses a risk of injection into the abdominal viscera. Pentobarbital, at 25 mg/kg IP, supplemented with ether anesthesia, was used successfully by investigators in England to anesthetize ferrets.[11] In another experiment the dose for pentobarbital alone was 36 mg/kg,[3] but unfortunately this dose prolongs recovery time. Because it is highly volatile and flammable, ether should be used with caution, and confined in a properly ventilated hood.

Smaller IP doses of pentobarbital or thiamylal sodium can also be supplemented with inhalant anesthetics, either methoxyflurane, halothane, or isoflurane, to allow for better control of anesthesia and a shorter recovery period.

INHALATION ANESTHESIA

Inhalation chambers can be used to induce anesthesia with volatile anesthetics, but preanesthetics or injectable anesthetics are often needed initially to sedate or anesthetize the ferrets when volatile compounds such as halothane (1–3%) supplemented with $N_2O:O_2$ and methoxyflurane with $N_2O:O_2$ (1:1) are used. A flow rate of 1 to 2 L/minute is used for maintenance through a mask or endotracheal tube and semiopen circuit.[1] Induction usually requires 1 to 2 minutes, during which the subject should be monitored carefully. After inhalation anesthetics are stopped, the ferret will regain consciousness in about 5 minutes. The depth of anesthesia can be monitored by evaluation of pedal and palpebral reflexes and heart and respiratory rates, using the same indices as those used for the cat.

Ferrets can be euthanized by an overdose of pentobarbital (120 mg/kg intraperitoneally) or euthanasia solution (except T-61) given intraperitoneally; use of CO_2 in a properly designed chamber is also acceptable. Animals can be exsanguinated by cardiac puncture if anesthetized.[11,12]

BLEEDING TECHNIQUES

Because the ferret's superficial veins are not readily discernible, venipuncture for blood withdrawal or IV dosing can be difficult.

RETRO-ORBITAL TECHNIQUE

Blood can be obtained by toenail clipping, but the yield will be minimal (0.5 ml). Lightly anesthetized ferrets can be bled using a retro-orbital blood collec-

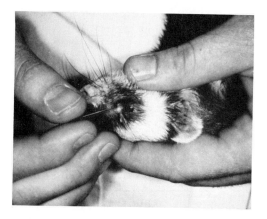

Fig. 16–2. Retro-orbital bleeding in an anesthetized ferret. The capillary tube is inserted into the medial canthus.

tion technique.[13] The animal is first anesthetized with ketamine hydrochloride (20–30 mg/kg) and xylazine (1–4 mg/kg), administered together IM.[10] Alternatively, volatile anesthetics (e.g., ether) may be used in a properly ventilated hood. The operator holds the animal's head downward, and supports its body with the hand and forearm (Fig. 16–2). The animal's eye partially protrudes if the eyelid is retracted, and mild digital pressure exerted periorbitally.

The procedure is as follows. Break a heparinized capillary tube in half, and place the irregular end into the medial canthus. Rotate and push the tube through the fat and fibrous tissue into the retro-orbital plexus with firm, gentle pressure. Direct blood flow from the capillary tube into an appropriate container. Hemostasis is achieved by digital pressure on the medial canthus. For young ferrets (100–300 g), 1 to 3 ml of blood can be collected safely. For adult animals (600–2000 g), 5 to 10 ml can be obtained without adverse side effects.

JUGULAR VEIN, CAUDAL VEIN OR ARTERY

Jugular veins and the caudal tail vein or artery can be used for blood collection.[14,15] Recently, Curl and Curl[14] described a restraining device that allows serial blood collection from the caudal tail artery (<1 ml) in unanesthetized ferrets (Fig. 16–3).[16] They used the restraining device and a 25-gauge needle, and obtained a maximum of 12 samples from the caudal arteries of seven ferrets within a 24-hour period. During the next 7 days, they successfully collected 10 additional samples.[16]

CARDIAC BLEEDING

Although not recommended, cardiac puncture in anesthetized ferrets can be used to obtain larger volumes of blood. This procedure is performed as follows, with

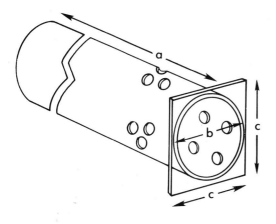

Fig. 16–3. Restraining device for caudal tail artery bleeding in a ferret (a, Length for males = 45.7 cm, females = 38.1 cm; b, Diameter (inner) for males = 10.2 cm, females = 7.6 cm; and c, Endplate for males = 12 cm, females = cm). (Curl, J.L., and Curl, J.S.: Restraint device for serial blood sampling of ferrets. Lab. Anim. Sci., *35*:296, 1985.)

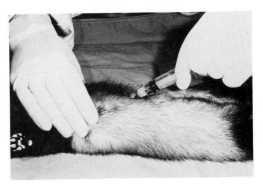

Fig. 16–4. Cardiac bleeding in an anesthetized ferret. A 1½-inch 18-gauge needle is inserted at a 30° angle cephalad near the xyphoid cartilage.

the animal in dorsal recumbency. Insert an 18-gauge 1½-inch needle cephalad near the xyphoid cartilage at a 30° angle, and collect the blood with a 5- or 10-ml syringe (Fig. 16–4). Only experienced personnel should perform this technique; if done incorrectly, life-threatening cardiac tamponade may result.[17]

INDWELLING CATHETER

A chronic indwelling catheter has been used for frequent and repeated blood collection or dosing of IV compounds, or both.[18–20] More recently, a simplified technique was developed for a jugular IV catheterization.[21]

Surgical Placement of Catheter

Following anesthesia with ketamine hydrochloride (30 mg/kg, IM), and xylazine (3 mg/kg, IM) in conjunction with atropine sulfate (0.05 mg/kg, SC) and presurgical shaving and scrubbing of the head and neck (using 70% isopropyl alcohol and povidone-iodine), the ferret is prepared for catheterization by the fol-

lowing procedure. It is placed in dorsal recumbency and draped. A 2-inch midline or paramedian skin incision is made on the ventral aspect of the neck, and the right jugular vein is exposed with blunt dissection. A looped section of 3-0 silk is passed underneath the vessel and cut, forming two separate sutures. Both sutures are loosely tied—one distal and one proximal to the site of phlebotomy. An 18-inch section of sterile polyethylene tubing (PE 50) filled with heparinized (5 U/ml) saline solution is fitted into the shaft of a 19-gauge needle. The distal suture is tied off and used to apply slight traction on the vessel by gently pulling the suture to stabilize the jugular vein for venotomy. Before tying off the distal suture, and during the phlebotomy, it is useful to apply pressure on the jugular vein on its proximal course to keep the vein engorged with blood. The 19-gauge needle is then inserted into the vessel. When the entire bevel of the needle is inside the lumen, the catheter is advanced about 2½ inches into the jugular vein lumen. Ensure the patency of the catheter before pulling the needle out and tie off the proximal suture. Further secure the catheter by looping the distal suture around several times and tying each loop with a square knot.

Next, the animal is placed in ventral recumbency and a small skin incision is made at the base of the pinna of the right ear. A thin-walled 17-gauge needle and matching stylet are inserted through the skin incision and directed subcutaneously in a caudo-ventral direction until the stylet tip emerges adjacent to the site of the phlebotomy. The stylet is removed, and the distal (or free) end of the catheter is disconnected from the stub adaptor and inserted retrograde into the 17-gauge needle until it emerges outside the skin. The needle is then removed gently, and the stub adaptor quickly refitted into the catheter to ascertain patency. The skin incisions are closed with 3-0 monofilament nylon. The suture used for closing the small head skin incision is further used to anchor the base of the free end of the catheter via several loops of the ligature (Fig. 16–5). Before its free end is heat-sealed, the patency of the catheter is again checked. Placing the polyethylene catheter inside the shaft of a 19-gauge hypodermic needle greatly facilitates intravascular catheterization of ferrets.

To minimize subcutaneous tissue trauma significantly when the catheter is brought to the exterior, use a sharp, 17-gauge thin-walled needle with a matching stylet. Wrap the sealed and coiled catheter under bandaging tape to provide additional protection. Seal the catheter by flaming and then crimping the tip of the free end to provide an airtight seal. This

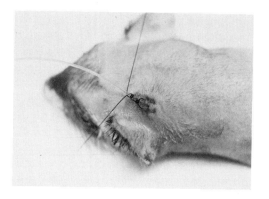

Fig. 16–5. Jugular catheter exteriorized and anchored at the base of the pinna.

sealing technique not only prevents infection through capillarity, but also helps to maintain the patency of the heparin-filled catheter.

Collection of Blood from Catheter

When the catheter is ready for blood collection, spray the sealed end with 70% isopropyl alcohol before cutting the tip with a pair of sterile scissors. Fit a sterile, blunted 23-gauge needle into the catheter. Next, a sterile three-way stopcock is connected to the hub of the 23-gauge stub needle adaptor. For blood withdrawal a 3-ml syringe, half-filled with heparinized (5 U/ml) saline solution, is attached to the horizontal port of the three-way stopcock, and used to fill the system with venous blood and to remove any air in the catheter. Blood sampling is performed with a second syringe attached to the vertical port of the stopcock. After each sampling, the catheter is flushed with heparinized saline solution. At the end of the last blood collection, the catheter is filled with heparinized (5 U/ml) saline solution and heat-sealed. Catheters are flushed with a heparinized (5 U/ml) solution of saline twice weekly. In the techniques described earlier, the authors did not find a single case of infection in 16 ferrets, who were subsequently necropsied.[21] Postmortem procedures included both gross and microscopic examination of all major organs, as well as bacterial cultures of blood samples. All catheterized animals were kept for a period of 4 weeks except for two ferrets, maintained for 10 and 12 weeks, respectively. At the time the ferrets were euthanized all the catheters were patent.[21]

HARVESTING FERRET PERITONEAL MACROPHAGES

Four- to five-month-old ferrets were stimulated with 3 ml of mineral oil administered IP.[22,23] Four days postinjection, the ferrets were anesthetized with a ketamine-xylazine combination, and the lower abdomen shaved and scrubbed with appropriate disinfectants. Two hundred ml of Eagle's Minimal Essential Medium with Earle's salts (MEM),* 200 ml, containing 10 U/ml of heparin, was then injected IP into the ferrets. The distended abdomen was massaged gently for 1 to 2 minutes. A 14-gauge needle with attached rubber tubing was inserted into the posterior abdomen, lateral to the midline. The peritoneal fluid containing the macrophages was collected in 50-ml polypropylene centrifuge tubes. Harvest of the macrophages in excess of 5×10^7 can be achieved with one peritoneal lavage.

Macrophages were centrifuged at 500 $\times$ g for 15 minutes and resuspended at 4×10^6 cells/ml in growth medium of MEM supplemented with 15% bovine fetal semen (BFS) and gentamicin sulfate. Purified macrophages were obtained by seeding tissue culture slides with 0.15 ml of the cell suspension/well, and washing vigorously with serum-free medium to remove unattached cells.[24] The cell population was fed with 0.3 ml of growth medium/well and incubated for variable periods, depending on the assay to be performed.

PREVENTIVE MEDICINE AND ELECTIVE SURGERY

QUARANTINE

If using ferrets in biomedical research, or, alternatively, if raising ferrets commercially, it is extremely important to institute strict quarantine and isolation procedures when new ferrets join the colony. Ferrets should be purchased only from reputable commercial sources. The animals should receive a thorough physical examination on delivery. Animals

---

* Available from Grand Island Biological Company, Grand Island, NY.

with any nasal discharge, skin infections, diarrhea, enlarged mesenteric lymph nodes, or unthrifty appearance should be rejected or placed in isolation for further diagnostic evaluation.

In addition, rectal temperatures should be recorded—normal is 101 to 102° F (38–39° C), with transient increases due to excitement or rough handling up to 104° F (40° C) occasionally recorded. If high temperatures are recorded, it is important to recheck them 2 or 3 hours later.[25] All newly purchased ferrets should be quarantined for a minimum of 2 weeks, and appropriate diagnostic tests undertaken to ascertain health status (Table 16–3). Depending on the use of the ani-

TABLE 16–3. PREVENTIVE MEDICINE AND ELECTIVE PROCEDURES IN FERRETS

Age	Procedure
6–8 weeks (postweaning)	Vaccination with *Clostridium* type C toxoid (optional)* Vaccination with canine distemper (CD) vaccine Spaying, castration, removal of anal gland (optional)† First fecal exam for oocytes, *Giardia* sp. and parasite ova
9–12 weeks	Culture for *Salmonella* and *Campylobacter*‡ Second vaccination of distemper vaccine Second fecal examination for oocytes, *Giardia* sp. and parasite ova
5–6 months	Spaying, castration, removal of anal gland (optional) Rabies vaccination not currently approved by USDA
15 months (1 year after CD vaccine)	Vaccination for CD, repeated every 3 years Physical examination

* For ferrets in commercial or fur farming operations.
† Often performed by commercial ferret suppliers prior to shipment of ferrets to pet stores or research facilities.
‡ Optional, depending on clinical status and risk of zoonotic spread, or potential impact on research being conducted.

mals, additional hematologic and clinical serum chemistries may be performed. When in doubt, the ferrets should be vaccinated against distemper.

If at all possible, place the newly introduced ferrets at the animal resource unit as far away as possible from random-source dogs. Even the technicians working with these dogs (whose distemper status is questionable) should not care for the ferrets. Technicians or other personnel working with ferrets should not keep puppies, particularly from pounds. Separate laboratory coats should be used by personnel working with ferrets, and those with upper respiratory infections should not be allowed into the ferret housing area. Also, because ferrets are susceptible to tuberculosis, personnel should be screened and declared free from that disease.

IMMUNIZATION

Ferrets must be vaccinated against canine distemper virus (CDV) with a modified live virus, preferably of chick embryo tissue culture origin. The first vaccination should be administered at 6 to 8 weeks of age if kits are from immune dams, and at 4 to 5 weeks if kits are from unvaccinated dams. A second vaccination is given at 9 to 12 weeks of age and subsequently every 3 years. The half-life of maternal antibody to distemper, 7.4 days, is very similar to the decline in dogs (8.5 days); the vaccination schedule against CDV in ferrets should follow the guidelines for dogs.[26] The polyvalent vaccines available to the veterinary practitioner are effective in protecting ferrets against challenge with virulent CDV.[27] Because the virus is not attenuated, distemper vaccine of ferret cell culture origin should never be used. Inactivated distemper vaccine provides only a short-lived, slow-developing immunity, if any.[28]

Ferrets are assumed to be susceptible to rabies and can transmit the virus, although oral administration of virulent rabies did not infect ferrets in a study done by Bell and Moore.[29] Nevertheless, rabies vaccination is not recommended because there is no licensed rabies vaccine for this species. At the insistence of some owners pet ferrets were given inactivated rabies vaccine, although neither modified live virus nor inactivated virus vaccine have been tested for efficacy in ferrets. In fact, in one clinical case of rabies, the ferret may have been previously vaccinated with modified live rabies virus.[30]

Ferrets are not susceptible to feline panleukopenia, enteritis mink virus, infectious canine hepatitis, feline rhinotracheitis, feline calcivirus, or canine parvovirus, although vaccination for these diseases (e.g., with a polyvalent vaccine) has shown no untoward effects.

Commercially raised ferrets should be vaccinated at weaning with type C botulism toxoid, which will protect them for 1 year. If they are fed only fresh or commercially processed pet food, ferrets do not require vaccination against botulism.

OVARIOHYSTERECTOMY

Similar to other carnivores, ferrets have a bicornate uterus (see Chap. 2). Spaying of female ferrets is performed using a midline ventral incision, the same as that described for the cat.[31] Because of heavy fat accumulations around the ovary, care must be exercised not to ligate the ureter during the procedure.[32] Nonbreeding females are spayed at 6 to 8 months of age, but ferret producers are now routinely spaying, castrating, and descenting ferrets at 8 to 10 weeks of age, prior to delivery of weanling ferrets to pet stores. Such procedures, when performed at this age and done with proper anesthesia and surgical techniques, are accomplished with low morbidity and mortality rates; tissue trauma and blood loss are minimal.

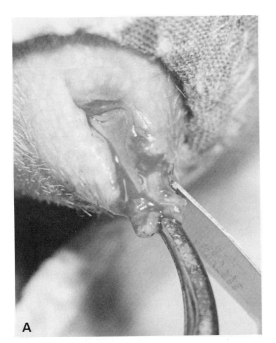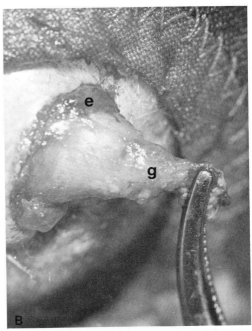

Fig. 16–6. Operative procedures for extirpation of the ferret's anal sacs. *A,* Skin and mucous membrane adjacent to the duct orifice are grasped with a mosquito forceps, and a circumferential incision is made. *B,* The glandular complex (*g*) has been dissected free, and a fascial plane has been located between the anal sac and the external and sphincter muscles (*e*). (Creed, J.E., and Kainer, R.A.: Surgical extirpation and related anatomy of anal sacs of the ferret. J. Am. Vet. Med. Assoc., *179*:575, 1981.)

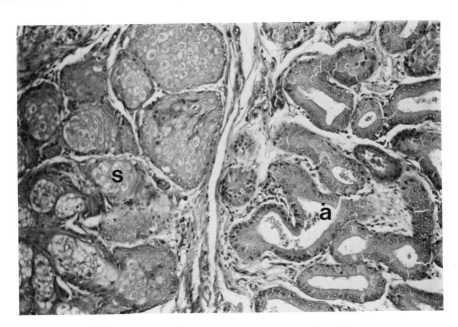

Fig. 16–7. Components of the glandular complex surrounding the duct of a ferret's anal sac (*s*, sebaceous gland; *a,* apocrine tubular gland; hematoxylin-phloxine-safran stain; × 40). (Creed, J.E., and Kainer, R.A.: Surgical extirpation and related anatomy of anal sacs of the ferret. J. Am. Vet. Med. Assoc., *179*:575, 1981.)

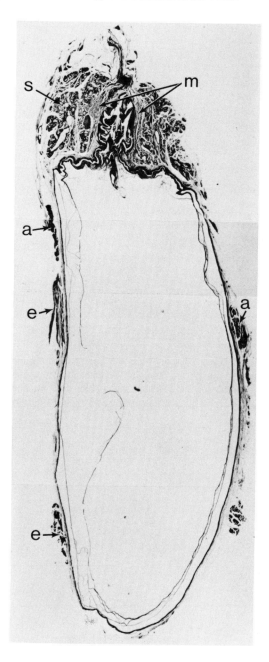

Fig. 16–8. Photomicrograph of longitudinal section from a surgically extirpated ferret's anal sac (*s,* sebaceous component of the glandular complex; *m,* sphincter muscle of the duct; *a,* remnants of the apocrine component; *e,* remnants of the external anal sphincter muscle; hematoxylin-phloxine-safran stain; × 4; montage). (Creed, J.E., and Kainer, R.A.: Surgical extirpation and related anatomy of anal sacs of the ferret. J. Am. Vet. Med. Assoc., *179:*575, 1981.)

CASTRATION

Nonbreeding males are castrated between 6 and 8 months of age or earlier, as indicated above. Castration reduces aggressive behavior and the musky odor from secretions of the sebaceous gland located in the skin. Surgical techniques used in cats (i.e., scrotal incision) are employed similarly in ferrets. Alternatively, the closed median approach used in dogs is sometimes employed.[31]

ANAL GLAND REMOVAL

Ferret anal glands are located lateral to the anus. When the animal is frightened or excited, the glands secrete a musk substance with a strong, noxious odor. Sometimes, the glands are removed at 8 to 10 weeks of age, but otherwise are usually removed when the animal is spayed or castrated. Some are opposed to removal of these glands because they believe it is a form of mutilation and deprives the animal of a defensive mechanism.[33] A surgical procedure describing removal of the scent glands was described.[34] This method is a modification of the procedure used to remove canine anal sacs, and is performed as follows.

A binocular loop magnifier will help to locate the minute end of each anal sac duct. The duct is grasped with mosquito forceps, taking care to include only a minimal amount of skin and mucous membrane (Fig. 16–6*A*). A circumferential skin incision is made with a No. 15 Bard-Parker scalpel blade immediately distal to the tip of the forceps. The skin and mucosa are reflected off the duct with gentle scraping. The glandular complex surrounding the duct for 3 to 4 mm makes dissection difficult. An attempt should be made to find a fascial plane. Dissection should be fairly superficial with respect to overlying tissue and, as the dissection proceeds beyond the glandular complex, a fascial plane is encountered (Fig. 16–6*B*). The anal sac can be removed readily by continuing to use a scraping action with the scalpel blade. Staying on the proper fascial plane will not only enhance removal of the anal sac, but will also minimize hemorrhage and damage to the internal and external anal sphincter muscles. The entire sebaceous component of the glandular complex is removed during surgery, but most of the apocrine component is either destroyed by the dissection or remains with the contiguous external and internal sphincter muscles (Figs. 16–7 and 16–8). Sutures are not required, and infusion of antimicrobial medication into the surgical wounds is unnecessary. Ferrets undergoing this procedure should not require any intensive postoperative care.

Other methods for removal of anal glands were described and proved satisfactory, according to the authors.[35,36]

ADRENALECTOMY

Adrenalectomy may be needed for experimental purposes or for the treatment of hyperadrenocorticism. The surgical incision is made either laterally or by a midline abdominal approach. In the lateral approach, a 1- to 2-inch incision is made just posterior to the last rib in the lateral abdominal wall.[37] The right adrenal gland lies on the inferior vena cava at the caval entry to the liver (see Chap. 2). Fascial tissue must be removed by blunt dissection, so extra care must be exercised when removing the fascia from the inferior vena cava. The adrenal vein is clamped with a hemostat before removing the gland. Once the adrenal has been removed, the vein is either sutured with 5-0 silk, or a Gelfoam sponge is placed on the stump of the adrenal vein.[37] The left adrenal gland lies in adipose tissue close to the cranial pole of the left kidney. Before removing the gland a lumbar vein, tranversing the gland, must be clamped and cut. Usually, minimal bleeding is encountered when removing the left adrenal. The peritoneum and muscle layer are closed with 4-0 chromic gut and the skin with 4-0 nylon sutures.

If bilateral surgery is required, a 1% saline solution instead of water is used to maintain sodium balance, and glucocorticosteroids may occasionally be required. Ferrets are sensitive to changes in salt concentrations in water, and will not drink solutions with greater than 1% concentration of salt.[37]

REFERENCES

1. Andrews, P.L.R., and Illman, O.: The ferret. *In* U.F.A.W. Handbook on the Care and Management of Laboratory Animals. 6th Ed., Edited by T. Poole. Longmans, London, 1987.
2. Korpas, J., and Widdicombe, J.G.: Defensive respiratory reflexes in ferrets. Respiration, 44:128, 1983.
3. Green, C.J.: Anesthetizing ferrets. Vet. Rec., 102:269, 1978.
4. Goodman, L.A., and Gilman, A.: The Pharmacological Basis of Therapeutics. New York, MacMillan, 1970.
5. Green, C.J., et al.: Ketamine alone and combined with diazepam or xylazine in laboratory animals: A 10-year experience. Lab. Anim., 15:163, 1981.
6. Moreland, A.F., and Glaser, C.: Evaluation of ketamine, ketamine-xylazine and ketamine-diazepam anesthesia in the ferret. Lab. Anim. Sci., 35:287, 1985.
7. Wright, M.: Pharmacologic effects of ketamine and its use in veterinary medicine. J. Am. Vet. Med. Assoc., 180:1462, 1982.

8. Sylvina, T.J., Hotaling, L.C., and Fox, J.G.: Effects of yohimbine on bradycardia and recovery time in ketamine/xylazine-anesthetized ferrets. Lab. Anim. Sci., *36*:583, 1986.

9. Ryland, L.M., and Gorham, J.R.: The ferret and its diseases. J. Am. Vet. Med. Assoc., *173*:1154, 1978.

10. Ryland, L.M., Bernard, S.L., and Gorham, J.R.: A clinical guide to the pet ferret. Compend. Cont. Educ. Pract. Vet., *5*:25, 1983.

11. Hammond, J., and Chesterman, F.C.: The ferret. *In* U.F.A.W. Handbook on the Care and Management of Laboratory Animals. 5th Ed. Edinburgh, Churchill Livingstone, 1976.

12. Clifford, D.H.: Preanesthesia, anesthesia, analgesia, and euthanasia. *In* Laboratory Animal Medicine. Edited by J.G. Fox, B.J. Cohen, and F.M. Loew. New York, Academic Press, 1984.

13. Fox, J.G., Hewes, K., and Niemi, S.M.: Retroorbital technique for blood collection from the ferret (*Mustela putorius furo*). Lab. Anim. Sci., *34*:198, 1984.

14. Buckland, M., et al.: A Guide to Laboratory Animal Technology. London, William Heinemann Medical Books, 1971.

15. Bleakley, S.P.: Simple technique for bleeding ferrets. Lab. Anim., *14*:59, 1980.

16. Curl, J.L., and Curl, J.S.: Restraint device for serial blood sampling of ferrets. Lab. Anim. Sci., *35*:296, 1985.

17. Baker, G.S., and Gorham, J.R.: The technique of bleeding ferrets and mink. Cornell Vet., *41*:235, 1951.

18. Florczyk, A.P., and Schurig, J.E.: A technique for chronic jugular catheterization in the ferret. Pharmacol. Biochem. Behav., *14*:255, 1981.

19. Greener, Y., and Gilles, B.: Intravenous infusion in ferrets. Lab. Anim., *14*:41, 1985.

20. Carroll, R.S., et al.: Coital stimuli controlling luteinizing hormone secretion and ovulation in the female ferret. Biol. Reprod., *32*:925, 1985.

21. Mesina, J., et al.: A simplified technique of jugular catheterization in the ferret. Lab. Anim. Sci., *38*:89, 1988.

22. Whetstone, C.A., Bunn, T.O., and Gourlay, J.A.: Canine distemper virus titration in ferret peritoneal macrophages. Cornell Vet., *71*:144, 1981.

23. Poste, G.: The growth and cytopathogenicity of virulent and attenuated strains of canine distemper virus in dog and ferret macrophages. J. Comp. Pathol., *81*: 1971.

24. Edelson, P.J., and Cohn, Z.A.: Purification and cultivation of monocytes and macrophages. *In* In Vitro Methods in Cell-Mediated and Tumor Immunity. Edited by B.R. Bloom and J.R. David. New York, Academic Press, 1976.

25. Rowlands, I.W.: The ferret. *In* U.F.A.W. Handbook on the Care and Management of Laboratory Animals. 3rd Ed. London, Baillière, Tindall and Cox, 1967.

26. Appel, M.J., and Harris, W.V.: Antibody titers in domestic ferret jills and their kits to canine distemper virus vaccine. J. Am. Vet. Med. Assoc., *193*:332, 1988.

27. Gorham, J.R.: Unpublished observations, 1985.

28. Ott, R.L., and Svehag, S.E.: Resistance to experimental distemper in ferrets following the use of killed tissue vaccine. West. Vet., *6*:107, 1959.

29. Bell, J.F., and Moore, G.J.: Susceptibility of carnivora to rabies virus administered orally. Am. J. Epidemiol., *93*:176, 1971.

30. Centers for Disease Control: Viral diseases: Pet ferrets and rabies. C.D.C. Vet. Publ. Health Notes, Oct. 1–2, 1980.

31. Randolph, R.W.: Preventive medical care for the pet ferret. *In* Current Veterinary Therapy, IX, p. 772. Edited by R.W. Kirk. Philadelphia, W.B. Saunders, 1986.

32. Nelson, W.B.: Hydronephrosis in a ferret. Vet. Med. Small Anim. Clin., *79*:516, 1984.

33. Cooper, J.E.: Ferrets. *In* Manual of Exotic Pets. Edited by J.E. Cooper, M.F. Hutchison, O.F. Jackson, and R.J. Maurice. West Sussex, England, British Small Animal Veterinary Association, 1985.

34. Creed, J.E., and Kainer, R.A.: Surgical extirpation and related anatomy of anal sacs of the ferret. J. Am. Vet. Med. Assoc., *179*:575, 1981.

35. Coleman, N.: A technique for descenting ferrets. Vet. Med./Small Anim. Clin., *77*:403, 1982.

36. Rowley, J.: A procedure for descenting ferrets. Med. Vet. Pract., *65*:389, 1984.

37. Filion, D.L., and Hoar, R.M.: Adrenalectomy in the ferret. Lab. Anim. Sci., *35*:294, 1985.

RESEARCH
APPLICATIONS

chapter 17

VIRAL DISEASE MODELS

R. C. Pearson

J. R. Gorham

CANINE DISTEMPER

Ferrets are used to study the etiology, transmission, pathogenesis, and immunization of canine distemper. Shen and Gorham[1] employed ferrets as sources of canine distemper virus (CDV) to study the ability of the virus to survive at 5° and 25°C. Other susceptible ferrets were inoculated with test viral suspensions to evaluate infectivity after the suspensions had been maintained at either 5° or 25°C for differing lengths of time. The CDV retained its virulence after being held in ferret lung suspension for 48 hours at 25°C and for 14 days at 5°C.

Transmission of distemper was studied by several groups. Gorham and Brandly[2] described the importance of fomites in the transmission of virulent CDV by demonstrating that the virus retains infectivity for 20 minutes (but not 30 minutes) on handling gloves. In another trial, they successfully infected ferrets with aerosolized CDV. Later, Shen and Gorham[3] demonstrated that CDV could be transmitted by direct contact of infected ferrets with susceptible ferrets.

They infected ferrets with pathogenic CDV by the aerosol route, and placed them with susceptible ferrets 6 to 11 days after exposure. The ferrets proved to be most infectious to the susceptible animals 9 to 11 days after aerosol exposure.

Gorham and Brandly[2] demonstrated that virus is present in the nasal exudate of ferrets 5 days after subcutaneous inoculation, in the conjunctival exudate 15 days postinoculation (DPI), and in the skin scurf later in the course of the disease. They noted that clinical signs do not appear until 10 to 11 DPI, and that virus persists for 11 to 15 days after ocular, nasal, and skin signs subside, or until death ensues.

The pathogenesis of distemper was studied by exposing ferrets either to intranasal[4] or aerosolized CDV,[5] and harvesting tissues from these animals at various intervals. Liu and Coffin[4] and Crook and colleagues[5] found that the respiratory tract is the preferred site for replication. Virus was recovered from the lungs, nasal tissues, cervical lymph nodes, and blood at 2 DPI. It was concluded that viremia is the means of dissemination, because virus is recovered from kidney, liver, urinary bladder, brain, muscle, and other tissues after its appearance in the blood. Viremia persists until death, or 12 DPI.

Shen and co-workers[6] successfully demonstrated viruria in CDV-infected ferrets. Virulent CDV was present in the urine from 10 to 13 DPI. Vaccine virus of chicken embryo tissue culture origin (CETCO) was not recovered from the urine of 20 ferrets after subcutaneous immunization. When 20 ferrets were vaccinated subcutaneously with modified live CDV and then challanged 12 days later with virulent Green's distemperoid, they remained clinically normal and did not shed pathogenic virus in their urine. They further demonstrated that aerosolized urine from CDV-moribund ferrets is infectious.

Distemper vaccines were evaluated in ferrets with regard to virus strain, onset of immunity, routes of administration, and effect on pregnant animals. Hansen and associates[7] tested various titrations of two different strains of canine distemper vaccine virus in mink and ferrets. They found that the two strains of modified live virus administered subcutaneously were comparable in their ability to protect the animals against challenge with virulent CDV.

Baker and colleagues[8] studied the onset of the immunity induced by egg-adapted attenuated CDV. They showed that ferrets can resist challenge with virulent virus as soon as 2 days after intramuscular vaccination, and attributed this ability in part to the phenomenon of interference. Cabasso and co-workers[9] found that a single intraperitoneal (IP) injection of avianized CDV vaccine afforded resistance to challenge as early as 24 to 72 hours later. This single vaccination protected ferrets against distemper for at least 2 years. Burger and Gorham[10] continued the study of interference and also evaluated the duration of immunity evoked by attenuated CDV. They found that they could effect interference by vaccinating with attenuated CDV 1 day before, simultaneously with, or 1 to 2 days after administering the challenge virus. A single dose of vaccine virus offered protection against challenge with virulent CDV at different intervals during a 6-year period.

Shen and others[11] compared subcutaneous and intramuscular administration of modified live CDV, and found that ferrets vaccinated by either route resist challenge with virulent virus. Gorham and colleagues[12] nebulized ferrets with attenuated CDV, finding that the animals are protected against challenge as early as 5 days later.

Ott and Gorham[13] tested the responses of neonatal and young ferrets to intranasal vaccination. They concluded that ferrets born to distemper-immune dams must be 7 weeks old before immunization is protective. Kits born to susceptible females, however, could be vaccinated successfully at 8 days and older. Farrell and co-workers[14] compared the aerosol and subcutaneous routes for vaccination of ferret kits with attenuated CDV. The ferret kits, all born to distemper-immune females, were refractory to immunization at 8 weeks old or younger by either route of vaccination.

Shen and associates[15] tested the efficacy of jet injection for rapid vaccination of mink and ferrets, which on commercial farms must sometimes be performed on as many as 800 animals per hour. They used three types of commercial vaccines: monovalent CDV; bivalent mink enteritis virus (MEV)-botulism, type C; and trivalent CDV-MEV-botulism, type C. The results indicated that immunogenicity of CDV and type C botulism toxoid is unimpaired by jet injection. They suggested that, because of the lower MEV neutralizing antibody titers elicited, the MEV component may have been unable to withstand the compressive and shearing forces of jet injection. They also added that the vaccines may have been weak in MEV antigen, suggesting that further study to determine the cause for the lower efficacy induced by this fraction is needed before jet injection can be recommended.

Complications arising from vaccines were noted and examined in ferrets. In 1976, Carpenter and colleagues[16] described fatal CETCO (or egg-adapted) vaccine-induced distemper in four female black-footed ferrets. In that same year, Goto and co-workers[17] reverted an attenuated CETCO distemper vaccine virus to high virulence for ferrets by 14 or more serial back passages. This study confirmed the frequently cited possibility that vaccine virus could revert to virulence for the host for which it was intended. This "newly created" virulent virus was again attenuated by four serial passages in fertile eggs by the same researchers.[17]

The effect of murine leukemia virus distemper vaccination on pregnant ferrets was studied by Hagen and colleagues.[18] Females were vaccinated subcutaneously with a CETCO distemper virus at different times during gestation. No attenuated virus was demonstrated in any of the fetuses sacrificed before term, nor were any abnormalities noted in the kits born to the immune dams.

Kauffman and others[19] studied the immunosuppressive effects of distemper virus in ferrets as an animal model for measles virus infection, because the two viruses are closely related antigenically. The effects on cell-mediated immunity occurred 5 days after viral inoculation and continued to day 30. Lymphopenia (of all lymphocyte subpopulations) was accompanied by suppression of lymphocyte transformation (to phytohemagglutinin, concanavalin A, and pokeweed mitogen) on day 5, reaching a nadir on days 8 to 11 and returning toward normal by 23 to 30 days after viral inoculation. They concluded that ferrets should be satisfactory models for studying the pathogenesis of measles virus-induced immunosuppression.

INFLUENZA

Recent experiments using the ferret are primarily in the field of human influenza research. Influenza infection in ferrets closely resembles that in humans with regard to signs, viral distribution, and immunity. Thus, ferrets are used as models for the study of virulence of influenza A strains, age-related susceptibility, and the pathogenesis of Reye's syndrome.

Husseini and associates[20] and Sweet and colleagues[21] found that, whereas nasal turbinates are the preferred site for viral replication, virulent strains of influenza A can infect lower respiratory tract tissues. In vivo infection of alveolar cells (pneumonia) is rare, but can be achieved through in vitro cell culture inoculation. Husseini and co-workers[20] hypothesized that the reasons that infection predominates in airways, especially bronchial epithelium, instead of in alveoli are the following: poor dissemination of the virus from intranasal inoculation; mucociliary action in airways; and phagocytosis of virus and virus-infected cells by alveolar macrophages.

Glathe and co-workers[22] produced virus replication in colonic mucosa by orogastric and/or rectal administration. They demonstrated virus antigen in the cytoplasm of colonic columnar epithelial cells by immunofluorescent staining. Enteritis was clinically observed as diarrhea lasting for 3 days in all ferrets. Although they did not measure antibody response, they suggested further study to evaluate oral administration of attenuated influenza virus as a route for vaccination in humans.

In 1982, Husseini and associates[23] demonstrated that, when the febrile response is suppressed (e.g., by sodium salicylate administration or by shaving) in influenza A-infected ferrets, virus shedding in nasal exudate is significantly greater and lasts longer than that in untreated ferrets. They discussed the agreement of their results with others who studied the effects of aspirin on pyrexia caused by herpesvirus, rabies virus, coxsackievirus B, and other virus infections. Recently, Coates and colleagues[24] studied the pyrogenicity of several strains of influenza in ferrets.

The immune response of the influenza virus-infected ferret was studied with regard to local and systemic humoral- and cell-mediated activities. From their work in 1978, Barber and Small[25] suggested that local immunity prevents influenza infection of the nasal mucosa, whereas systemic immunity does not prevent infection but influences the recovery from infection. McLaren and Butchko[26] measured B- and T-lymphocyte responses within regional lymph nodes and spleens of intranasally infected ferrets. Specific antibody-secreting B cells were identi-

fied in both lymph nodes and splenic tissue 3 DPI, when virus shedding was high, and remained to day 43. Serum hemagglutination-inhibiting (HI) antibody was first detectable 6 DPI; T-cell assays showed response of lymph node cells to the specific strain from days 6 to 43. Virus was no longer shed from the respiratory tract after day 7. Kauffman and co-workers[27] found that, unlike certain viruses, influenza does not cause suppression of systemic cell-mediated immunity (CMI), because T lymphocytes remained responsive to phytohemagglutinin (PHA) during influenza infection of ferrets.

The use of ferrets provides important guidelines in influenza epidemiology. Work with inactivated and attenuated vaccines[28,29] contributed additional evidence that local immunity is protective, and that modified live virus (MLV) vaccines are more efficacious in inducing local response. Unlike that for attenuated viruses, local antibody was not detected, nor was a mixed inflammatory response noted histologically in the tracheas of ferrets inoculated with inactivated virus. Several strains of influenza A virus were inoculated into ferrets simultaneously[30] or sequentially.[31,32] The phenomenon of interference observed between two different influenza A strains given simultaneously led Potter and colleagues[30] to recommend singular vaccination of humans with two MLV, even in the instance of a dual epidemic. Serial infection of ferrets with several influenza strains[31,32] illustrated the occurrence of cross-reactive antibodies and heterotypic immunity. In addition to the above, many studies have used ferrets in testing virulence and/or attenuation of influenza virus strains in the quest for superior vaccine viruses.[33-39]

Ferrets were used in the study of antiviral compounds. Husseini and associates[40] tested the induction of interferon in nasal washes of ferrets infected with either a virulent (clone 7a) or attenuated (clone 64d) strain of influenza. They found that both clones elicit the onset of interferon production at the same time, and both are equally sensitive to interferon. They concluded that this host defense mechanism cannot be used to differentiate the level of virulence between two strains of influenza virus. Steffenhagen and colleagues[41] tested 6-azauridine and 5-iododeoxyuridine for their potential antiviral activity against ten different viral infections in five species. Although some antiviral activity was suggested against four viruses, most of the animal models experienced either enhanced disease or intoxication from the two compounds. In 1973, Haff and Pinto[42] described the decongestant activity of aspirin given intranasally at a low concentration to ferrets with influenza infection. Grunberg and Prince[43] used ferrets and several other species to test the antiviral potential of 3,4-dihydro-1-isoquinolineacetamide (DIQA). They found that DIQA exhibits in vivo activity against both RNA and DNA viruses but only a narrow range of in vitro activity.

The occurrence of infant deaths during influenza epidemics prompted Collie and co-workers[44] to study influenza infection in neonatal ferrets, because adult ferrets and humans respond similarly to influenza. Intranasal infection of 1-day-old ferret kits resulted in the death of all animals. Causes of mortality were influenza pneumonia, airway and esophageal obstruction, which produced difficulty in breathing and feeding, and aspiration pneumonia. Later, in two separate studies, Coates and associates[45,46] compared the response of 1-day-old neonates to that of 15-day-old suckling ferrets. They confirmed the results of Collie's group[44] when the neonatal ferrets succumbed and 15-day-old ferrets suffered only mild respiratory tract infection, having nearly the same resistance as adults. They suggested that the reasons for this difference in susceptibility are based on the stage of lung development and on the susceptibility of various respiratory tract cells. They reported that the deaths of many newborn ferrets are attributed to lower respiratory tract infection, and added that neonates have a higher proportion of ciliated airway epithelium, narrower diameter airways, and lower amounts of alveolar tissue than do suckling or adult ferrets. In one study,[46] it was shown by in vivo infection and by cell culture that airway and alveolar epithelial cells are more susceptible to infection by influenza virus than the same cells in older animals. Epithelial cell debris and inflammatory exudate were seen to plug the lumens of bronchi and bronchioles of the younger ferrets.[45]

Husseini and colleagues[47] offered encouraging results when they immunized ferret dams intranasally in midgestation with either virulent or attenuated influenza virus. All ferret neonates born to immunized dams were resistant to challenge with virulent influenza at 1 day of age. It was suggested that the protection is antibody mediated, passively transferred in the colostrum, because neonates born to nonimmune dams and fostered onto immune dams are also protected against virulent influenza challenge. They recommended vaccinating human mothers during pregnancy so that specific IgG antibody may be passed transplacentally to the fetus. Although they did not specify MLV or killed virus, they cited others who stated that vaccination is not detrimental to the developing fetus. They also recommended breast feeding, although the human infant is probably less efficient at absorbing IgG across the gut mucosa than are other species.

In previous work by others with ferrets, intranasal inoculation[48,49] of pregnant ferrets resulted in neither infection nor detrimental effects on the fetuses, whereas intracardiac inoculation[48–50] of pregnant ferrets resulted in fetal resorption, smaller litters,[48,50] and infection of the fetus and fetal membranes.[49] Rushton and co-workers[50] described the histo-logic findings in the hemophagous organ (fetal part of the placenta) and in the fetal liver and respiratory tract. Collie and associates[51] directly inoculated the am-niotic fluid surrounding embryo ferrets with influenza virus soon after implanta-tion. Fetal death was apparent 4 days later, followed by resorption.

Finally, use of the ferret as a model has led to much important information on the etiology and pathogenesis of Reye's syndrome. Deshmukh and Thomas[52] and Deshmukh and colleagues[53] found that young ferrets fed an arginine-free diet (i.e., they were unable to meet their orni-thine requirements) develop hyperam-monemia and encephalopathy. Ferrets subjected to concurrent administration of aspirin, human influenza virus, and an arginine-free diet experience rapidly developing hyperammonemia and enceph-alopathy, progressing to coma and, usu-ally, death.[52,53] They discussed the ability of aspirin and ammonia to disrupt hepatic mitochondrial activity, and ex-plained the importance of using ferrets for the study of Reye's syndrome; be-cause human patients ingest aspirin be-fore the disease is diagnosed, making the study of pathogenesis difficult in human patients.

INFECTIOUS BOVINE RHINOTRACHEITIS

In 1975 Porter and co-workers[54] reported the isolation of infectious bovine rhino-tracheitis (IBR) virus in ferret splenic cell culture. They obtained the ferret from a commercial breeder who fed a diet con-taining 5% raw beef by-products. The fer-ret was clinically normal, although a cytopathic effect was observed in some of the cell culture bottles.

In 1979, Smith[55] induced acute and chronic IBR infections of the respiratory tract of ferrets by intranasal and intraper-itoneal inoculations. The infection was clinically manifested by sneezing, cough-ing, and anorexia from days 3 to 7 after exposure. The virus was isolated from the upper and lower respiratory tracts, and the retropharyngeal lymph nodes, in ferrets sacrificed on day 4, but virus was recovered only from the pharyngeal epi-thelium of ferrets euthanatized on days 8 and 12 after exposure. Administration of dexamethasone to some ferrets caused re-crudescence of virus shedding. Smith suggested that ferrets are an excellent model for IBR vaccine evaluation, be-cause their responses to the virus are similar to those of cattle. Von Abraham and Straub,[56] however, did not elicit similar results, and concluded that fer-rets are not suitable for this function.

PSEUDORABIES

Natural outbreaks of pseudorabies have not been reported for ferrets, although they are susceptible to experimental in-fection. Ohshima and associates[57] and Goto and colleagues[58] demonstrated that pseudorabies will cause death in ferrets if administered by oral, nasal, subcutane-ous, intramuscular, or intracardiac routes. They discussed the clinical signs, patho-genesis, and pathology of the disease.[57]

SUBACUTE SCLEROSING PANENCEPHALITIS

Subacute sclerosing panencephalitis (SSPE) is caused by a defective measles virus, and onset usually occurs 6 to 7 years after measles infection. It is a slowly progressing central nervous sys-tem disease, typically affecting children 5 to 14 years old. Symptoms begin with a decrease in intellectual function, fol-lowed by myoclonus and incoordination. Complete loss of cerebral function and death result in 1 to 2 years after onset. It is not possible to study the pathogenesis in human SSPE patients, so the ferret has been used as an animal model. Cells infected with wild-type measles virus release infectious particles by cell membrane budding. The SSPE isolates are nonproductive, however, and spread from cell to cell by syncytia formation (i.e., fusion of cell membranes).[59] Brown and co-workers[60] inoculated ferrets with SSPE virus intracerebrally. When animals became ill, they were sacrificed and their brains examined by an immunolabeling technique. Brown and associates[60] were impressed that measles virus antigen is especially apparent in postsynaptic regions.

VESICULAR STOMATITIS VIRUS

The widespread use of vesicular stomatitis virus (VSV) in the laboratory, because of the ease with which it can be grown in cell culture, led Suffin and colleagues[61] to test its effects on ferret fetuses. This research group inoculated pregnant ferrets by intranasal, intramuscular, intracardiac, and intraperitoneal routes. Although no clinical illness was observed in the jills, transplacental infection caused fetal death and abortion. They cited a report of infection of 40 laboratory workers, and recommended consideration of the safety of women of child-bearing years working with this virus.

RESPIRATORY SYNCYTIAL VIRUS

In 1976, Prince and Porter[62] described the susceptibility of the neonatal ferret to infection with respiratory syncytial virus (RSV). They found that infections of nasal tissues occur independent of age, whereas lower respiratory tract infections decrease with age. Suffin and co-workers[63] found that neonatal ferrets born to dams immunized during gestation are protected from infection by RSV when they are 3 days old. Adult immune ferret serum did not confer immunity to neonates when given either intraperitoneally or orally, however, so they concluded that passive immunization of the neonatal ferret is not entirely antibody-mediated.

TRANSMISSIBLE MINK ENCEPHALOPATHY

Transmissible mink encephalopathy (TME) agent was experimentally inoculated into ferrets to define the host range of the agent and to study the pathogenesis of the disease.[64,65] Scrapie in sheep (and presumably TME in mink) is caused by an unusually small infectious agent that may not contain a nucleic acid, which is sometimes called a prion (proteinaceous infectious particle). There were no reported natural outbreaks of TME on commercial ferret farms. This disease, occurring occasionally in commercial mink, is identified by a long incubation period, progression of clinically abnormal central nervous system function, and spongiform encephalopathy.[66,67] Marsh and associates[65] inoculated ten ferrets (nine sable and one albino) subcutaneously with varying dilutions of TME agent. The nine sable ferrets remained normal for 3 years and, following euthanasia, no neurologic lesions were observed at necropsy. The albino ferret had dysphagia and difficulty with mastication 10 months after exposure. The ferret lost weight and experienced incoordination by 13 months, but later gained weight and appeared to recover neurologic function.

The albino ferret was sacrificed at 15 months and examined. Histopathologic findings included multiple large vacuoles (5–70 μ in diameter) in the cerebral cortex, with no evidence of neuroglial response. Ten percent brain and spleen suspensions from this ferret produced signs of disease and similar lesions in mink and in eight albino ferrets (four sable ferrets remained unaffected for 28 months) 14 to 15 months after intracerebral subinoculation. Four of the albino ferrets were sacrificed during clinically apparent disease, and the other four experienced remission and remained clinically normal through month 28.

Eckroade and colleagues[64] induced lesions in albino and sable ferrets when they inoculated 15 ferret fetuses in 2 jills 1 week before parturition. The inoculum was injected through the uterine wall into the body below the head of each fetus. The animals experienced no clinical disease for 2 years after exposure, when they were sacrificed. All had cerebral cortical vacuolization. Eckroade and co-workers[64] suggested that signs of disease might have occurred later, and remarked that the pigmented ferrets are as susceptible as the albino ferrets. They also noted that full recovery from clinical disease with TME has never been reported in mink or primates.

REFERENCES

1. Shen, D.T., and Gorham, J.R.: Survival of pathogenic distemper virus at 5°C and 25°C. Vet. Med. Small Anim. Clin., 75:69, 1980.
2. Gorham, J.R., and Brandly, C.A.: The transmission of distemper among ferrets and mink. Proc. 90th Mtg. Am. Vet. Med. Assoc., 90:141, 1953.
3. Shen, D.T., and Gorham, J.R.: Contact transmission of distemper virus in ferrets. Res. Vet. Sci., 24:118, 1978.
4. Liu, C., and Coffin, D.L.: Studies on canine distemper infection by means of fluorescein-labeled antibody. I. The pathogenesis, pathology, and diagnosis of the disease in experimentally infected ferrets. Virology, 3:115, 1957.
5. Crook, E., Gorham, J.R., and McNutt, S.H.: Experimental distemper in mink and ferrets. I. Pathogenesis. Am. J. Vet. Res., 19:955, 1958.
6. Shen, D.T., Gorham, J.R., and Pedersen, V.: Viruria in dogs infected with canine distemper. Vet. Med. Small Anim. Clin., 76:1175, 1981.
7. Hansen, M, Jacobsen, P., and Lund, E.: Comparative distemper vaccine titrations in ferrets and minks. Nord. Vet. Med., 25:1, 1973.
8. Baker, G.A., Leader, R.W., and Gorham, J.R.: Immune response of ferrets to vaccination with egg-adapted distemper virus. 1. Time of development of resistance to virulent distemper virus. Vet. Med., 47:463, 1952.
9. Cabasso, V.J., Stebbins, M.R., and Cox, H.R.: Onset of resistance and duration of immunity to distemper in ferrets following a single injection of avianized distemper vaccine. Vet. Med., 48:147, 1953.
10. Burger, D., and Gorham, J.R.: Response of ferrets and mink to vaccination with chicken embryo-adapted distemper virus. II. Interference phenomenon and duration of resistance. Arch. Ges. Virusforsch., 14:449, 1964.
11. Shen, D.T., Gorham, J.R., Evermann, J.F., and McKeirnan, A.J.: Comparison of subcutaneous and intramuscular administration of a live attenuated distemper virus vaccine in ferrets. Vet. Rec., 114:42, 1984.
12. Gorham, J.R., Leader, R.W., and Gutierrez, J.C.: Distemper immunization of ferrets by nebulization with egg-adapted virus. Science, 119:125, 1954.
13. Ott, R.L., and Gorham, J.R.: The response of newborn and young ferrets to intranasal administration with egg-adapted distemper virus. Am. J. Vet. Res., 16:571, 1955.
14. Farrell, R.K., Skinner, S.F., Gorham, J.R., and Lauerman, L.H.: The aerosol and subcutaneous administration of attenuated egg-adapted distemper vaccine to ferret kits from distemper-immune females. Res. Vet. Sci., 12:392, 1971.
15. Shen, D.T., Gorham, J.R., Ryland, L.M., and Strating, A.: Using jet injection to vaccinate mink and ferrets against canine distemper, mink virus enteritis, and botulism, type C. Vet. Med. Small Anim. Clin., 76:856, 1981.
16. Carpenter, J.W., Appel, M.J.G., Erickson, R.C., and Novilla, M.N.: Fatal vaccine-induced canine distemper virus infection in black-footed ferrets. J. Am. Vet. Med. Assoc., 169:961, 1976.

17. Goto, H., Shen, D.T., and Gorham, J.R.: Reversion to virulence of an attenuated distemper virus vaccine strain induced by rapid serial passage in ferrets. Fed. Proc., 35:391, 1976.

18. Hagen, K.W., Goto, H., and Gorham, J.R.: Distemper vaccine in pregnant ferrets and mink. Res. Vet. Sci., 11:458, 1970.

19. Kauffman, C.A., Bergman, A.G., and O'Connor, R.P.: Distemper virus infection in ferrets: An animal model of measles-induced immunosuppression. Clin. Exp. Immunol., 47:617, 1982.

20. Husseini, R.H., et al.: Distribution of viral antigen within the lower respiratory tract of ferrets infected with a virulent influenza virus: Production and release of virus from corresponding organ cultures. J. Gen. Virol., 64:589, 1983.

21. Sweet, C., et al.: Differential distribution of virus and histological damage in the lower respiratory tract of ferrets infected with influenza viruses of differing virulence. J. Gen. Virol., 54:103, 1981.

22. Glathe, H., et al.: The intestine of ferret—a possible site of influenza virus replication. Acta Virol., 28:287, 1984.

23. Husseini, R.H., Sweet, C., Collie, M.H., and Smith, H.: Elevation of nasal viral levels by suppression of fever in ferrets infected with influenza viruses of differing virulence. J. Infect. Dis., 145:520, 1982.

24. Coates, D.M., Sweet, C., and Smith, H.: Severity of fever in influenza: Differing pyrogenicity in ferrets exhibited by H1N1 and H3N2 strains of differing virulence. J. Gen. Virol., 67:419, 1986.

25. Barber, W.H., and Small, P.A., Jr.: Local and systemic immunity to influenza infections in ferrets. Infect. Immun., 21:221, 1978.

26. McLaren, C., and Butchko, G.M.: Regional T- and B-cell responses in influenza-infected ferrets. Infect. Immun., 22:189, 1978.

27. Kauffman, C.A., Schiff, G.M., and Phair, J.P.: Influenza in ferrets and guinea pigs: Effect on cell-mediated immunity. Infect. Immun., 19:547, 1978.

28. Fenton, R.J., Clark, A., and Potter, C.W.: Immunity to influenza in ferrets. XIV: Comparative immunity following infection or immunization with live or inactivated vaccine. Br. J. Exp. Pathol., 62:297, 1981.

29. McLaren, C., Potter, C.W., and Jennings, R.: Immunity to influenza in ferrets. XI. Cross-immunity between A/Hong Kong/68 and A/England/72 viruses: Serum antibodies produced by infection or immunization. J. Hyg., 73:389, 1974.

30. Potter, C.W., Jennings, R., Clark, A., and Ali, M.: Interference following dual inoculation with influenza A (H3N2) and (H1N1) viruses in ferrets and volunteers. J. Med. Virol., 11:77, 1983.

31. Yetter, R.A., Barber, W.H., and Small, P.A., Jr.: Heterotypic immunity to influenza in ferrets. Infect. Immun., 29:650, 1980.

32. Masurel, N., and Drescher, J.: Production of highly cross-reactive hemagglutination-inhibiting influenza antibodies in ferrets. Infect. Immun., 13:1023, 1976.

33. Hinshaw, V.S., Webster, R.G., Easterday, B.C., and Bean, W.J., Jr.: Replication of avian influenza A viruses in mammals. Infect. Immun., 34:354, 1981.

34. Fenton, R.J., Jennings, R., and Potter, C.W.: Differential response of ferrets to infection with virulent and avirulent influenza viruses: A possible marker of virus attenuation. Arch. Virol., 55:55, 1977.

35. Toms, G.L., Sweet, C., and Smith, H.: Behavior in ferrets of swine influenza virus isolated from man. Lancet, 1:68, 1977.

36. Maassab, H.F., Kendal, A.P., Abrams, G.D., and Monto, A.S.: Evaluation of a cold-recombinant influenza virus vaccine in ferrets. J. Infect. Dis., 146:780, 1982.

37. Campbell, D., et al.: Genetic composition and virulence of influenza virus: Differences in facets of virulence in ferrets between two parts of recombinants with RNA segments of the same parental origin. J. Gen. Virol., 58(Pt. 2):387, 1982.

38. Matsuyama, T., Sweet, C., Collie, M.H., and Smith, H.: Aspects of virulence in ferrets exhibited by influenza virus recombinants of known genetic constitution. J. Infect. Dis., 141:351, 1980.

39. Campbell, D., Sweet., C., and Smith, H.: Comparisons of virulence of influenza virus recombinants in ferrets in relation to their behaviors in man and their genetic constitution. J. Gen. Virol., 44:37, 1979.

40. Husseini, R.H., Sweet, C., Collie, M.H., and Smith, H.: The relation of interferon and nonspecific inhibitors to virus levels in nasal washes of ferrets infected with influenza viruses of differing virulence. Br. J. Exp. Pathol., 62:87, 1981.

41. Steffenhagen, K.A., Easterday, B.C., and Galasso, G.J.: Evaluation of 6-azauridine and 5-iododeoxyuridine in the treatment of experimental viral infections. J. Infect. Dis., 133:603, 1976.

42. Haff, R.F., and Pinto, C.A.: The nasal decongestant action of aspirin in influenza-infected ferrets. Life Sci., 12:9, 1973.

43. Grunberg, E., and Prince, H.N.: The antiviral activity of 3,4-dihydro-1-isoquinolineacetamide hydrochloride in vitro, in ovo, and in small laboratory animals. Proc. Soc. Exp. Biol. Med., 129:422, 1968.

44. Collie, M.H., Rushton, D.I., Sweet, C., and Smith, H.: Studies of influenza virus infection in newborn ferrets. J. Med. Microbiol., 13:561, 1980.

45. Coates, D.M., et al.: The role of lung development in the age-related susceptibility of ferrets to influenza virus. Br. J. Exp. Pathol., 65:543, 1984.
46. Coates, D.M., et al.: The role of cellular susceptibility in the declining severity of respiratory influenza of ferrets with age. Br. J. Exp. Pathol., 65:29, 1984.
47. Husseini, R.H., Sweet, C., Overton, H., and Smith, H.: Role of maternal immunity in the protection of newborn ferrets against infection with a virulent influenza virus. Immunology, 52:389, 1984.
48. Collie, M.H., Sweet, C., Cavanagh, D., and Smith, H.: Association of fetal wastage with influenza infection during ferret pregnancy. Br. J. Exp. Pathol., 59:190, 1978.
49. Sweet, C., Toms, G.L., and Smith, H.: The pregnant ferret as a model for studying the congenital effects of influenza virus infection in utero: Infection of fetal tissues in organ culture and in vivo. Br. J. Exp. Pathol., 58:113, 1977.
50. Rushton, D.I., et al.: The effects of maternal influenzal viremia in late gestation on the conceptus of the pregnant ferret. J. Pathol., 140:181, 1983.
51. Collie, M.H., et al.: Ferret fetal infection with influenza virus at early gestation. Br. J. Exp. Pathol., 63:299, 1982.
52. Deshmukh, D.R., and Thomas, P.E.: Arginine deficiency, hyperammonemia and Reye's syndrome in ferrets. Lab. Anim. Sci., 35:242, 1985.
53. Deshmukh, D.R., Maassab, H.F., and Mason, M.: Interactions of aspirin and other potential etiologic factors in an animal model of Reye's syndrome. Proc. Natl. Acad. Sci., 79:7557, 1982.
54. Porter, D.D., Larsen, A.E., and Cox, N.A.: Isolation of infectious bovine rhinotracheitis virus from Mustelidae. J. Clin. Microbiol., 1:112, 1975.
55. Smith, P.C.: Experimental infectious bovine rhinotracheitis virus infection of English ferrets (*Mustela putorius furo* L.). Am. J. Vet. Res., 39:1369, 1978.
56. Von Abraham, A., and Straub, O.C.: Über die Eignung von Frettchen für die Impfstoffprufung von IBR-IPV-Vakzinen. Berl. Munch. Tierarztl. Wochenschr., 94:431, 1981.
57. Ohshima, K., Gorham, J.R., and Henson, J.B.: Pathologic changes in ferrets exposed to pseudorabies virus. Am. J. Vet. Res., 37:591, 1976.
58. Goto, H., Burger, D., and Gorham, J.R.: Quantitative studies of pseudorabies virus in mink, ferrets, rabbits and mice. Jap. J. Vet. Sci., 33:145, 1971.
59. Thormar, H., Mehta, P.D., Barshatzky, M.R., and Brown, H.R.: Measles virus encephalitis in ferrets as a model for subacute sclerosing panencephalitis. Lab. Anim. Sci., 35:229, 1985.
60. Brown, H.R., Thormar, H., Barshatzky, M., and Wisniewski, H.M.: Localization of measles virus antigens in subacute sclerosing panencephalitis in ferrets. Lab. Anim. Sci., 35:233, 1985.
61. Suffin, S.C., Muck, K.B., and Porter, D.D.: Vesicular stomatitis virus causes abortion and neonatal death in ferrets. J. Clin. Microbiol., 6:437, 1977.
62. Prince, G.A., and Porter, D.D.: The pathogenesis of respiratory syncytial virus infection in infant ferrets. Am. J. Pathol., 82:339, 1976.
63. Suffin, S.C., Prince, G.A., Muck, K.B., and Porter, D.D.: Immunoprophylaxis of respiratory syncytial virus infection in the infant ferret. J. Immunol., 123:10, 1979.
64. Eckroade, R.J., ZuRhein, G.M., and Hanson, R.P.: Transmissible mink encephalopathy in carnivores: Clinical light and electron microscopic studies in raccoons, skunks and ferrets. J. Wildl. Dis., 9:229, 1973.
65. Marsh, R.F., et al.: A preliminary report on the experimental host range of the transmissible mink encephalopathy agent. J. Infect. Dis., 120:713, 1969.
66. Hartsough, G.R., and Burger, D.: Encephalopathy of mink. I. Epizootiologic and clinical observations. J. Infect. Dis., 115:387, 1965.
67. Burger, D., and Hartsough, G.R.: Encephalopathy of mink. II. Experimental and natural transmission. J. Infect. Dis., 115:393, 1965.

chapter 18

USE OF THE FERRET IN BEHAVIORAL RESEARCH

M. J. Baum

Rabe and colleagues[1] recently published an excellent review of research literature in which ferrets served as subjects for behavioral studies utilizing several different learning paradigms. These included spatial maze learning, delayed response, visual discrimination, learning set formation, learning of operant schedules of reinforcement, and shock avoidance learning. Clearly, the ferret is ideally suited to behavioral studies of this sort. This review will be limited to an overview of the research literature in which the regulation of various species-specific behaviors was studied in ferrets, including locomotor activity, sexual behavior, and play behavior. It should become evident that, as in the case of learned behaviors, ferrets are highly appropriate subjects for this type of research.

LOCOMOTOR ACTIVITY

Scientists who work with ferrets have speculated for years about whether or not this species exhibits a circadian rhythm in sleep-activity. Recently, however, Dono-

ACKNOWLEDGMENT

Preparation of this review was supported by Research Scientist Development Award MH00392. I thank my colleagues Mary Erskine and Stuart Tobet for helpful discussions.

van[2] recorded wheel-running activity in female ferrets who were either in estrus or anestrus. He found that anestrous females ran in the wheels only during the light period of the daily 8L:16D lighting regimen. By contrast, when the photoperiod was switched to long days (e.g., 16L:8D), females came into estrus and exhibited wheel running during both the daylight and dark hours of each day. As a result, the total distance run each day was considerably greater in estrous than in anestrous females. In contrast to these findings, Stockman and co-workers,[3] using a different method to measure ferrets' activity, found no evidence of a daily rhythm in locomotor activity in either males or females. Capacitative sensors placed beneath each ferret's home cage provided a reliable index of movement; in fact, hamsters kept in the same apparatus reliably showed a circadian rhythm in activity. Whereas Donovan found that estrous ferrets were more active in running wheels than anestrous females, Stockman's group observed no effect of estrogen treatment on home cage activity in gonadectomized ferrets of either sex.

The methods used to monitor ferrets' activity were very different in these two studies. Thus, the display of a predominantly diurnal period of activity may be revealed only when ferrets can run vigorously, as when a running wheel is provided. The fact that Donovan fed his ferrets canned dog food each morning at about 10:00 (although dry food was available at all times) may have provided his ferrets with a *zeitgeber*, which they used to synchronize their daily period of activity. Stockman and associates[3] provided dry cat food and water continuously, with replenishment of the food and cleaning of the cages occurring every several days. More work will be needed to reconcile these different results.

It is worth noting that, in a field study,[4] female ferrets were trapped over a smaller range during the breeding season than at other times of the year. Thus, their activity was presumably restricted during this period. It should be noted, however, that these workers did not distinguish between estrous, unmated females, and females who had mated and become pregnant. Had they done so, they might have found that estrous females are more active than anestrous animals. In this same field study males expanded their range of movement during the breeding season, presumably to maximize the chances of encountering estrous females insofar as the two sexes are normally segregated throughout the year.

MASCULINE SEXUAL BEHAVIOR

The male ferret's sexual responses include neck gripping, mounting, pelvic thrusting, and penile intromission with the estrous female. A pair of copulating ferrets is shown in Figure 18–1. As described in Chapter 19, the sequence of masculine coital behaviors, culminating in intromission and ejaculation, not only ensures that sperm are transmitted to the female, but also that ovulation and activation of the corpora lutea occur.

The expression of masculine sexual behavior is strongly influenced by the exposure of the male's brain to circulating testicular hormones at two different times in the male's life. In adulthood the male exhibits sexual behavior only during the breeding season, when the testes are secreting testosterone (T). Typically, plasma T levels in breeding males may range from 10 to 40 ng/ml,[5–7] and males' coital performance seems to be directly proportional to the amount of circulating T.[5,8] After castration in adulthood, sexual behavior can be activated by SC injections of T[9] or by SC implantation of Silastic capsules containing this steroid.[10] Interestingly, administration of estradiol (E) to castrated male ferrets also causes a highly significant increase in all aspects

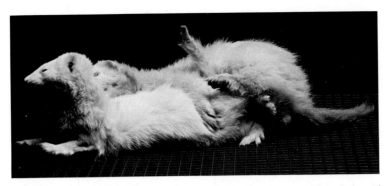

Fig. 18–1. Receptive behavior exhibited by an ovariectomized, estrogen-treated female ferret in response to a neck grip and mount by a gonadally intact male in breeding condition.

of masculine coital performance.[9, 10] Aromatization of androgen to estrogen occurs in the hypothalamic and preoptic regions of the adult male ferret brain,[11] and both estrogen and androgen receptors are present in these regions.[12] The metabolism of T to an estrogen, therefore, may normally play some role in the steroidal activation of mating in the male ferret, just as it does in several rodent species.[13] In the castrated male ferret,[14] as in the male rat,[15] administration of the 5α reduced metabolite of T, 5α-dihydrotestosterone (DHT), concurrently with E, activates masculine sexual behavior more intensely than E alone, suggesting that both E and DHT, formed in the male ferret brain from circulating T, normally contribute to the activation of masculine sexual behavior.

Exposure of the brain to T during perinatal development is also required for the male ferret to exhibit masculine sexual behavior in adulthood. As shown in Figure 18–2, if the male ferret is castrated soon after birth (e.g., postnatal day 5), he later exhibits low levels of masculine sexual behavior in response to adult treatment with T.[16] When castration is delayed to postnatal day 20, or later, males exhibit normal levels of masculine coital behavior when tested in adulthood while receiving T. This implies that testicular secretions act between days 5 and 20 to masculinize the brain mechanisms that control this aspect of coital performance. This impression was confirmed (Fig. 18–3) by a study in which female ferrets were implanted SC with Silastic capsules containing either a high or low dosage of T over postnatal days 5 to 20 or days 20 to 35. Only implantation of the high dosage of T over days 5 to 20 caused an increase in females' coital performance when they received T in adulthood. Interestingly, the plasma levels of T that resulted from implantation over days 5 to 20 of this behaviorally effective dose of T into females were five to six times higher than comparable T levels in gonadally intact male ferrets.[7, 16] This suggests that the developing male brain is more sensitive than the female brain to the neonatal masculinizing action of T.

In addition to masculinizing ferrets' ability to express coital behavior, neonatal exposure to T also alters the inclination to approach conspecific males versus females. In one such study,[17] neonatal administration of T to female ferrets led them to spend less time in the vicinity of stimulus males than did control females, when tested as adults in a large open field apparatus that had various stimulus ferrets housed behind wire mesh on each of the four sides. In another study,[18] ferrets with different endocrine histories were allowed to approach and interact with

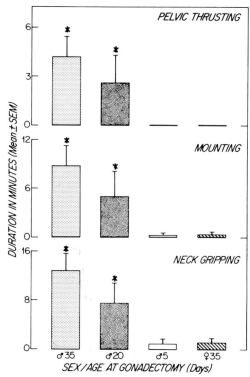

Fig. 18–2. Parameters of masculine sexual behavior displayed by male and female ferrets gonadectomized at different neonatal ages and tested in adulthood with an estrous female. All subjects were tested after being implanted subcutaneously with a Silastic capsule containing testosterone. (Baum, M.J., and Erskine, M.S.: Effect of neonatal gonadectomy and administration of testosterone on coital masculinization in the ferret. Endocrinology, *115*:2440, 1984.)

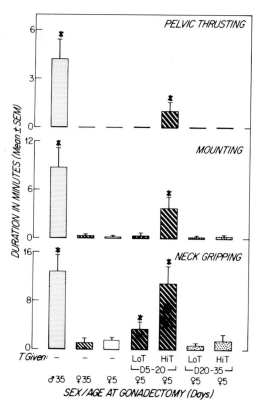

Fig. 18–3. Parameters of masculine sexual behavior displayed by female ferrets ovariectomized at postnatal day 5 and implanted subcutaneously with Silastic capsules containing either low (Lo T) or high (Hi T) dosages of testosterone over postnatal days 5 to 20 (D5–20) or days 20 to 35 (D20–35). In adulthood all subjects were implanted subcutaneously with a Silastic capsule containing testosterone prior to being tested with an estrous female. (Baum, M.J., and Erskine, M.S.: Effect of neonatal gonadectomy and administration of testosterone on coital masculinization in the ferret. Endocrinology, *115*:2440, 1984.)

either a sexually active male or female housed in a goal chamber in the arms of a T maze. After castration on postnatal day 5 (a treatment that greatly attenuated their ability to exhibit mascular coital behaviors in later life), male ferrets significantly reduced their approach responses toward sexually receptive stimulus females. Thus, the "sexual orientation" of the male ferret was found to change as a result of neonatal steroid hormone deprivation. It can be inferred from these data that neonatal exposure to T normally enhances the male ferret's inclination to approach and mate with an estrous female.

Studies were conducted to determine whether either neural metabolite of T (e.g., E or DHT) is required for the process of coital masculinization. It was found that neonatal administration of either DHT or E, or the combination of E + DHT, failed to duplicate the masculinizing action of T itself.[10, 19] In another study,[14] male ferrets were treated neonatally with drugs that either inhibited the synthesis of E or of DHT. Neither treatment attenuated the normal course of coital masculinization, further suggesting that T itself (and not some metabolite) acts neonatally in the male ferret brain to promote coital masculinization.

An additional study[20] was conducted to assess the possible contribution of prenatal exposure to testicular steroids on the occurrence of coital masculinization in ferrets. Treatment of pregnant ferrets with different doses of T caused significant masculinization of the external genital organs of female offspring; these females, however, displayed no significant augmentation in masculine sexual behavior when tested after T treatment in adulthood. This finding suggests that prenatal T exposure, by itself, cannot masculinize the ferret brain, but it does not rule out the possibility that prenatal exposure of the male brain to T, or to a metabolite, augments its sensitivity to the T that circulates in males neonatally. Prenatal deprivation of estrogenic stimulation to the male ferret brain (via maternal ovariectomy and treatment with an aromatase inhibitor) caused a significant reduction in masculine coital behavior, tested in adulthood after treatment with T. No such deficit was found in males whose brains were deprived prenatally of androgenic stimulation via maternal treatment with an antiandrogen, flutamide. These results raise the possibility that E, formed prenatally in specific brain regions of the male ferret from circulating T, "sensitizes" the brain to the later actions of T. More research will be needed to test this hypothesis directly.

FEMININE SEXUAL BEHAVIOR

The estrous female ferret exhibits the limp acceptance posture portrayed in Figure 18–1 when neck-gripped and mounted by a male. When not in estrus, the female refuses to tolerate neck gripping from a male, biting him viciously to avoid his advances. The degree of acceptance be-

havior exhibited by individual ferrets maintained under different endocrine conditions can be quantified in standard tests of sexual receptivity.[9] Typically, during a standard 8-minute test, the investigator records the amount of time that the female exhibits the receptive posture in response to a male's neck grip. The ratio of the duration of the female's receptive posture:duration of the male's neck grip ($\times$ 100) is defined as the female's acceptance quotient. Ovariectomized ferrets displayed dose-dependent increments in acceptance quotients in response to daily SC injections of E,[21] irrespective of whether the animals were housed under short or long photoperiods. Also, there was no effect of these photoperiods on the content of estrogen receptors present in brain cytosols from these same groups of female ferrets.[22] In a wide variety of vertebrate species in which the female ovulates "spontaneously," sequential exposure to estradiol and progesterone is required for the full activation of feminine receptive behavior. Ovulation in the female ferret occurs only after mating, and thus it is perhaps not surprising that progesterone plays no role in the hormonal induction of sexual receptivity. In fact, progesterone was shown to antagonize the stimulatory effect of E on both vulval edema[23] and on acceptance behavior.[24] Estrogen readily induces progestin receptor synthesis in the ovariectomized female ferret's hypothalamus and pituitary gland,[24] just as it does in several other species, including the rat, guinea pig, hamster, and rhesus monkey. There is, however, no relationship among these various species in the distribution of estrogen-inducible progestin receptors in the brain and the ability of progesterone either to facilitate or inhibit feminine sexual behavior.

In nonprimate mammalian species, the male typically exhibits very little feminine receptive behavior, even after castration and treatment with E and progesterone.[25]

The male may be described as being "defeminized." It was therefore surprising to discover[9, 26] that administration of E to male ferrets castrated in adulthood results in the full activation of receptive behavior in response to neck gripping and mounting by a stud male. The receptive behavior displayed by these males is qualitatively and quantitatively indistinguishable from the behavior shown by an estrous female. In fact, during the breeding season, I noted that male ferrets housed together, or brought together temporarily,[27, 28] exhibit receptivity in response to the neck gripping of other males.

In nonprimate mammals, perinatal exposure of females to T causes a dramatic reduction in their later ability to exhibit receptive behavior, even after treatment with estrogen and progesterone. Again, in ferrets, it has been very difficult to "defeminize" females by prenatal or neonatal administration of T.[9, 10, 29] As shown in Figure 18–4, acceptance quotients were equivalent in groups of male ferrets castrated at different postnatal ages and in control females in response to increasing dosages of estrogen. It should be noted that more recent work[30] suggests that exposure of female fetuses to pharmacologic dosages of T over the last 10 days of

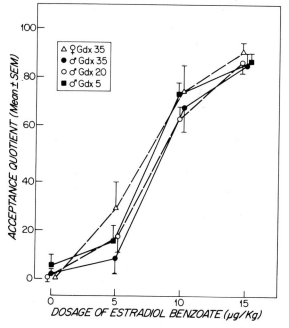

Fig. 18–4. Equivalent acceptance of neck gripping by a stud male (index of sexual receptivity) in male and female ferrets gonadectomized at different neonatal ages and tested in adulthood while receiving daily subcutaneous injections of different dosages of estradiol benzoate in sesame oil. Groups include control females gonadectomized at day 35 (♀ Gdx 35), control males gonadectomized at day 35 (♂ Gdx 35), males gonadectomized at day 20 (♂ Gdx 20), and males gonadectomized at day 5 (♂ Gdx 5). (Copyright 1988 by the American Psychological Association. Reprinted by permission of the publisher and authors. Baum, M.J., Stockman, E.R., and Lundell, L.A.: Evidence of proceptive without receptive defeminization in male ferrets. Behav. Neurosci., *99*:742, 1985.)

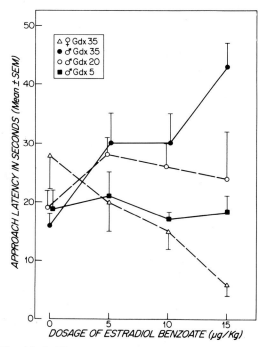

Fig. 18–5. Divergent approach latencies to a stud male (index of sexual proceptivity) in male and female ferrets gonadectomized at different neonatal ages and tested in adulthood in an L-shaped runway while receiving daily subcutaneous injections of different dosages of estradiol benzoate in sesame oil. See caption to Figure 18–4 for group definitions. (Copyright 1988 by the American Psychological Association. Reprinted by permission of the publisher and authors. Baum, M.J., Stockman, E.R., and Lundell, L.A.: Evidence of proceptive without receptive defeminization in male ferrets. Behav. Neurosci., *99*:742, 1985.)

gestation can cause a slight, statistically significant degree of receptive defeminization. In rhesus monkeys, as in ferrets, there is very little evidence that perinatal exposure to testicular hormones consistently causes receptive defeminization.[31] This similarity with primates makes the ferret an especially attractive model for use in studies concerning the neuroendocrine control of brain and behavioral sexual differentiation.

Feminine sexual behavior is comprised of motivated "proceptive" responses, in addition to the receptive postures already discussed.[32] In response to estrogen, female ferrets show evidence of this proceptive behavior by approaching sexually active males. In one study,[29] gonadectomized females and males were allowed to approach a stud male restrained in a goal chamber at the end of a 2-m long runway. Control females, ovariectomized on postnatal day 35, showed a linear dose-dependent reduction in approach latencies to the stud male in response to increasing dosages of E (Fig. 18–5). By contrast, males castrated on postnatal day 35 ran progressively more slowly to the stud male as the dosage of estrogen was raised. Males castrated on postnatal days 20 and 5 had approach latencies that were intermediate to the extremes of the males and females gonadectomized on day 35. This finding suggests that testicular hormones act neonatally in male ferrets to cause proceptive defeminization. In rhesus monkeys T acts prenatally in a similar fashion.[31] It is clear from the data shown in Figure 18–5 that males castrated on postnatal day 5 exhibit approach latency profiles that, although differing from those of males castrated at later ages, are not identical to those of control females. More recent research[30] showed that prenatal exposure of females to T causes proceptive defeminization. Furthermore, prenatal inhibition of estrogen biosynthesis blocked this process in male ferrets, whereas exposing fetal males to antiandrogen had no such consequence. This suggests that proceptive defeminization in male ferrets, like coital masculinization (see above), depends on the prenatal production of estrogen from androgen precursor in the male brain. More work is needed to identify sites in the male brain in which this hormonal action occurs.

PLAY BEHAVIOR

The young of many mammalian species exhibit exuberant play behavior during certain periods prior to the onset of puberty. Such behavior, not surprisingly, also occurs in the ferret.[33] More recent studies have shown that the intensity of this play behavior during adolescent life is greater in males than in females.[34, 35] As would be expected from the results of experiments on the ontogeny of sex differences in sexual behavior, the sex difference in play behavior also results from the action of T (or a metabolite of this steroid) in the developing male. The critical period during which testicular steroids cause coital masculinization in male ferrets appears to end by postnatal day 20. By contrast, no such restriction on the timing of T's action in affecting play behavior was found. Manipulation of circulating T concentrations as late as 70 days after birth had significant effects on the expression of play behavior by male ferrets.[35] This finding implies that the mechanism of action of T, at least in those parts of the brain that control play, may be similar across a range of perinatal ages.

ADDITIONAL CONSIDERATIONS

Although a steady number of studies involving behavior-dependent variables is published each year, it is surprising that more work of this nature is not being conducted using ferrets as subjects. Investigators who do use ferrets in their behavioral studies have come to appreciate the ease of working with this species in situations in which the animals must readily learn a task or perform species-specific behaviors in social situations. Unlike rodents, ferrets are fearless subjects who never freeze for long periods of time with what appears to be no real provocation, and who readily engage in social interaction while being observed. They are ideal for studies involving the ontogeny of behavior, given their relatively short gestation (42-day) and lactation periods, and their large litter size (6 to 10 kits/litter). Finally, manipulations of the ferret brain are easily carried out, both neonatally and later in adulthood, prior to the subsequent evaluation of any long-term behavioral consequences of such manipulation. Obviously, the choice of an animal model for any research question involves weighing numerous theoretic and practical factors. When a phylogenetically more advanced mammal is required for behavioral studies, however, the ferret, not the cat, dog, or monkey, will often be the appropriate choice.

REFERENCES

1. Rabe, A., Haddad, R., and Dumas, R.: Behavior and neurobehavioral teratology using the ferret. Lab. Anim. Sci., 35:256, 1985.
2. Donovan, B.T.: Wheel-running during anestrus and estrus in the ferret. Physiol. Behav., 34:825, 1985.
3. Stockman, E.R., Albers, H.E., and Baum, M.J.: Activity in the ferret: estradiol effects and circadian rhythms. Anim. Behav., 33:150, 1985.
4. Moors, P.J., and Lavers, R.B.: Movements and home range of ferrets at Pukepuke Lagoon, New Zealand. N. Z. J. Zool., 8:413, 1981.
5. Baum, M.J., and Schretlen, P.: Neuroendocrine effects of perinatal androgenization in the male ferret. *In* Progress in Brain Research, Vol. 42. Edited by W.H. Gispen, T. van Wimersma Greidanus, B. Bohus, and D. deWied. Amsterdam, Elsevier, 1975.
6. Neal, J., Murphy, B.D., Moger, W.H., and Oliphant, L.W.: Reproduction in the male ferret: Gonadal activity during the annual cycle; recrudescence and maturation. Biol. Reprod., 17:380, 1977.
7. Erskine, M.S., and Baum, M.J.: Plasma concentrations of testosterone and dihydrotestosterone during perinatal development in male and female ferrets. Endocrinology, 111:767, 1982.
8. Baum, M.J., Tobet, S.A., and Erskine, M.S.: Unpublished observations, 1985.
9. Baum, M.J.: Effects of testosterone propionate administered perinatally on sexual behavior of female ferrets. J. Comp. Physiol. Psychol., 90: 399, 1976.
10. Baum, M.J. Gallagher, C.A., Martin, J.T., and Damassa, D.A.: Effect of testosterone, dihydrotestosterone, or estradiol administered neonatally on sexual behavior of female ferrets. Endocrinology, 111:773, 1982.
11. Tobet, S.A., et al.: Androgen aromatization and 5-alpha reduction in ferret brain during perinatal development: Effects of sex and testosterone manipulation. Endocrinology, 116:1869, 1985.
12. Vito, C.C., Baum, M.J., Bloom, C., and Fox, T.O.: Androgen and estrogen receptors in perinatal ferret brain. J. Neurosci., 5:268, 1985.
13. Baum, M.J., and Vreeburg, J.T.M.: Differential effects of the anti-estrogen MER-25 and of three 5-alpha-reduced androgens on mounting and lordosis behavior in the rat. Horm. Behav., 7:87, 1976.
14. Baum, M.J., Gallagher, C.A., Shim, J.H., and Canick, J.A.: Normal differentiation of masculine sexual behavior in male ferrets despite neonatal inhibition of brain aromatase or 5-alpha-reductase activity. Neuroendocrinology, 36: 277, 1983.
15. Baum, M.J., and Vreeburg, J.T.M.: Copulation in castrated male rats following combined treatment with estradiol and dihydrotestosterone. Science, 182:283, 1973.
16. Baum, M.J., and Erskine, M.S.: Effect of neonatal gonadectomy and administration of testosterone on coital masculinization in the ferret. Endocrinology, 115:2440, 1984.

17. Martin, J.T., and Baum, M.J.: Neonatal exposure of female ferrets to testosterone alters social preference in adulthood. Psychoneuroendocrinology, 11:167, 1986.

18. Stockman, E.R., Callaghan, R.S., and Baum, M.J.: Effect of neonatal castration and testosterone treatment on sexual partner preference in the ferret. Physiol. Behav., 34:409, 1985.

19. Baum, M.J., and Tobet, S.A.: Unpublished data, 1985.

20. Tobet, S.A., and Baum, M.J.: Role for prenatal estrogen in the development of masculine sexual behavior in the male ferret. Horm. Behav., 21:419, 1987.

21. Baum, M.J., and Schretlen, P.: Oestrogenic induction of sexual behavior in ovariectomized ferrets housed under short or long photoperiods. J. Endocrinol., 78:295, 1978.

22. Baum, M.J., and Schretlen, P.: Cytoplasmic binding of estradiol in several brain regions, pituitary, and uterus of ferrets ovariectomized while in or out of estrus. J. Reprod. Fertil., 55:317, 1979.

23. Marshall, F.H.A., and Hammond, J., Jr.: Experimental control by hormone action of the estrous cycle in the ferret. J. Endocrinol., 4:159, 1946.

24. Baum, M.J., Gerlach, J.L., Krey, L.C., and McEwen, B.S.: Biochemical and autoradiographic analysis of estrogen-inducible progestin receptors in female ferret brain and pituitary: Correlations with effects of progesterone on sexual behavior and Gn-RH-stimulated secretion of luteinizing hormone. Brain Res., 368:296, 1986.

25. Baum, M.J.: Differentiation of coital behavior in mammals: A comparative analysis. Neurosci. Biobehav. Rev., 3:265, 1979.

26. Baum, M.J., and Gallagher, C.A.: Increasing dosages of estradiol benzoate activate equivalent degrees of sexual receptivity in gonadectomized male and female ferrets. Physiol. Behav., 26:751, 1981.

27. Poole, T.B.: Aspects of aggressive behavior in polecats. Z. Tierpsychol., 24:351, 1967.

28. Poole, T.B.: Some behavioral differences between the European polecat, *Mustela putorius*, the ferrets, *M. furo*, and their hybrids. J. Zool. [Lond.], 166:25, 1972.

29. Baum, M.J., Stockman, E.R., and Lundell, L.A.: Evidence of proceptive without receptive defeminization in male ferrets. Behav. Neurosci., 99:742, 1985.

30. Baum, M.J., and Tobet, S.A.: Effect of prenatal exposure to aromatase inhibitor, testosterone, or antiandrogen on the development of feminine sexual behavior in ferrets of both sexes. Physiol. Behav., 37:111, 1986.

31. Pomerantz, S.M., Roy, M.M., Thornton, J.E., and Goy, R.W.: Expression of adult female patterns of sexual behavior by male, female and pseudohermaphroditic female rhesus monkeys. Biol. Reprod., 33:878, 1985.

32. Beach, F.A.: Sexual attractivity, proceptivity, and receptivity in female mammals. Horm. Behav., 7:105, 1976.

33. Poole, T.B.: Aggressive play in polecats. Symp. Zool. [Lond.], 18:23, 1966.

34. Biden, M.: Sex differences in the play of young ferrets. Biol. Behav., 7:303, 1982.

35. Stockman, E.R., Callaghan, R.S., Gallagher, C.A., and Baum, M.J.: Sexual differentiation of play behavior in the ferret. Behav. Neurosci., 100:563, 1986.

chapter 19

USE OF THE FERRET IN REPRODUCTIVE NEUROENDOCRINOLOGY

M. J. Baum

Ferrets have been domesticated for centuries.[1] Thus, it must be presumed that people who kept ferrets came to realize that both males and females breed only when the days are lengthening, and that the female stays in estrus for weeks or even months until a male mates with her. Scientific investigation of these matters began in this century, when Marshall[2] conducted a systematic study of the occurrence of estrus in female ferrets. This work included an analysis of ovarian and uterine histology, and an unambiguous demonstration that ovulation occurs in this species only after mating.

This study, which was later followed by similar, more detailed analyses,[3–5] heralded the beginning of what is now nearly a century of research on various aspects of reproductive neuroendocrinology in ferrets. The usefulness of ferrets to reproductive neuroendocrinologists derives from several characteristics of the species. First and foremost, the ferret is a domesticated species—easily kept, bred, and handled. Second, the female's estrous cycle is very easy to monitor because of the dramatic external swelling

ACKNOWLEDGMENT

This review is dedicated to Prof. J.J. van der Werff ten Bosch, of the Department of Endocrinology, Growth, & Reproduction, Erasmus University, Rotterdam, The Netherlands, who first introduced me to ferrets as experimental subjects in 1969. I thank my colleagues Rona Carroll, Mary Erskine, and Stuart Tobet for helpful discussions. Preparation of this review was supported by Research Scientist Development Award MH00392.

(edema) of the vulvar tissues in response to estrogen secretion by the ovaries. The occurrence of vulval edema was especially important in the early days of research, prior to the advent of techniques for monitoring cyclic changes in vaginal cell characteristics and of assays for circulating hormones. Another attractive attribute of the ferret for neuroendocrinologists is its seasonal reproductive cycle, which is synchronized by changes in the prevailing photoperiod. This fact, plus the fact that the female ovulates only after being mated, meant that ferrets were recognized early on as useful subjects for understanding how neural signals (resulting from changes in photoperiod or from the somatosensory stimulation associated with mating) are transduced into endocrine signals, which ultimately stimulate gamete production, sexual behavior, and pituitary gonadotropin secretion in both sexes.

Most recently, the need to collect blood samples frequently (i.e., every 5 minutes for many consecutive hours) to monitor the pulsatile secretion of pituitary luteinizing hormone (LH) and follicle-stimulating hormone (FSH), as well as gonadal steroids, has again made the ferret an attractive model. Its relatively large body size (average body weight of males, 1500 g; females, 750 g) and blood volume mean that investigators can withdraw considerable amounts of blood at frequent intervals via indwelling jugular catheters, which are well tolerated.[6]

It is obvious that ferrets (both male and female) have a secure niche in the history of reproductive neuroendocrinology. More importantly, however, it is clear the ferret is ideally suited to studies on the neuroendocrine mechanisms that control seasonal reproduction, sexual differentiation, puberty, ovulation, and the control of corpus luteum function, as shown by the reviews that follow.

PHOTOPERIODIC CONTROL OF SEASONAL REPRODUCTION

The first scientists who kept ferrets for experimental purposes housed them in outdoor sheds, in which natural daylight provided the only source of illumination. In England and the northeastern part of the United States, where such studies were originally conducted, female ferrets typically all come into estrus within a 1- to 2-week period, beginning at the end of March. Males show testicular development at the same time. If mating is allowed, females become pregnant, deliver a litter approximately 42 days later, and nurse the litter for an additional 42 days. After weaning a litter, females usually come back into estrus, provided this occurs in early summer. Occasionally even a third estrus pregnancy occurs, but most female ferrets kept under natural photoperiods breed only twice yearly. The close synchrony of the onset of estrus in female ferrets and testicular maturation in males led Bissonnette[7–9] to study the effects of providing additional artificial lighting in the fall months on the initiation of reproductive activity. His studies showed clearly that exposure to long days (i.e., more than 12 hours of light/day) causes an onset of estrus and testicular activity within 4 to 6 weeks in the late fall, several months earlier than the time when these events normally occur in ferrets of both sexes housed under natural daylight. More recently, changes in steroid hormone secretion that accompany light-induced gonadal development were documented in both female[10] and male ferrets.[11]

Some researchers concentrated on the role of light intensity[12,13] and on the duration of the daily phases of light and dark[14] in attempting to specify how photoperiod promotes reproductive activity in the ferret. Others concentrated their efforts on the mechanism whereby a physical stimulus (light) is translated into an endocrine signal (secretion of pituitary gonadotropins, which stimulate estrus). It was quickly shown[15] that blinded ferrets failed to come into premature estrus in response to lengthened photoperiods. Furthermore, large lesions of various portions of the primary visual projections to occipital cortex in ferrets failed to block the effect of long days on estrus.[16] These data imply that, although some retinal projection to the brain is required for the endocrine effect of light to occur, the pathway involved is not the classic one that underlies visual perception. It was several decades before the identity of this pathway was discovered (see below).

In the early 1950s, Harris and co-workers suggested that the secretion of hormones by the anterior pituitary gland is actually controlled by chemical signals released from neurons in the hypothalamus into the portal vessels of the median eminence. From here, it was suggested, these factors are conducted the short distance down to the anterior pituitary gland, where they either stimulate or inhibit the secretion of various tropic hormones. The stimulation of estrus in ferrets by long-day photoperiods provided these workers with an ideal model in which to test their hypothesis. They found that sectioning of the pituitary stalk prevented light-induced estrus in most ferrets; a small percentage persisted in showing the response, however, regardless of the stalk section.[17] It was quickly shown that regrowth of the portal vessels had occurred in those females who showed the response to light, and that insertion of a piece of wax paper into the site of stalk section prevented this regrowth and the occurrence of estrus in all females tested. Although some of these results were for a time bitterly contested,[18] it soon became apparent that Harris and colleagues were correct. A hypothalamic neuropeptide, gonadotropin-releasing hormone (Gn-RH), is released into the portal vessels and

stimulates the secretion of both FSH and LH by the anterior pituitary gland. When synthetic Gn-RH became available, Donovan and Ter Haar[19] showed that exogenous administration of this peptide facilitates LH and FSH secretion differentially in female ferrets, depending on the endocrine condition prevailing at the time of treatment. More recent studies[20] specified the distribution of Gn-RH-containing cell bodies and nerve terminals in the female ferret brain. Gn-RH-containing cell bodies are located rostrally in the preoptic area in the region of the organum vasculosum of the lamina terminalis, projecting back to the median eminence. Other Gn-RH-containing neurons can be found more caudally distributed along the midline. Labeled cells were even seen in the pituitary stalk; these cells projected to the posterior pituitary gland.[21] The functional significance of this rather unique distribution of Gn-RH-containing neurons in the female ferret remains to be elucidated.

Although it was clear that information about the daily duration of night and day was somehow translated by the retina and the nervous system into a signal that promoted the secretion of Gn-RH and then of FSH and/or LH, little progress was made for quite some time in understanding the pathways that mediated this response to light. In the early 1960s, several investigators, including Wurtman and Axelrod,[22] showed that the secretion of an indole amine, melatonin, by the pineal gland occurs each night as the result of neural inputs from the superior cervical ganglion. The work of Reiter and Fraschini,[23] using hamsters, first showed unambiguously that the response of the male hamsters pituitary-gonadal axis to changes in photoperiod depends on the integrity of the sympathetic-pineal system. Shortly thereafter Herbert,[24] working with ferrets, reported that pinealectomy blocks the ability of long-day photoperiods to advance estrus. Much earlier studies[25,26] had shown that bilateral removal of the superior cervical ganglia has a similar effect in female ferrets, although these workers were not yet aware of the role of the pineal in the effect they observed. Thorpe and Herbert[27] later showed that imposition of a short daily photoperiod (e.g., less than 12 hours of light per day) leads to the termination of estrus in female ferrets, and that this response to photoperiod is also blocked by pinealectomy. Finally, Herbert and colleagues[28] compared the long-term effects of blinding and pinealectomy on the yearly occurrence of estrus in female ferrets who were housed (in England) under natural lighting conditions. As can be seen in Figure 19–1, both procedures eventually caused estrous periods to fall out of synchrony with the yearly lengthening of photoperiod in the spring.

Thorpe and Herbert[29] demonstrated that a direct retinohypothalamic pathway exists in the ferret, which terminates in the suprachiasmatic nucleus of the hypothalamus. Evidence from the ferret and from several other species suggest that changes in the activity of neurons of the suprachiasmatic nuclei (SCN) are responsible for changes in the activity of the sympathetic nerves that innervate the pineal gland. Increments in neuronal firing lead to increased release of norepinephrine in the pineal gland and to an activation of the enzymes that control melatonin synthesis by pineal cells. Information about day and night is apparently transmitted to the SCN by the retinohypothalamic pathway, where the activity of neurons is synchronized so that the highest level of neuronal activity occurs during the dark hours of each day. In the ferret, as in every other species studied, the nocturnal period of melatonin secretion follows the duration of the daily period of darkness.[30] Thus, as shown in Figure 19–2, melatonin is secreted for a longer period in ferrets kept under a short

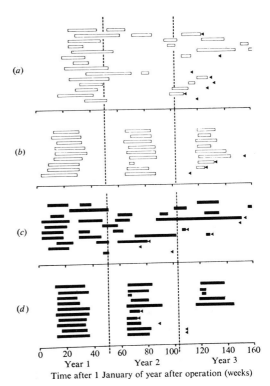

Fig. 19–1. Recurrent estrus over 3 consecutive years in female ferrets who in the summer prior to the onset of year 1 were pinealectomized (*a*), sham-pinealectomized (control; *b*), optic nerve-sectioned (blinded; *c*) or given no surgical treatment (control; *d*). Occurrence of vulval edema (estrus) for each animal is indicated by an open or shaded bar. Closed triangles indicate death of individual ferrets from unspecified causes. (Herbert, J., Stacey, P.M., and Thorpe, D.H.: Recurrent breeding seasons in pinealectomized or optic-nerve sectioned ferrets. J. Endocrinol., *78*:389, 1978.)

photoperiod as opposed to a long photoperiod. It seems likely that daily exposure to different durations of melatonin stimulation account for the eventual activation and termination of activity in the ferret's hypothalamic-pituitary-gonadal axis.[31]

It should be obvious from the data reviewed thus far that the ferret is a useful model for studies on the mechanism whereby an environmental factor (light) influences seasonal reproductive activity.

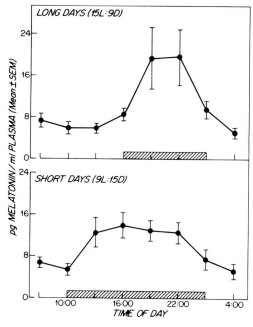

Fig. 19–2. Plasma melatonin concentrations in ovo-hysterectomized female ferrets housed under either long or short days. Plasma samples from 6 to 12 ferrets were analyzed at each time point. The samples collected under long days at 16:00 h and under short days at 10:00 h were taken just before the colony lights went off. The samples collected at 01:00 h under both long and short days were taken just before the colony lights went on. The hatched bars indicate period of darkness. (Baum, M.J., Lynch, H.J., Gallagher, C.A., and Deng, M.-H.: Plasma and pineal melatonin levels in female ferrets housed under long or short photoperiods. Biol. Reprod., *34*:96, 1986.)

CONTROL OF PUBERTY

The studies described above were among the first to suggest that neural factors control the secretion of anterior pituitary hormones. In ferrets, as in all mammalian species, the establishment of the adult pattern of gonadal function (puberty) is delayed for some time after birth. In ferrets born in late spring or summer, and housed under natural lighting conditions, the onset of gonadal activity is normally delayed until the spring of the next year. Much early evidence, however, suggested that both the pituitary and the gonads can attain adultlike levels of function many

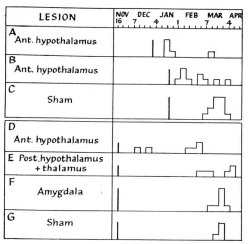

Fig. 19–3. The onset of vulval edema (estrus) in female ferrets after direct current lesions of the anterior hypothalamus, the posterior hypothalamus plus thalamus, or the amygdala. Additional females received sham operations in these brain regions. Each unit square indicates occurrence of estrus in a single ferret. Vertical lines indicate time of brain operation for ferrets in panels *A* through *G*. (Donovan, B.T., and van der Werff ten Bosch, J.J.: Physiology of Puberty. London, Edward Arnold, 1965.)

months prior to the normal onset of activity (witness the profound acceleration of estrus/testis function in ferrets exposed to artificial long days in the fall). Studies with ferrets[32] were among the first to show that destructive lesions of the anterior hypothalamus in prepubertal females accelerate the onset of reproductive activity (Fig. 19–3). Despite an initial report to the contrary,[33] it is now well established that lesions in other parts of the hypothalamus do not exert such an action. More recent studies[34] showed that similar lesions of the anterior hypothalamus also accelerate gonadal maturation in males. Finally, bilateral lesions of the medial amygdaloid regions accelerated pubertal development in female but not in male ferrets.[35]

The mechanism whereby brain lesions accelerate sexual maturation is still not completely resolved. One hypothesis is that the lesions destroy the neurons that mediate the inhibitory feedback effects of circulating gonadal steroids on Gn-RH release (and thereby on the secretion of pituitary FSH and LH). It was suggested that, prior to puberty, this "gonadostat" is exquisitely sensitive to the inhibitory feedback effect of very low levels of sex steroids secreted by the prepubertal gonads, whereas after puberty the gonadostat is considerably less sensitive to circulating steroid levels.[36] In one study,[37] female ferrets in whom hypothalamic lesions induced precocious puberty, still showed evidence of strong inhibitory feedback action on pituitary gonadotropin secretion, suggesting that the effective lesions do not eliminate all sources of inhibitory feedback.

A major advance in the study of puberty was the advent of assays for measuring pituitary and gonadal hormones. A detailed analysis of developmental changes in the pulsatile secretion of LH and estradiol that occur in female ferrets in which puberty was accelerated by exposure to long days was published by Ryan and Robinson.[38] Control of pulsatile LH secretion was also studied in male ferrets.[39] Donovan[40] showed that prepubertal and anestrous female ferrets show compensatory ovarian hypertrophy after unilateral ovariectomy, suggesting that in such animals some low level of estradiol is secreted that tonically inhibits pituitary gonadotropin secretion.

More recently, Ryan[41] provided evidence that the sensitivity of the brain gonadostat, which mediates the inhibitory effect of estradiol, becomes less sensitive at puberty (Fig. 19–4). She ovariecto-

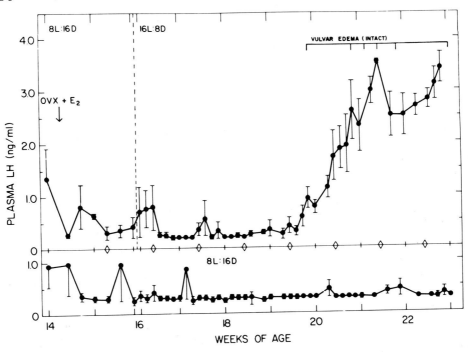

Fig. 19–4. Plasma luteinizing hormone (LH) concentrations (mean + SEM) for two groups of immature female ferrets who were ovariectomized and implanted subcutaneously with a Silastic capsule containing estradiol while being kept on a short-day photoperiod (8L:16D). Animals whose LH values are given in the top panel were switched to a long-day photoperiod (16L:8D) when they were 16 weeks old (*vertical dashed line*). Animals whose LH values are given in the bottom panel were left in short days. Note that for animals in the top panel the estradiol implants lost their ability to restrain LH secretion at about the time after the imposition of long days when vulval edema first occurred in a third group of gonadally intact females (*upper right*). (Ryan, K.D.: Hormonal correlates of photoperiod-induced puberty in a reflex ovulator, the female ferret. Biol. Reprod., *31*:925, 1984.)

mized prepubertal female ferrets and implanted them SC immediately with a Silastic capsule that released a low level of estradiol. Half of the females were housed under long days, which stimulates precocious puberty in gonadally intact females; the other ferrets were kept under a short-day photoperiod. Shortly after ovariectomy, plasma LH levels were kept very low by the inhibitory action of the implanted estradiol on the hypothalamic-pituitary axis. Approximately 4 weeks after introduction of the long-day (stimulatory) photoperiod, however, when gonadally intact control females begin to display vulvar edema, LH levels rose despite the presence of estrogen-secreting capsules. No such increase occurred in females kept under a short-day photoperiod. It appears that, in response to long days, the potential of a fixed dose of estradiol to inhibit LH secretion is reduced. Similar events occur in prepubertally castrated male ferrets given exogenous testosterone.[42] There is no indication at the molecular level of the changes in the neural gonadostat that account for the pubertal changes in the inhibitory feedback potential of estrogen and androgen in the two sexes. The possibility that nutritional factors or some set point in body weight or composition contribute to pubertal development in female ferrets appears unlikely.[43] More work is needed to identify the specific neurons that constitute the ferret gonadostat before it will be possible to understand how changes in the feedback potential of sex steroids occur in these cells.

BEHAVIORAL INDUCTION OF OVULATION AND CORPUS LUTEUM ACTIVITY

The earliest observations on the female ferret's reproductive life[2] established that periods of estrus last for weeks, even months, until mating occurs. Hill and

Parkes[44] later showed that hypophysectomy carried out within hours after mating blocks ovulation, further suggesting that the act of mating is responsible for the ovulatory secretion of LH by the pituitary gland. Only recently, however, has direct measurement of postcoital surges in circulating LH been made in the female ferret.[45] Estrous females were implanted with jugular catheters from which blood samples could be taken before, during, and after mating. Normally, the male ferret's pattern of mating behavior includes a period of neck gripping and mounting of the female, with intermittent bouts of pelvic thrusting behavior.[46] Eventually the male achieves a penile intromission, whereupon all thrusting ceases. The intromission may be maintained for periods of 2 to 150 minutes. Intromission is an absolute requirement for the occurrence of an LH surge in the estrous female ferret. As shown in Figure 19–5, a female who received an intromission showed an LH surge and later was found to have corpora lutea in the ovaries (a sign that ovulation had in fact occurred). By contrast, a female who received neck grips, mounts, and pelvic thrusting from a male (without intromission) showed no LH surge or histologic indication that ovulation had occurred. Although these data show that penile intromission is required for the induction of ovulation in estrous ferrets, it seems likely that the stimuli associated with the male's neck grip, mounting, and pelvic thrusting behaviors may contribute to the female's LH responsiveness. Preliminary work[47] suggests that stimulation of the vaginal cervix of an estrous ferret using a glass rod, by itself, fails to induce an LH surge leading to ovulation. Glass rod stimulation carried out on an estrous female while she is being neckgripped and mounted by a male, however, successfully induces ovulation.

The mating stimulus, in addition to inducing an LH surge, promotes the se-

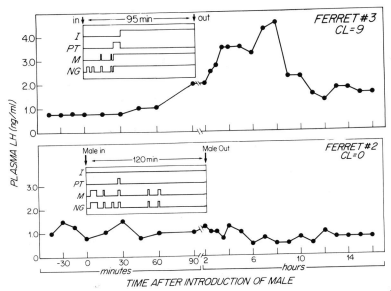

Fig. 19–5. Plasma concentrations of luteinizing hormone (LH) in two estrous female ferrets before and after exposure to a sexually active male. A continuous record is shown for the occurrence of neck gripping (NG), mounting (M), pelvic thrusting (PT), and penile intromission (I) during the time that each female was with a male. Note that a surge in plasma LH occurred only in ferret 3, which received an intromission from the male. This animal subsequently was found to have nine corpora lutea (CL) in the ovaries, indicating that ovulation had occurred. No LH surge or CL formation occurred in ferret #2, which received neck gripping, mounting, and pelvic thrusting from the male without intromission. (Carroll, R.S., et al.: Coital stimuli controlling luteinizing hormone and secretion and ovulation in the female ferret. Biol. Reprod., *32*:925, 1985.)

cretion of a luteotropic factor from the anterior pituitary. This factor promotes the secretion of progesterone by the corpora lutea within 2 to 3 days after mating, with peak levels of secretion being attained by postcoital day 12, when implantation of the blastocysts occurs.[48–50] Progesterone secretion is sustained until the last 10 days of the 42-day pregnancy, when levels gradually decline. Mating an estrous ferret with a vasectomized male results in a pseudopregnancy that lasts for 42 days,[3] during which the pattern of progesterone secretion is essentially identical to that of pregnant animals. This suggests that the ferret placenta secretes little, if any, progesterone.

Much evidence indicates that the secretion of prolactin by the pituitary gland promotes the secretion of progesterone by the corpora lutea. Thus, Hill and Parkes[44] first showed that hypophysectomy car-

ried out several days after mating causes a regression of corpora lutea in the ovaries of pregnant ferrets. More recently, Donovan[51] showed that severing the pituitary stalk in pregnant ferrets causes no disruption in luteal function, presumably because prolactin secretion continues unabated from the pituitary gland in the absence of any inhibitory factors of neural origin reaching the gland by way of the portal blood vessels. In addition, Donovan[52] and Murphy[53] reported that corpus luteum function could be adequately maintained in hypophysectomized pregnant ferrets during the first half of pregnancy by daily injections of ovine and bovine prolactin, respectively. Recent evidence[54] suggests that prolactin may exert its stimulation of progesterone synthesis in the ferret corpora lutea by increasing the uptake of lipoprotein-borne cholesterol, thereby providing the main substrate for steroid hormone biosynthesis. More studies are required to determine whether prolactin, either alone or in concert with some other hypophyseal factor, is responsible for the maintenance of luteal function during the second half of pregnancy in ferrets.

Implantation of the fertilized blastocysts normally occurs in the ferret 12 days after mating. The precise identity of the endocrine secretions required for this event, however, remains uncertain. Wu and Chang[55, 56] reported that ovariectomy of pregnant ferrets 6 days after mating blocked implantation, even if progesterone were injected. Implantation did occur in ferrets ovariectomized 8 days after mating, provided progesterone was given. This finding, along with other data,[57] showed that the corpora lutea secrete some factor in addition to progesterone on days 6 to 8 after mating, which is essential for the process of implantation. Other research[58, 59] showed that this critical factor is not estradiol. Kintner and Mead[60] compared the in vitro synthesis of steroids from labeled pregnenolone, progesterone, or dehydroepiandrosterone by corpora lutea dissected from ovaries of ferrets killed on either day 6 or 8 of pregnancy. No striking differences in product formation were detected, raising the possibility that some nonsteroidal hormone is secreted by the corpora lutea on days 6 to 8 that acts in the uterus to promote implantation. At this writing the identity of this hormone remains undetermined.

CONTROL OF BRAIN SEXUAL DIFFERENTIATION

Tobet and co-workers[61] studied the role of gonadal steroids in controlling sex differences in the organization of the ferret brain. The adult male ferret possesses a discrete nucleus in the dorsomedial location at the border of the preoptic area and anterior hypothalamus (POA/AH).[61] This nucleus, henceforth referred to as the male nucleus of the POA/AH (Mn-POA/AH), is absent in females. The somal areas of cells in the Mn-POA/AH increase in size in adult castrated males after systemic administration of testosterone (T) or either of the two primary metabolites of T, estradiol (E) or dihydrotestosterone (DHT), but not progesterone. In no instance did adult administration of these steroids organize a Mn-POA/AH in female ferrets, raising the possibility that this sexually dimorphic nucleus develops in males under the influence of sex steroids secreted either prenatally or neonatally.

Deanesley[62, 63] used histologic methods to compare ovarian and testicular development in female and male ferrets. She observed lipid in the interstitial cells of the testis as early as gestational day 30, whereas in females lipid was first seen in the ovarian interstitium on postnatal day 14. Direct measurement of plasma concentrations of testosterone revealed that levels are significantly higher in males than in females prenatally (e.g., gestational day 37) and neonatally (postnatal days 10 and 15).[64] Also, within a few hours after birth, plasma T concentrations rise dramatically, so that T levels are two- or threefold higher in males than in females over the first several postnatal hours.[65] Administration of T prenatally to female ferrets (by implanting the mothers with T pellets over gestational days 30–42) caused a Mn-POA/AH to differentiate, whereas neonatal castration failed to disrupt Mn-POA/AH development in male ferrets.[66]

These results suggest that testicular hormones normally act prenatally in the male to organize a Mn-POA/AH. Additional studies were conducted to determine whether this action of T results from activation of estrogen or androgen receptors in the developing male brain. Plasma levels of estradiol and estrone were equivalent in males and females at the prenatal and neonatal ages sampled,[67] suggesting that circulating estrogens are not responsible for the observed sex dimorphism in neural organization. The activity of hypothalamic aromatase, which converts androgen to estrogen, was, however, significantly higher in male than in female ferrets on gestational days 34 and 37.[68] This fact, coupled with the presence of higher circulating concentrations of T in males, raises the possibility that significantly more estrogen is synthesized in local regions of the hypothalamus and in the preoptic area of males than females.

Additional work[69,70] showed that both estrogen and androgen receptors exist in male and female ferrets in hypothalamic and preoptic tissues collected prenatally and neonatally. The development of the Mn-POA/AH appears to depend on the action of E formed prenatally in the male ferret POA/AH. Males born of pregnant ferrets who had been ovariectomized and implanted with an aromatase inhibitor on gestational day 30 (along with a progesterone capsule to maintain pregnancy) lacked a Mn-POA/AH in adulthood. This treatment effect was reversed in one surviving male derived from a litter that received a high dosage of E in addition to the aromatase inhibitor.[66] Prenatal exposure of males to a potent antiandrogenic drug (flutamide) failed to disrupt development of the Mn-POA/AH, although anogenital distances were significantly reduced in these males, suggesting that the antiandrogen did reach the developing fetuses. Other research using the rat, guinea pig, and zebra finch had implicated estrogen in the control of sexually dimorphic forebrain development, but this study using the ferret is the first to suggest that such events also occur in higher mammals.

REFERENCES

1. Thompson, A.P.D.: A history of the ferret. J. Hist. Med. Allied Sci., 6:471, 1951.
2. Marshall, F.H.A.: The estrous cycle in the common ferret. Q. J. Micr. Sci., 48:323, 1904.
3. Hammond, J., and Marshall, F.H.A.: Estrus and pseudopregnancy in the ferret. Proc. R. Soc., Lond. [Biol.], 105:607, 1930.
4. Hammond, J., and Walton, A.: Notes on ovulation and fertilization in the ferret. J. Exp. Biol., 11:307, 1934.
5. Hamilton, W.J., and Gould, J.H.: The normal estrous cycle of the ferret. Trans. R. Soc. Edin., 60:12, 1939–1940.
6. Florczyk, A.P., and Schurig, J.E.: A technique for chronic jugular catheterization in the ferret. Pharmacol. Biochem. Behav., 14:255, 1981.
7. Bissonnette, T.H.: Modification of mammalian sexual cycles; reactions of ferrets of both sexes to electric light added after dark in November and December. Proc. R. Soc. Lond. [Biol.], 110:322, 1932.
8. Bissonnette, T.H.: Modification of mammalian sexual cycles: Effects upon young male ferrets of constant eight and one-half hour days and six hours of illumination after dark between November and June. Biol. Bull., 68:300, 1934.
9. Bissonnette, T.H.: Modification of mammalian sexual cycles: Reversal of the cycle in male ferrets by increasing periods of exposure to light between October second and March thirtieth. J. Exp. Zool., 71:341, 1935.
10. Donovan, B.T., Matson, C., and Kilpatrick, M.J.: Effect of exposure to long days on the secretion of estradiol, estrone, progesterone, testosterone, androstenedione, cortisol and follicle-stimulating hormone in intact and spayed ferrets. J. Endocrinol., 99:361, 1983.
11. Neal, J., Murphy, B.D., Moger, W.H., and Oliphant, L.W.: Reproduction in the male ferret: Gonadal activity during the annual cycle; recrudescence and maturation. Biol. Reprod., 17: 380, 1977.

12. Marshall, F.H.A.: Effect of light intensity on the timing of estrus in female ferrets. J. Exp. Biol., 17:139, 1940.

13. Vincent, D.S.: Modification of the annual estrous cycle of the ferret by various regimes of artificial light. J. Endocrinol., 48:iii, 1970.

14. Hart, D.S.: Photoperiodicity in the female ferret. J. Exp. Biol., 28:1, 1951.

15. Bissonnette, T.H.: Effect of enucleation on the induction of estrus in ferrets by artificial light. J. Comp. Psychol., 22:93, 1936.

16. Le Gros Clark, W.E., McKeown, T., and Zuckerman, S.: Visual pathways concerned in gonadal stimulation in ferrets. Proc. R. Soc. Lond. [Biol.], 126:449, 1939.

17. Donovan, B.T., and Harris, G.W.: Effect of pituitary stalk section on light-induced estrus in the ferret. Nature, 174:503, 1954.

18. Thomson, A.P.D., and Zuckerman, S.: Functional relations of the adenohypophysis and hypothalamus. Nature, 171:970, 1953.

19. Donovan, B.T., and Ter Haar, M.B.: Effects of luteinizing hormone releasing hormone on plasma follicle-stimulating hormone and luteinizing hormone levels in the ferret. J. Endocrinol., 73:37, 1977.

20. King, J.C., and Anthony, E.L.P.: LHRH neurons and their projections in humans and other mammals: Species comparisons. Peptides, 5[Suppl. 1]:195, 1984.

21. Anthony, E.L.P., King, J.C., and Stopa, E.G.: Immunocytochemical localization of LHRH in the median eminence, infundibular stalk, and neurohypophysis. Cell Tiss. Res., 236:5, 1984.

22. Wurtman, R.J., and Axelrod, J.: The pineal gland. Sci. Am., 213:50, 1965.

23. Reiter, R.J., and Fraschini, F.: Endocrine aspects of the mammalian pineal gland: A review. Neuroendocrinology, 5:219, 1969.

24. Herbert, J.: The pineal gland and light-induced estrus in ferrets. J. Endocrinol., 43:625, 1969.

25. Abrams, M.E., Marshall, W.A., and Thomson, A.P.D.: Effect of cervical sympathectomy on the onset of estrus in ferrets. Nature, 174:311, 1954.

26. Donovan, B.T., and van der Werff ten Bosch, J.J.: The cervical sympathetic system and light-induced estrus in the ferret. J. Physiol., 132:123, 1956.

27. Thorpe, P.A., and Herbert, J.: Studies on the duration of the breeding season and photorefractoriness in female ferrets pinealectomized or treated with melatonin. J. Endocrinol., 70:255, 1976.

28. Herbert, J., Stacey, P.M., and Thorpe, D.H.: Recurrent breeding seasons in pinealectomized or optic-nerve sectioned ferrets. J. Endocrinol., 78:389, 1978.

29. Thorpe, P.A., and Herbert, J.: The accessory optic system of the ferret. J. Comp. Neurol., 170:295, 1976.

30. Baum, M.J., Lynch, H.J., Gallagher, C.A., and Deng, M.-H.: Plasma and pineal melatonin levels in female ferrets housed under long or short photoperiods. Biol. Reprod., 34:96, 1986.

31. Carter, D.S., Herbert, J., and Stacey, P.M.: Modulation of gonadal activity by injections of melatonin in pinealectomized or intact ferrets kept under two photoperiods. J. Endocrinol., 93:211, 1982.

32. Donovan, B.T., and van der Werff ten Bosch, J.J.: The relationship of the hypothalamus to estrus in the ferret. J. Physiol., 147:93, 1959.

33. Herbert, J., and Zuckerman, S.: Ovarian stimulation following cerebral lesions in ferrets. J. Endocrinol., 17:433, 1958.

34. Baum, M.J., and Goldfoot, D.A.: Effect of hypothalamic lesions on maturation and annual cyclicity of the ferret testis. J. Endocrinol., 62:59, 1974.

35. Baum, M.J., and Goldfoot, D.A.: Effect of amygdaloid lesions on gonadal maturation in male and female ferrets. Am. J. Physiol., 228:1646, 1975.

36. Donovan, B.T., and van der Werff ten Bosch, J.J.: Physiology of Puberty. London, Edward Arnold, 1965.

37. Baum, M.J., and van der Werff ten Bosch, J.J.: Hypothalamic lesions, estrogen and precocious puberty in the female ferret. J. Endocrinol., 48:xi, 1970.

38. Ryan, K.D., and Robinson, S.L.: A rise in tonic luteinizing hormone secretion occurs during photoperiod-stimulated sexual maturation of the female ferret. Endocrinology, 116:2013, 1985.

39. Sisk, C.L., and Desjardins, C.: Pulsatile release of luteinizing hormone and testosterone in male ferrets. Endocrinology, 119:1195, 1986.

40. Donovan, B.T.: The feedback action of ovarian hormones in the ferret. J. Endocrinol., 38:173, 1967.

41. Ryan, K.D.: Hormonal correlates of photoperiod-induced puberty in a reflex ovulator, the female ferret. Biol. Reprod., 31:925, 1984.

42. Sisk, C.L.: Evidence that a decrease in testosterone negative feedback mediates the pubertal increase in luteinizing hormone pulse frequency in male ferrets. Biol. Reprod., 37:73, 1987.

43. Donovan, B.T.: Is there a critical weight for estrus in the ferret? J. Reprod. Fertil., 76:491, 1986.

44. Hill, M., and Parkes, A.L.: Studies on the hypophysectomized ferret. III. Effects of postcoitus hypophysectomy in ovulation and development of the corpus luteum. Proc. R. Soc. Lond. [Biol.], 112:153, 1932.

45. Carroll, R.S., et al.: Coital stimuli controlling luteinizing hormone and secretion and ovulation in the female ferret. Biol. Reprod., *32*:925, 1985.

46. Baum, M.J., and Schretlen, P.: Neuroendocrine effects of perinatal androgenization in the male ferret. *In* Progress in Brain Research, Vol. 42. Edited by W.H. Gispen, van Wimersma Greidanus, B. Bohus, and D. deWied. Amsterdam, Elsevier, 1975.

47. Tobet, S.A., et al.: Unpublished observations, 1985.

48. Heap, R.B., and Hammond, J., Jr.: Plasma progesterone levels in pregnant and pseudopregnant ferrets. J. Reprod. Fertil., *39*:149, 1974.

49. Blatchley, F.R., and Donovan, B.T.: Progesterone secretion during pregnancy and pseudopregnancy in the ferret. J. Reprod. Fertil., *46*:455, 1976.

50. Daniel, J.C., Jr.: Plasma progesterone levels before and at the time of implantation in the ferret. J. Reprod. Fertil., *48*:437, 1976.

51. Donovan, B.T.: The effect of pituitary stalk section on luteal function in the ferret. J. Endocrinol., *27*:201, 1963.

52. Donovan, B.T.: The control of the corpus luteum function in the ferret. Arch. Anat. Microsc. Morphol. Exp., *56*(Suppl. 3–4):315, 1967.

53. Murphy, B.D.: The role of prolactin in implantation and luteal maintenance in the ferret. Biol. Reprod., *21*:517, 1979.

54. McKibbin, P.E., Rajkumar, K., and Murphy, B.D.: Role of lipoproteins and prolactin in luteal function in the ferret. Biol. Reprod., *30*:1160, 1984.

55. Wu, J.T., and Chang, M.C.: Effects of progesterone and estrogen on the fate of blastocysts in ovariectomized pregnant ferrets: A preliminary study. Biol. Reprod., *7*:231, 1972.

56. Wu, J.T., and Chang, M.C.: Hormonal requirements for implantation and embryonic development in the ferret. Biol. Reprod., *9*:350, 1973.

57. Foresman, K.R., and Mead, R.A.: Luteal control of nidation in the ferret. Biol. Reprod., *18*:490, 1978.

58. Murphy, B.D., and Mead, R.A.: Effects of antibodies to estrogens on implantation in ferrets. J. Reprod. Fertil., *46*:261, 1976.

59. Mead, R.A., and McRae, M.: Is estrogen required for implantation in the ferret? Biol. Reprod., *27*:540, 1982.

60. Kintner, P.J., and Mead, R.A.: Steroid metabolism in the corpus luteum of the ferret. Biol. Reprod., *29*:1121, 1983.

61. Tobet, S.A., Zahniser, D.J., and Baum, M.J.: Sexual dimorphism in the preoptic/anterior hypothalamic area of ferrets: Effects of adult exposure to sex steroids. Brain Res., *364*:249, 1986.

62. Deanesly, R.: Oogenesis and the development of the ovarian interstitial tissue in the ferret. J. Anat., *107*:165, 1970.

63. Deanesly, R.: Testis differentiation in the fetal and postnatal ferret. J. Anat., *123*:589, 1977.

64. Erskine, M.S., and Baum, M.J.: Plasma concentrations of testosterone and dihydrotestosterone during perinatal development in male and female ferrets. Endocrinology, *111*:767, 1982.

65. Erskin, M.S., Tobet, S.A., and Baum, M.J.: Effect of birth on plasma testosterone, brain aromatase activity, and hypothalamic estradiol in male and female ferrets. Endocrinology, *122*:524, 1988.

66. Tobet, S.A., Zahniser, D.J., and Baum, M.J.: Differentiation in male ferrets of a sexually dimorphic nucleus of the preoptic/anterior hypothalamic area requires prenatal estrogen. Neuroendocrinology, *44*:299, 1986.

67. Erskine, M.S., and Baum, M.J.: Plasma concentrations of estradiol and estrone during perinatal development in male and female ferrets. J. Endocrinol., *100*:161, 1984.

68. Tobet, S.A., et al.: Androgen aromatization and 5-alpha reduction in ferret brain during perinatal development: Effects of sex and testosterone manipulation. Endocrinology, *116*:1869, 1985.

69. Vito, C.C., Baum, M.J., Bloom, C., and Fox, T.O.: Androgen and estrogen receptors in perinatal ferret brain. J. Neurosci., *5*:268, 1985.

70. Holbrook, P.G., and Baum, M.J.: Characterization of estradiol receptors in brain cytosols from perinatal ferrets. Dev. Brain Res., *7*:1, 1983.

INDEX

Numerals in italics indicate a figure, "t" following a page number indicates tabular matter.